Errata

On page 512, the authors of "Recurrent Large-Group Phenomena: Studies of an Adolescent Therapeutic Community," should be listed as LOREN H. CRABTREE, JR., and DOUGLAS F. LEVINSON.

On page 513, the section "Oscillatory Cycles of Tension," which continues on page 514 through the paragraph beginning "Using Rapoport's (1960) description. . . ," should be read after the paragraph beginning, "We gradually became aware. . . ," on page 516.

ADOLESCENT PSYCHIATRY

DEVELOPMENTAL AND CLINICAL STUDIES

VOLUME VIII

Annals of the American Society for Adolescent Psychiatry

ADOLESCENT PSYCHIATRY

DEVELOPMENTAL AND CLINICAL STUDIES

VOLUME VIII

Edited by
SHERMAN C. FEINSTEIN
PETER L. GIOVACCHINI
JOHN G. LOONEY
ALLAN Z. SCHWARTZBERG
ARTHUR D. SOROSKY

University of Chicago Press
Chicago and London

The University of Chicago Press, Chicago 60637
The University of Chicago Press, Ltd., London

International Standard Book Number: 0-226-24053-3
Library of Congress Catalog Card Number: 70-147017

CONTENTS

PART II. DEVELOPMENTAL RESEARCH
AND ADOLESCENT PROCESS

VULNERABLE YOUTH: HOPE, DESPAIR, AND RENEWAL
MIRIAM ELSON AND JOHN F. KRAMER, Special Editors

PREFACE

The beginning of a new decade with the end of a century in sight leads to appraisals of the past and perspectives for the future. The themes of appraisal and perspective are found throughout this present volume and are dealt with in a wide variety of approaches, always emphasizing the multidimensional manner in which adolescence may be considered by a growing number of observers.

By this time, most clinicians concerned with adolescent psychiatry are convinced that adolescence is a unique phase concerned with special developmental tasks, requiring special training and therapeutic approaches. It is a time of character consolidation that leads to the formation of the adult sense of identity. Emotional disturbances occurring during this period manifest themselves in particular forms of psychopathology, such as the identity diffusion syndrome which is the outcome, roughly speaking, of the breakdown of the self-representation.

The teenage years are characterized by structural homogeneity. That is to say, the minds of adolescents, their psychic structure, are in a formative developmental stage. In terms of psychosexual stages, they are in a postoedipal state, attempting to integrate their biologically based sexual drives in the general ego organization. Generally, they are acquiring adaptive techniques to cope with the external world at an adult level. These tasks seem to be constants in the adolescent context.

At the more superficial behavioral level, the situation admits considerable variability. There have been marked changes in the general behavior of adolescents during the past several decades, but as far as our clinical experiences can ascertain their underlying psychic states are more or less the same. In view of the fact that there is practically no homogeneity to adolescent behavior, some investigators question whether adolescence, as a phenomenon, does, in fact, exist.

The articles in this volume do not restrict themselves to surface phenomena. Although various facets that have been considered characteristic of adolescence, for example, rebellion, are challenged, the overall concept of an adolescent evolving character structure is not abandoned; actually, it is reinforced. What is being stressed, however, is how the interplay of various frames of reference, the external world and inner drives, affect the adolescent process and reciprocally how adolescents contribute to the shaping of the world they live in. This may include psychopathology. Psychopathological adaptations may undergo sufficient modifications that they may become workable and determine particular life-styles.

Modern youth today have shown little need to become isolated and set themselves up as a separate group as was the situation in the past. Cults and mystical religions still exist but, by and large, there has been considerable integration of adolescents into the general world. This makes them more accessible than they have ever been. For the most part, teenagers are willing to share their thoughts and feelings with adults, and this has been a mutually enriching and rewarding experience.

We are pleased to announce the addition of new senior editors to the editorial group of this volume. John G. Looney, Allan Z. Schwartzberg, and Arthur D. Sorosky have already made their presence known.

SHERMAN C. FEINSTEIN
PETER L. GIOVACCHINI
JOHN G. LOONEY
ALLAN Z. SCHWARTZBERG
ARTHUR D. SOROSKY

PART I

ADOLESCENCE:
GENERAL
CONSIDERATIONS

EDITORS' INTRODUCTION

Our Western society is currently going through its own stage of sociological adolescence which only further complicates the lives of its youngsters attempting to grow and develop through role models provided by parents, teachers, and governmental leaders. Parental confusion, familial fragmentation, societal unrest, and increasing peer pressures have led to an upsurge in narcissistic and impulse control disorders. The adolescents' attraction to religious cults and missionary groups provides an illuminating symbol of the times: a search for the structure, limit setting, impulse controls, and affection not provided in their homes and communities.

The subjects of the chapters in this part range from the historical, social, and cultural factors affecting adolescent development to psychiatric aspects of cult membership, and finally to the dynamics of narcissism and the narcissistic personality. Adolescent growth and development does not occur in a vacuum. It is profoundly influenced by psychosocial, cultural, and historical processes. As our society becomes increasingly anomic and fragmented, there is a corresponding weakening of family cohesiveness, loss of authority and shared value systems, and the rise of alternative life-styles exemplified by cults and communes. The increase of cultural narcissism contributes to and in turn is influenced by rising numbers of narcissistic and borderline personalities. Our increased understanding of these personality types may lead to more effective intervention.

Peter Blos continues his modifications of traditional psychoanalytical theory with a review of female adolescent development (see *Adolescent Psychiatry* 7:6–25). Freud's original formulations of female development have been challenged by experiences from treatment and direct observation of children and adolescents. He believes that revision of the theory of female

3

development could become an expedient factor in changing woman's place in the minds of modern man and woman as well as social institutions. Blos discusses certain modifications, including a reemphasis on parental and social influences on gender identity; revision of temporal aspects of biological development; a redefinition of penis envy as a universal metaphor for a general sense of loss; further considerations of oedipal resolution in female adolescents; and the influence of contemporary culture on female adolescent development.

Leon Eisenberg, honoring Albert Einstein's centenary and theory of relativity, emphasizes the relativity of adolescence as a set of developmental phenomena which are shaped by what has been up to now blind social change. He defines adolescence from a contemporary perspective as a critical period of human development marking the end of childhood and establishing the foundation for maturity. Eisenberg sees adolescence as a series of constructs, each varying with culture, history, class, and caste, arising from the human need to make coherent sense of and to control what occurs during the transformation. He furthur believes that it is within our power as citizens to construct a society in which the potential for healthy growth of personality will be enhanced—just as social conditions have permitted physical maturation to flower.

Ernest S. Wolf, on the occasion of the 1979 William S. Schonfeld Distinguished Service Award to Heinz Kohut, reviews Kohut's contributions to adolescent psychiatry and psychoanalysis. Wolf discusses the studies on empathy in which Kohut shifted the emphasis in psychoanalytic research from investigation of the external world with one's sense organs to an emphasis on investigating the inner world through introspection and empathy. This introspective-empathic method led eventually to the realization that certain transference-like phenomena were not manifestations of unconscious conflicts but were manifestations of a deficiency in psychic structure. This placed the patient's self at the core of the observed field, and a psychology of the self emerged.

Kohut, a student of Aichhorn, has paid a great deal of attention to the vicissitudes of the self during adolescence. He wrote that much of the sexual activities of adolescents serve narcissistic purposes—to enhance self-esteem especially when exposed to the revival of frightening childhood experiences of self-depletion and fragmentation. Adolescent sexual activity, therefore, may be understood to be a secondary manifestation of self-pathology. He described certain types of adolescent delinquents who loudly proclaim their grandiosity and warned against the utilization of any artificial activity which might encourage idealization of the therapist while allowing the transference to develop spontaneously. Adolescent turmoil may be considered a traumatic state of the self, overburdened by excessive stimuli and, therefore, unable to contain its fragmented constituents safely within the boundaries of cohesion. The overstimulation and sexuality may then be self-induced as a desperate attempt to escape the unbearable experience of apathy that accompanies depletion of the self.

Sol Nichtern pursues the missing adolescent. He traces the attitudes toward the teenage group through history—their position in the family, their value to labor through servitude and apprenticeship, and the various religions' expectations. He finds that adolescence did not exist in social and economic institutions and that the young were denied a separate identity from the family for thousands of years. The adolescent was born from a class of youth who at first existed outside the family. Gradually this age group acquired characteristics determined as much by social and economic factors as biological and psychological. In visits to developing countries he found the historical hidden adolescent still exists. When the society becomes industrialized the children are relegated to community institutions rather than the family. The missing adolescent then emerges.

Peter L. Giovacchini examines the effects of sociocultural factors and lifestyle on the formation of adolescent psychopathology. Comparing ghetto, middle-income, and affluent families he concludes that the sociocultural environment is a factor in determining health or psychopathology, but that the early life experiences of the mother and her own emotional development outweigh all other factors as determinants of motherliness. When the methods of being soothed and nurtured and the character adaptations acquired do not function smoothly in a changing environment, as illustrated by the second-generation immigrant, psychopathology develops. Giovacchini believes that this psychopathology now influences cultural norms and has become incorporated into the behavior and ideologies of many adolescents.

Otto Pollak examines the impact of social change on family life, its expression in the structure and function of the marital relationship, and its effect on child development. Among the changes analyzed are the growing equality between the sexes, the new assertiveness and self-realization in women, the presence of optional life-styles in lieu of ordinary marriage, and the existential search for authenticity and a loss of faith. Pollak believes that these social changes lead to internal stress on children as well as adults and that this stress may be one of the most significant aspects of modern middle-class life.

Vivian M. Rakoff traces the effects of historical forces on adolescent process as well as its manifestations in adolescent disorders. He believes that the notion of the right to individual personality and identity was an aristocratic privilege that became a democratic option. At the same time, the task of establishing a sense of identity established its opposite—the danger of social alienation and the loss of a sense of moral significance. Many families in our culture are restless movers, detached from the contexts of place, history, religion, and similar communal customs. Even their children's names reflect the lack of family history, ethnic group, or ethical community. Language, communal context, a shared sense of ethical values, and social rituals are seen as necessary components of the self within the world, something akin to Winnicott's transitional object concept.

Philip Katz compares the problems in education and, eventually, work for adolescents struggling with cultural conflicts or psychopathology. He reviews the significance of work and points out the important role it plays in identity formation. He then describes various cultural attitudes of certain Indian tribes toward work and shows how differences with Western culture may have the same effect as psychopathology on adjustment.

Sherman C. Feinstein considers the psychiatric aspects of middle-class youth joining fringe religious groups and exotic cults. He does not find the converts essentially pathological but rather vulnerable from the transitional demands of their developmental stage. Of great concern is the relief they report after joining a cult. He believes this is the result of massive repression of drive impulses. On leaving the cult the young may be in a fragile emotional state, the result of regression and drive resurgence. Deprogramees may manifest a regressive state which resembles a psychotic alteration of consciousness.

Saul V. Levine considers the role of the psychiatrist in dealing with cult members and their families. He found that most young people joined the cult movement because of personal dissatisfaction with their life situation at a critical period in their lives. At this point they were vulnerable to simplistic solutions owning to feelings of alienation and demoralization. Levine, however, did not find them a particularly disturbed group. Joining a religious group provided them with opportunities for believing and belonging. Levine suggests techniques to be considered prior to conversion, during cult membership, and after leaving a cult. He recommends the psychiatrist act as a facilitator helping to maintain communcation; as an adviser to families concerning strategies; as an educator clarifying the mysteries of the group; and as a consultant to institutions, groups, and authorities regarding specific approaches to the phenomenon. As a psychotherapist he discusses the approaches to be considered at different stages of the process. And, finally, he suggests the psychiatrist play a developmental role which requires availability, flexibility, sensitivity, and directive prodding of the young person in order to exploit the seeds of doubt which may manifest themselves.

Edward M. Levine looks at the social experiment aspect of middle-class youth joining noncreedal rural communes and urban religious cults. He believes that they manifest certain narcissistic personality characteristics and do not understand limits and the meaning of freedom and responsibility. He traces the development of narcissistic character disorders to developmental defects in the families of origin and an anomic society. Permissive parenting stems from the inability of adults to use their authority with assurance and assertiveness. It fails to assist children to adopt and use values and standards that are central to sound development. An anomic society emphasizes impulse gratification, self-centeredness, and a disregard for the future. Professor Levine is concerned about the vulnerability of such a society and its people.

1   MODIFICATIONS IN THE TRADITIONAL
     PSYCHOANALYTIC THEORY OF FEMALE
     ADOLESCENT DEVELOPMENT

PETER BLOS

To the clinician who works with the adolescent, particularly to the one who works with the adolescent girl, it has become increasingly clear over the last decades that the classical psychoanalytic theory on which the clinical work with the adolescent girl is founded requires a considered alignment with those developmental findings which we have at our disposal today. Many makeshift and patchy revisions in female adolescent psychology have only succeeded in muddling the field. We easily recognize two major trends that have cast clouds of incredulity on the classical psychoanalytic view of female psychosexual development. One lies in the fact that the original formulations by Freud were derived entirely from the psychoanalytic treatment of adult women rather than from work with children or adolescents. Freud's reconstruction of early female development was soon met by deviating opinions like those of Klein, Jones, and Horney. A second challenge came from the confrontation of the classical theory by direct infant and child observation; research in this rapidly expanding field imbued the whole controversy with a revisionist fervor. The accumulation of divergent and contradictory data as well as their variegated explanations forced upon us the urgent need to cast a fresh look at the traditional psychoanalytic schema of female psychological development.

An accelerating influence on the many revisionist elaborations issued from the worldwide burgeoning movement of women's liberation. The champions of this movement proposed and demanded sweeping reorientations in issues of the socioeconomic politics concerning women. These reforms were timely and overdue. Unfortunately, the movement became entangled in the ideological conviction that the psychoanalytic view of female development is not only scientifically antiquated and "sexist" but also serves as an insidious pseudointellectual tool for preserving the status quo of women in society.

There is ample justification in the request for a revision of the theory of female development; such a revision could indeed become an expedient factor in changing woman's place in the minds of modern men and women as well as in social institutions. However, there is no place for Lysenkoism, namely, the accommodation of scientific facts to programmatic ideologies. I stand on the side of an evolutionary approach which has served psychoanalysis well and has established it as an open-ended system of scientific thought. In the spirit of this tradition, the rich harvest derived from direct child observation, as well as from research in adolescent and adult female psychology, is slowly but steadily assimilated in the framework of psychoanalysis—even though groans of resistance and fractional animosities remain audible. The continued open-endedness of the psychoanalytic system confirms my expectation that it can adopt into its realm new observations of human behavior, regardless of their challenge to some of its established or cherished tenets.

Before I approach the topic of this presentation I wish to point out two delimitations of this chapter; both are intentional. One concerns the fact that I have focused my attention on those issues which are particularly relevant for the revision of the theory of female adolescence. Consequently, my historical review remains incomplete and selective. Second, I shall not present a comparative view of girl and boy, because such an expansion of the topic within the framework of this chapter would only blur the central issue.

Defining the Issue

Dusting off the accumulation of years, we readily admit that the question which Ernest Jones asked in 1935 is still relevant and provocative, even though it still remains unanswered to everybody's satisfaction. In his paper on "Early Female Sexuality," Jones took issue with Freud's view of penis envy and its role in the development of femininity. His closing sentence reads, "The ultimate question is whether a woman is born or made." However, he was sure of three facts, namely, that a woman is not an *homme manqué;* that preoedipal little boys and girls are not, psychologically speaking, both masculine; and, last but not least, that femininity is not a defensive formation at its origin. "On the contrary, her [the little girl's] femininity

9

develops progressively from the promptings of an instinctual constitution'' (Jones 1935, p. 495). Whether a primary femininity exists is still a controversial issue, but contemporary evidence leans strongly toward the conclusion that woman is born and not made, and, certainly, that femininity cannot be defined or understood by its negative apposition to the male.

At this point our investigation will best be served by stating briefly the classical Freudian concept of female development before we turn our attention to modifications of the psychoanalytic psychology of the adolescent girl. This detour into the early years of life, into the origins of what is to follow later, is essential for an understanding of female adolescence. Obviously, the psychosexual component of development stands in the center of our attention, when the psychological differentiation in the development of boy and girl is under scrutiny. In Freud's view, infantile female and male psychosexual development initially follow an identical course, namely, one of male valence; in other words, there is only one genital for both sexes, namely, the male one. The phallic phase of the girl is one of complete concordance of genital orientation in the little boy and girl. I shall quote the opinion Freud (1933) adhered to throughout his life: "With their entry into the phallic phase the differences between the sexes are completely eclipsed by their agreements. We are now obliged to recognize that the little girl is a little man" (p. 118). Freud goes on to say that masturbation during this phase is carried out on the "penis equivalent," that is, the clitoris. When the girl discovers her "genital inferiority" (as it was called then), the masturbation of boy and girl follows different lines. With the advent of this critical divergence in psychosexual development arises the division into "male equals active" and "female equals passive." This point of view has led to much confusion, simplification, and acrimonious debate. To quote a key sentence from Freud: "Along with abandonment of clitoral masturbation a certain amount of activity is renounced. Passivity now has the upper hand . . . " (Freud 1933, p. 128).

Up to this stage in Freud's psychosexual development the vagina remains undiscovered by both sexes. Indeed, Freud (1933) was of the opinion that the girl does not discover her vagina until puberty; therefore—so the argument goes—a full sense of femaleness cannot exist at any earlier age. At puberty the leading role of the clitoris recedes with the ascendancy of the vagina as the excitable organ, thus ushering in feminity. In order to accomplish this progression in psychosexual development, "The clitoris should wholly or in part hand over its sensitivity and, at the same time, its importance to the vagina" (p. 118). In the very next sentence, Freud states that "the more fortunate man'' does not have anything analogous to the ''handing-over'' with which the would-be woman has to contend. What the disadvantage of possessing two organs of sexual sensitivity and excitability might be is never considered or debated. At any rate, the little girl remains a little boy until she discovers that she does not possess a penis. The realization of her sexual identity is supposed to occur at the decline of the phallic phase.

The ensuing castration complex consolidates penis envy which, in turn, becomes the ultimate propellant force toward a female body image and the girl's acceptance of her physical state as castrated. Consequently, femininity supposedly has its origin in a defensive position; it is not genuine but constitutes a secondary formation. With the ascendancy of the reality principle the little girl transcends the inescapable disappointment in her body—and her mother's as well—by turning to the father. Thus, in a jealous identification with the mother she obtains the paternal phallus and by proxy gives a baby to the father just as her mother had done. This procreative achievement must be left dormant in wishful thinking due to her physical immaturity. The oedipal experience brings penis envy to a relative decline because the oedipal baby supposedly represents a restitution of the penis which she had either lost or never possessed.

These internal events are eloquently expressed in doll play; in this common activity of the little girl we note the significant fact that the baby doll of the little girl is always female—from time immemorial and the world over. Doll play reestablishes the little girl's sense of bodily completeness as well as the awareness of the female procreative faculties which she shares with her mother.[1]

I am prepared to hear the complaint that I have drawn too scant a sketch of Freud's views, leaving out those modulating elaborations which give his presentation of the subject a far larger and more profound scope and complexity. I can only reply that I have intentionally focused on those of Freud's formulations which have become subject to reconsideration in the light of new findings. However, we must guard against throwing out the baby with the bathwater because there is much worth saving. As you might have noticed, I broke off the summary of Freud's schema before I came to discuss how the little girl shifts her primary attachment to the mother over to the oedipal father. I postpone this topic, which is of singular importance in adolescence, because I intend to discuss it when I come later to the exploration of clinical observations in female adolescence. At this point I shall subject the basic and pivotal assumptions of classical psychoanalysis as outlined to a critical review.

Toward New Definitions

This intention brings us back immediately to the question we had considered, namely, is gender identity due to innate (biological-genetic) or learned (cultural-environmental) factors or what combination of both is of determinative valence? Let us start with the much discussed Freudian dictum, "Anatomy is destiny." This declaratory statement removes the influence of social factors on the shaping of femininity into the realm of almost trivial epiphenomena. We must admit that this classical psychoanalytic position has been slowly turned around, and today many of its aspects stand quite securely on their heads. This is to say that, on the basis of clinical evidence, we can attribute to parental and wider social influences and attitudes toward the female baby and young child a significance for gender-identity formation that tends to outweigh biological givens (Stoller 1976; Ticho 1976). Paraphrasing Freud's dictum, Stoller (1974) adds an elegant twist to it, indeed a most convincing one, by saying; "Anatomy is not destiny; destiny comes from what people make of anatomy."

Gender-identity formation seems to occur much earlier than previously thought. Stoller has advanced the plausible opinion that core gender identity[2] has its roots in the first year of life. Child observation supports the assumption that an innate male-female dimorphism is a biological given which permits us to speak of a primary femininity and masculinity. Sex differences can be observed in the neonate before we can speak of learned behavior, even though we do not know exactly when and how learning, imprinting, and conditioning affect decisively and lastingly the process of differentiation within the core gender identity. At any rate, there exists an appreciable body of data which lend weight to the opinion that neonates show observable differences linked to their sex (Green 1976; Hamburg and Lunde 1966).

Any unprejudiced observer of young children has no difficulty in noticing early manifestations of sex differences in behavior, be this in motility, posture, play patterns, investigative curiosity, and fantasies. Additional support has been derived through studies of sex differences in the fields of physiology (fetal hormonal research) and psychology as, for example and mentioning just one of many, in the study of fear of visual novelty (Bronson 1973). Observation of young children has also altered our knowledge of the timing of genital awareness and excitability, clitoral and vaginal; they have to be dated much earlier—during the second half of the second year of life—than the classical timetable had made us believe (Galenson and Roiphe 1976; Roiphe 1968). The child's recognition of sexual differences also occurs at a younger age, contradicting Freud's view that little boys and little girls register the genital sex differences only with the decline of the phallic phase.

It seems far closer to the truth that penis envy is aroused defensively to ward off regression to and aggression against the early mother, that is, any "good enough mother" who, under normal circumstances of life, is bound to repeatedly frustrate and disappoint her child. It is in the nature of growing toward autonomy that the child is confronted with a general sense of loss. This kind of early penis envy exists harmoniously within the matrix of primary femininity. We might then conceive of penis envy as a universal metaphor (Grossman and Stewart 1976), specific for the immature female, encompassing and reifying the various defeated desires and sensory frustrations which every child experiences early in life. This vast and varied infantile experience of incompleteness leads in boy and girl to different mental representations of self and object. We know, for instance, that the little boy resists more aggressively than the girl the demand for sphincter control and behavioral restraints in general. He is usually more difficult to train and to manage than the girl, who tends to contain her aggression toward the mother more globally by deflecting it toward the acquisition or possession of a body part, the penis, which merges symbolically with the representation of the lost breast; both body parts gain the nature of perfection through idealization. The little boy's wish for a baby in his attempt to achieve body completeness is seldom as concretely expressed as the girl's wish for a penis. The adolescent boy's defensive reaction toward passive homosexual strivings or fantasies far exceeds in intensity anything we witness in an adolescent girl who might sense or become aware of lesbian feelings. Two observations shall complement what has been proposed.

1. Freud (1909, pp. 86–87) records the following dialogue between the five-year-old Hans and his father:

HANS: I am going to have a little girl.

I: Where will you get her, then?

HANS: Why, from the stork. . . .

I: You'd like to have a little girl.

HANS: *Yes, next year, I am going to have one* . . . .

I: But why isn't Mummy to have a little girl?

HANS: Because *I* want to have a little girl for once.

I: But you can't have a little girl.

HANS: Oh yes, boys have girls and girls have boys.

I: Boys don't have children . . . .

HANS: But why shouldn't I?

The little boy's envy of the female procreative function will in time yield to the reality principle by way of the transmuting processes of substitution, sublimation, and the symbolic sharing in parturition.

2. A three-year-old girl went to the toilet of her nursery school with a boy her age. When she saw his penis she demanded, "Give it to me," repeating her request in threatening crescendo. The boy took to his heels in fright but the girl pursued him while shouting, "Give it to me." At home she berated her mother to buy her the "little toy" which the boy possessed. The mother's explanation that she could not buy it at a store left the little girl unconvinced and unconsoled.

Such observations, even if less dramatic, are so common that we look at them as typical. Penis envy appears as a two-layered phenomenon: The girl's wish for the mother's breast becomes shunted onto a masculine track in her effort to avoid regression to primary passivity; in this process she deflects the aggressive impulse from harming the mother by directing it greedily toward the male genital. Should a fixation on this level occur, the foundation for the development of a masculinity complex is prepared. This constellation often appears in full bloom at adolescence and never fails to reveal in treatment an unresolved and severe ambivalence conflict with the preodipal mother.

For an example, I refer to an analytic patient, an adolescent girl with wildly untamed masculine wishes. She furiously brushed my reference to "penis envy" aside by saying, "Nonsense, I don't want my brother's penis; I don't want *him* to have one." Needless to say, the brother was the mother's admired and favored child. What she desired was the mother's exclusive attention and love, both intrinsically associated with the possession of a penis or the imputed superiority of boys.

I recall another patient, a late-adolescent girl who used to assign to all physical objects in the world a male or female designation. For example, big books were male, pictures were female, and so forth. During a college course this girl once made a comment which was responded to by the teacher as being extremely intelligent. At this moment she had the hallucinatory physical sensation of having a penis. Being a dedicated member of the women's liberation movement she reported this experience with fury, disgust, and a sense of humiliation. I mention this incident because it occurred at a time in her analysis when the analytic work had reached the repressed and frustrated childhood cravings for her mother's physical affection which, at this juncture in her late adolescence, surfaced in fantasies of a lesbian relationship and the thought of playing with the breast of her girlfriend. Since the resolution of preoedipal fixations and of the negative oedipus complex constitutes one of the obligatory tasks of adolescence, the emergence of so-called penis envy in conjunction with lesbian trends should be considered a transient but normal, though quantitatively and qualitatively variant, epiphenomenon of the process of psychic restructuring during female adolescence.

As we know from Freud's writings about femininity, he was never convinced that any of his developmental propositions were telling the whole story. He had come early to the conclusion that the course by which the oedipal stage is reached and the Oedipus complex resolved is not analogous for the male and female child. Contemplating the girl's resolution of the Oedipus complex, Freud (1924) was struck by the fact that "at this point our material—for some incomprehensible reason—becomes far more obscure and full of gaps." In the perplexing pursuit of this problem Freud came to realize that the preoedipal period exerts an influence on the emotional development of women that equals or even exceeds the influence of the oedipal stage. He finally went so far as to throw doubts on one of the cornerstones of psychoanalytic theory when he wrote, "It would seem as though we must retract the universality of the thesis that the Oedipus complex is the nucleus of the neurosis" (1931, p. 226).[3] The relentless study of the adolescent girl over the last decade has thrown new light on this bewildering subject. We shall now direct our attention to female adolescence.

Modifications in the Theory of Female Adolescence

From my work with adolescents I came to realize that in the realm of object relations the most profound and obdurate complex resides in the boy's oedipal attachment to his father and in the girl's preoedipal bond with her mother. Both these complexes represent usually quite formidable obstacles in the course of analytic work with adolescents. It is a major task of adolescence to settle this crucial issue because the attainment of emotional maturity remains out of reach if the resolution of the negative Oedipus complex is not accomplished at this period of life. I stress these aspects of early object relations because we tend to overstress the positive oedipal constellation and its resuscitation in the life of the adolescent boy and girl. I am aware that my proposition overstates the case, but not without reason; I intend to emphasize the tenacious nature of the negative Oedipus complex which I find enmeshed in the etiology of every adolescent emotional disturbance, regardless of its particular nature.

I have dealt extensively with this problem as it concerns the male adolescent and have postulated on that occasion a biphasic resolution of the male oedipal conflict: one at the entry into latency and one at the closing phase of adolescence (Blos 1974, 1979a). It has long been taken for granted that there is no parallel between the resolutions of the male and female Oedipus complex. One difference has always struck me, namely, the requisite of a radical extinction of the positive and negative Oedipus complex in the adolescent boy before his progressive development toward adulthood moves vigorously ahead. In contrast, the adolescent girl tolerates—within limits, to be sure— a far greater fluidity between the infantile attachments to both parents and her adult personality consolidation, without being necessarily encumbered in her advance toward emotional maturity.

The girl's normal ambivalence toward the preoedipal mother, the mother of the dyadic period of infancy, reaches a dramatic and intense reactivation during adolescence proper and late adolescence. In her past, the little girl had once rescued herself from this early and intense ambivalence by a flight to the father. Her need for nurturance and love turned—in direct and unaltered descent from her maternal attachment—to the father who bears the distinction of never having been contaminated by the chaotic-archaic ambitendencies which burdened her relationship with the early mother. Behind the emotional closeness to and partial identification with the father looms lastingly and dreamlike the realm of the preodipal mother and the yearning to regain it. This constellation becomes particularly virulent in adolescence when the girl, under the powerful sway of the regressive pull to the early mother, turns passionately and frantically to the other sex. Attachments of this kind are of a defensive nature and should be looked at as prestages on the path to mature femininity.

The defensive emotional thrust to which I have just alluded flourishes within the realm of fantasy and emotional attitudes but not infrequently finds expression in sexual involvements; they are, to a large extent, devoid of personal-effective closeness despite the intense passion the girl experiences. They might be described as the concretized yet ethereal bearers of blissful infantile emotions. Beyond the girl's genuine personal liking of her boyfriend we can observe the rise and fall of a transient and global object hypercathexis. The girl seems to be involved in a frenzied search for a refuge from an overwhelming regressive need for the early mother, expecting to find it through heterosexual object possession. For these reasons I have called the (pseudo) heterosexuality of female early adolescence the "oedipal defense." The dynamics of this constellation are apparent, indeed obvious, to any therapist who is not totally prejudiced in favor of oedipal interpretations as the master key that opens at this stage of adolescence all the gateways to emotional maturity. In fact, early adolescence precedes the turn to femininity; this turn can only occur after the ambivalence to the preoedipal mother is resolved—optimally rather than totally—by the girl's postambivalent identification with the maternal function. Then and only then can the girl's ambivalent self-image as female be transcended and a cohesive harmony in the self be attained. I should hastily add that the maternal function I speak of should not be taken literally, because any identification of this kind always remains subject to transformations in consonance with the individual's emotional disposition and ego-ideal propensities. In other words, the emotional maturity of a woman is not necessarily contingent on being a mother or bringing up a child.

How seriously this developmental forward step of the adolescent girl can be interfered with by her mother's need for closeness and sharing—couched usually in the benevolent desire to understand her daughter more fully and more deeply—was well worded by an adolescent girl's outcry, "My mother took my inner life away from me by always wanting to share it." In every successful analysis of an adolescent girl we observe that the ambivalence toward the early mother, as perceived and acted on in the present, has markedly declined. Concurrently, there appears a definitive move toward femininity and mature object relations. A reconciliation of this nature does not, by any means, imply that a warm, loving, and conflictless relationship between daughter and mother has been established; but it does mean that a loosening of preoedipal fixations has occurred, thus liberating the daughter from a confining, emotional bondage and insidious dependency. This internal liberation sets the daughter free to seek fulfillment of her own choosing in the realm of her own body and mind. Their ownership is thereby established; concomitantly, the sense of identity acquires its ultimate solidity and clarity. I will mention one further clinical observation which belongs to this adolscent struggle for liberation. Whenever the little girl has failed to transcend the normal infantile split into the "good" and the "bad" mother, she finds herself hampered in the progression to the stage of whole-object representation. This structural deficit appears in later life, grossly manifest in adolescence, in the chronic need for idealization as a restorative affect. Repetitive, abortive love relations are the typical misfortunes we observe in the lives of these infantile personalities; they, indeed, suffer from a syndromal condition which brings many late-adolescent girls to our professional attention.

Having observed these various adolescent constellations of daughter-mother conflicts and their decline in the course of analytic treatment, I feel justified in summarizing my observations in a general way. The anxiety due to internal rage toward the mother imago, when misplaced to the actual mother of the adolescent girl, rises in intensity with the degree of imminent emotional helplessness which the adolescent girl experiences under the impact of the regressive pull to preoedipality. We can even go one step further in the relative consideration of oedipal feelings and remind ourselves of Freud's comment that "where the woman's attachment to her father was particularly intense, analysis showed it has been preceded by a phase of exclusive attachment to her mother which had been equally intense and passionate" (1931, p. 225). The case history of Dora offers an eloquent example of this fact.[4] If we think of the dyadic and preoedipal periods of female development and of their attenuated extension into adolescence and, beyond that, into normal femininity, we must admit that there is nothing analogous in the life of the adolescent boy.

It must have become apparent from my comments that I look at many of Freud's inferences, which he drew from adult analysis about early female development, as still valid, even though not all of his extrapolations have stood the test of time. Take, for example, the issue of the female superego as contrasted with that of the male.[5] Freud attributed the difference to the fact that the male oedipal child, being in fear of castration, constructs a protective bulwark in the form of a rigorous and exacting superego, while the girl remains more yielding and open to revisions due to her realization of being castrated; this condition then rules out the necessity for an equally forceful and uncompromising superego as is the case in the male. Since the particular preconditions implicit in Freud's reasoning about female superego consolidation have given way to reformulations, we might attribute the observed difference in matters of male and female superego to the fact that the girl has never abandoned her preoedipal attachment to the mother as fully as the boy has. When blending these earliest attachments with oedipal passions, the girl's range of empathy broadens and her fluid potential for identification unfolds, going far beyond anything available to the male. We encounter here again the well-known face that bisexuality is more stringently repressed in men than in women and that the boy's repression of the negative oedipal attachment is more rigorous and definitive than what we can ascertain in the girl. This assertion fits together with some clinical findings, namely, that daughter-father incest occurs far more frequently than son-mother incest; in fact, the latter is almost nonexistent. Speaking in a lighter vein, I mention the so-called pajama party, a social gathering popular among preadolescent girls but quite unthinkable in the life of the preadolescent boy.

What has just been said about the male-female superego characteristics might serve as a paradigm of the psychoanalytic revision that pertains not only to early development of object relations but also to the divergence in sex and gender schematization and, consequently, to male-female body- and self-image differentiation. We speak readily today of a primary, nondefensive femininity, and we also speak of sociocultural influences as outweighing the anatomical determinants pertaining to definitive gender differentiation. These facts have altered radically our view of female adolescence. Where once we inferred penis envy, today we are ready to discover behind this concept the vast region of preoedipal vicissitudes in object relations and in early ego development. Where once we considered it phase adequate for the little girl to be ignorant of her genitals, especially of her vagina, we now recognize fantasies or sensations, as reported from clinical and research work with children, the derivatives of such prephallic awarenesses. Indeed, today we attribute a far more specifically feminine psychological development to the first year of the girl's life than was the case in the past. One remarkable consequence of the constitutional, nondefensive differentiation between male and female can be observed in the role which orality plays in female adolescent symptomatology. The clinician of female adolescence is familiar with the frequency of the depressive syndrome as well as with the ubiquitous struggle over dietary problems, epitomized by obesity and anorexia. Furthermore, I should mention the source of conflict attached to oral aggression which plays such a profound role in the etiology of some forms of frigidity. The insidious influence of infantile object idealization has to be emphasized in this connection as a severe encumbrance in the path toward postadolescent emotional maturity. To this list should be added the hysteria symptomatology which Freud (1931), late in his life, came to attribute to the girl's early attachment to the mother.[6]

From my experience I can report that undisguised and pleasurable daydreams or thoughts about the mother's breast are not uncommon among adolescent girls, especially older adolescent girls. Such mental images are accompanied by a deeply felt sense of bliss which, for the moment, alters the view of the world as physically and emotionally perceived. Should this regressed state arouse fright or panic, we observe withdrawal or distancing behavior, nightmares or anxiety attacks. One late-adolescent girl, affectively frozen, socially scared to the point of isolation, perceived the world around herself in an opaque and dreamy way. She reported an image that came to her while riding on a bus; she was holding and sucking her mother's breast. As long as this image lasted, her vision was momentarily clear and sharp, her mood one of hopefulness and confidence. Metaphorically speaking, this fantasy expressed in condensed form her expectations from the world around her on every level of present-day living. Slight wonder that the affect dominating her life was one of silent rage, despair, and depressive immobility, physical and emotional.

The Influence of Contemporary Culture

In discussing the psychology of the adolescent girl we cannot ignore the contemporary, history-bound adolescent milieu. Therefore, I shall now take a brief look at influences which are of a different order from those of a constitutional or developmental nature. The adolescent girl of today's Western world grows up almost totally unsupported by traditions or rites of passage. She is called upon to act as an individual in making choices regarding work, education, and residence, as well as erotic and sexual alternatives, from holding hands to coitus. She is expected to do this at an evolutionary stage when the female body matures earlier than was the case in antecedent generations. It does not follow from the alteration in the timetable of menarche that the girl's social, emotional, and cognitive development advances at a parallel rate. The technological ingenuity that produced "the pill" offered the ill-conceived hope that adolescent pregnancies would be controlled by the intervention of mature self-determination. We came to realize that the sexual act in and of itself is no indicator of maturity in judgment and thought nor does it guarantee the advance toward these mental capabilities. The attainment of emotional maturity is contingent on the synchronization and integration of physical and emotional experiences. The normal adolescent emotional disengagement from family ties is frequently preempted today by the fact that such ties, still woefully needed for sound psychic restructuring, are abruptly abandoned before the developmental task has had time to be completed within the confines of a facilitating environment. Peer and cultural ("the media") influences rush in to fill the void by holding out rewards of success and happiness which the sexual act or sexuality in general will assure. Equating adultomorphic behavior with adulthood itself tends to become the source of confusion and identity disturbances. Clinical work has shown that for many adolescent girls submission to the conventionality of the unconventional, namely, "having sex," negates glibly her attentiveness to the most personal motives and emotions; thus, she stunts her emotional growth and

20

settles for what Deutsch (1967) has called an "infantile personality." The cultural ambience of sexual freedom is reflected in the flood of instructively detailed magazine articles, films, and illustrated sex guides which become an insidious *vade mecum* for those adolescent girls whose pain and challenge of normal adolescent conflict is blown away, at least temporarily, by the sexual act. As a result, no succinctly personal accommodation to the slow process of growing up is lived through.

In order not to be misunderstood I hasten to say that sexual experimentation during adolescence has been with us from time immemorial. What has changed is the form which the expression of sexual urges has taken in the contemporary adolescent generation, namely, its conventionality and social conformity as well as the obliviousness to a personal sense of emotional style and readiness for new experiences. To this has to be added the widespread belief that sex is the magic gateway to a world as wished for, whatever that might be at this age of youthful expectations and uncertainties.

We might ask ourselves how these matters just touched upon will affect the next generation since the future mothers are today's adolescent girls. Many of them are ashamed or made ashamed by their peers if they harbor maternal yearnings and aspirations of domesticity or, worse still, if they prefer to put off an active sex life to the future. In their quandary they often settle for regressive gratifications in the act of lovemaking. Then the most desired sensation of the act itself is frequently called by the girl—especially the young adolescent girl—"cuddling," reflecting a stage of object relation which is far removed from mature intimacy. Thus, sex becomes a peculiarly isolated pleasure experience, unintegrated into the total life of the personality. A conflict of singular importance for the contemporary girl lies in the polarity of motherhood versus work or career. New styles of marriage have emerged which promise to eliminate these tradition-bound exclusivities of roles. We must remember that personality growth and psychological differentiation come about only through the elaboration of conflict and its transformation into adult personality structures; from these novel configurations issue, over time, new life-styles and, ultimately, sociocultural innovations and traditions by which the generations to come will be strengthened and renewed (Blos 1976).

Conclusions

The definitive teasing out of the many specific factors which, in their intermeshing dynamics, compose the whole panorama of female adolescent development is a task not yet completed. The factors I am talking about are of a most heterogeneous nature; a grasp of their synergic organization and function remains the object of our search. The science of human development aims at coordinating the influences of constitutional givens, of earliest irreversible imprintings, of object relations and their effect on psychic patterning, and, last but not least, of sociocultural determinants in their ceaseless changeability over history. I have succeeded only partially in doing justice to this task. However, I hope I succeeded in sharpening our awareness of those still-obscure regions where investigative work is waiting impatiently for our attentive presence.

NOTES

1. A question never elucidated in Freud's writing pertains to the fact that the wished-for oedipal baby in doll play is always female, while the commonly wished-for baby of the mature woman is a boy: "A mother is only brought unlimited satisfaction by relation to a son" (Freud 1933, p. 133). We cannot but ponder whether the so-called oedipal baby (female doll) is not an amalgam of the experience of preoedipal mothering in its active and passive forms and, secondarily, of oedipal strivings which contain earliest feminine wishes. The fact that mature women usually, but not always, prefer a baby boy contains powerful sociocultural influences, but beyond this, we recognize in this preference for the penis bearer an effort of the mature woman to stem the everlasting regressive pull to the preoedipal mother imago, a pull and counterpull to which the doll-playing little girl has once in the past given herself over with such abandon.

2. "Core identity develops first and is the central nexus around which masculinity and feminity gradually accrete" (Stoller 1976, p. 61).

3. To make this "correction" is, however, not necessary—Freud continues—if we include in the Oedipus complex the negative component of the girl's exclusive attachment to the mother and realize that the girl reaches the positive position only after "she has surmounted a period before it that is governed by the negative complex" (p. 226).

4. I have discussed elsewhere the preoedipal etiology of Dora's hysterical symptomatology (see Blos 1979b).

5. "Their [women's] superego is never so inexorable, so impersonal, so independent of its emotional origins as we require it to be in men" (Freud 1925).

22

6. "This phase of attachment to the mother is espeically intimately related to the aetiology of hysteria . . . the neurosis characteristically feminine . . . " (Freud 1931, p. 227).

REFERENCES

Blos, P. 1974. The genealogy of the ego ideal. *Psychoanalytic Study of the Child* 29:43 – 88.

Blos, P. 1976. When and how does adolescence end: structural criteria for adolescent closure. *Adolescent Psychiatry* 5:3–17.

Blos, P. 1979a. Modifications in the classical psychoanalytic model of adolescence. *Adolescent Psychiatry* 7:6 – 25.

Blos, P. 1979b. Preoedipal factors in the etiology of female deliquency: postscript 1976. *The Adolescent Passage*. New York: International Universities Press.

Bronson, G. W. 1973. Fear of visual novelty: developmental patterns in males and females. In L. J. Stone, H. T. Smith, and L. B. Murphy, eds. *The Social Infant*. New York: Basic.

Deutsch, H. 1967. Selected problems of adolescence. *Psychoanalytic Study of the Child*. Monograph no. 3. New York: International Universities Press.

Freud, S. 1909. Analysis of a phobia in a five-year-old boy. *Standard Edition* 10:5–149. London: Hogarth, 1955.

Freud, S. 1924. The dissolution of the Oedipus complex. *Standard Edition* 19:171–179. London: Hogarth, 1961.

Freud, S. 1925. Some consequences of the anatomical distinction between the sexes. *Standard Edition* 19:248–260. London: Hogarth, 1961.

Freud, S. 1931. Female sexuality. *Standard Edition* 21:225–243. London: Hogarth, 1961.

Freud, S. 1933. Femininity. *Standard Edition:* 22:112–135. London: Hogarth, 1964.

Galenson, E., and Roiphe, H. 1976. Some suggested revisions concerning early female development. *Journal of the American Psychoanalytic Association* 24(5): 29 – 57.

Green, R. 1976. Human sexuality: research and treatment frontiers. In S. Arieti, ed. *American Handbook of Psychiatry*. New York: Basic.

Grossman, W. I., and Stewart, W. A. 1976. Penis envy; from childhood wish to developmental metaphor. *Journal of the American Psychoanalytic Association* 24(5): 193–212.

Hamburg, D. A., and Lunde, D. T. 1966. Sex hormones in the development of sex differences in human behavior. In E. E. Maccoby, ed. *The Development of Sex Differences*. Stanford, Calif.: Stanford University Press.

Jones, E. 1935. Early female sexuality. *Papers on Psychoanalysis*. Boston: Beacon, 1961.

Roiphe, H. 1968. On an early genital phase: with an addendum on genesis. *Psychoanalytic Study of the Child* 23:348–365.

Stoller, R. 1974. Facts and fancies: an examination of Freud's concept of bisexuality. In J. Strouse, ed. *Women and Analysis*. New York: Grossman.

Stoller, R. 1976. Primary femininity. *Journal of the American Psychoanalytic Association* 24(5): 59–78.

Ticho, G. R. 1976. Female autonomy and young adult women. *Journal of the American Psychoanalytic Association* 24(5): 139–155.

2

THE RELATIVITY OF ADOLESCENCE:
EFFECTS OF TIME, PLACE, AND PERSONS

LEON EISENBERG

Adolescence is not a thing "out there" or "in itself," a "fact" of human development or a biological "reality." Adolescence, like beauty, is in the eye of the beholder; as with beauty, eye and object gazed upon modify each other. Adolescence is a construct—or, rather, many constructs, each varying with culture, history, class, and caste. Such social constructs arise from the human need to make coherent sense of and to control what occurs during the transformation from child into adult.

Let me not be misunderstood. I do not worship at the altar of Bishop Berkeley's solipsism. Children do become adults, however culture conceptualizes the process. What I wish to stress is that there is no culture without a mythology about the transformation and that the mythology influences the process itself. That mythology is so thoroughly embedded in consciousness that it comes to be regarded as part of nature rather than as a human construct.

Hence stems such justification as I can provide for the use of the word "relativity" in the title of this chapter. Because Albert Einstein was the hero of my own adolescent years (and remains one into my senium), I want to honor the centenary of his birth by tying these remarks to that celebration.

In 1907, while Einstein was struggling to make the special theory of relativity, which applied only to systems moving with constant velocity, broad enough to accommodate accelerating systems and, hence, gravity, he had what he termed "the happiest thought of my life." As he wrote later,

Just as is the case with the electric field produced by electromagnetic induction, the gravitational field has similarly only a relative existence. *For if one considers an observer in free fall, e.g., from the roof of a house, there exists for him during his fall no gravitational field*—at least in his immediate vicinity. For if the observer releases any objects, they will remain relative to him in a state of rest, or in a state of uniform motion. . . . The observer therefore is justified to consider his state as one of "rest."

The extraordinarily curious, empirical law that all bodies in the same gravitational field fall with the same acceleration received through this consideration at once a deep physical meaning. For if there is even a single thing which falls differently into a gravitational field than do the others, the observer would discern by means of it that he is in a gravitational field, and that he is falling into it. But if such a thing does not exist—as experience has confirmed with great precision—the observer lacks any objective ground to consider himself as falling in a gravitational field. Rather, he has the right to consider his state as that of rest, and his surroundings (with respect to gravitation) as field-free. The fact of experience concerning the independence of acceleration in free-fall with respect to the material is therefore a mighty argument that the postulate of relativity is to be extended to coordinate systems that move non-uniformly relative to one another. [Einstein 1979, pp. 156–157]

By analogy, we are blind to the "gravitational field" effects on the phenomenology of adolescence insofar as we function within a cultural "coordinate system," like the observer in free-fall. We only become aware of the coordinates of our own social system when we correct for our ethnocentrism by studying other cultures, other times of history, and other social classes. Relativity, as I employ it, lacks the "deep physical meaning" it has in physics but, nonetheless, serves heuristic purposes by emphasizing the mutability of adolescent phenomena and by acknowledging the extent to which those phenomena are shaped by the belief systems and the social institutions of each community in which children become adults.

The concept of adolescence is taken as a given by twentieth-century Americans. But neither it nor childhood, to say nothing of the current interest in the later stages of adult development (Levinson 1978), are immanent in the human life cycle. Aries (1962) has argued persuasively that the idea of childhood is a relatively recent cultural invention. In the Middle Ages, only infancy was recognized as a separate stage. It lasted until the age of seven, when the child was assimilated into the adult world by apprenticeship, with little or no formal education for the vast majority of children. The concept of childhood as a separate stage of human development was first advanced in the educational writings of the French philosophers of the Enlightenment.

As infant mortality began to decrease, and as the amount of leisure time began to increase, the experience of childhood was transformed. With the growth of industrialization and its need for a better-trained working class, the education of children and their segregation from adult society in the special institutions appropriate to the new concept of childhood became the norm for an ever-larger percentage of the world's children.

Kenniston (1971) has carried the argument one step further; he suggests that the concept of adolescence is a twentieth-century invention resulting from further social evolution. Freud, writing at the turn of the century, spoke of puberty as a biological event and had relatively little to say about it, in contrast to the profusion of publications on adolescence which flourished in the post–World War II period. Mandatory schooling to the age of eighteen has become the rule; the period of being assigned formal educational tasks and of being denied work roles has been extended to an increasingly larger percentage of the twelve- to eighteen-year-old population, for whom the job market has, in any event, no openings. With 11 million young Americans in postsecondary education, Kenniston suggests that the ground has been set for a new stage of psychological development: the postadolescent stage of youth. The point I make is simply this: though there is a programmed sequence of biological changes in the transition from child to adult, today's conception of adolescence has resulted from societal changes and, in turn, has shaped the experience of the individual undergoing that transition.

Thus, from a contemporary perspective, adolescence may be defined as a critical period of human development manifested at the biological, psychological, and social levels of integration, of variable onset and duration but marking the end of childhood and establishing the foundation for maturity. Biologically, its onset is signaled by the acceleration of somatic growth and by the beginnings of secondary sexual development, its termination by the fusion of the osseous epiphyses and by the completion of sexual maturation. Socially, it is a period of intensified preparation for the assumption of an adult role, and its termination is signaled when the individual is accorded full adult prerogatives, the timing and nature of which vary widely from society to society. The interaction of biological maturation and social experience determines its psychological attributes: an acceleration of cognitive growth, the formation of a personal identity, the renegotiation of relationships with parents and peers, and the crystallization of gender role, all of them attributes that become problematic precisely in a society undergoing unparalleled social transformations. Such is not the case in traditional or "static"

27

societies where roles are sharply defined, choices few, and places available for all. In our world, adolescence is indeed a "critical period" for development because of the rapid and profound changes in mental and physical development during adolescence and because their effective resolution is a necessary, though not sufficient, condition for full maturation in adulthood.

The relativity of adolescence is evident even at the biological level of organization. Consider puberty, the one developmental sequence which is relatively invariant across cultures in the ordering of its steps, though not in their timing, duration, or outcome. For Americans, the median ages for the major growth spurts are twelve to fifteen for boys and ten to thirteen for girls (National Center for Health Statistics 1973b); but puberty's onset in either sex may be as early as seven or as late as seventeen, its termination as early as fifteen or as late as twenty-five.

The timing of onset and termination is a function of both internal factors (sex and heredity) and external factors (nutrition and health status). Severe malnutrition markedly retards growth; if repaired early enough, catch-up growth is possible within limits. In the presence of chronic disease (renal failure), growth retardation is marked and permanent. With the improvement in the standard of living of our population over the past century, there has been a substantial increment in the final height of young Americans. Nisei growing up in California before World War II were several inches taller than children raised in Japan; with postwar gains in the Japanese economy, the difference between Japanese and Nisei is no longer evident. The role of genetic factors remains decisive in controlling growth potential; Japanese do not attain the height of Watusi and males remain taller than females.

Similar sensitivity to environmental factors is evident in sexual maturation. The current mean age at menarche in the United States is 12.8 years of age, earlier than it was at the turn of the century (National Center for Health Statistics 1973a). Data collected from European sources indicate a progressive lowering of the age of menarche, by as much as four years over the past century (Tanner 1962). Yet, among the !Kung bushmen in the Kalihari Desert, the average menarchial age had, until very recently, remained unchanged for millennia but is beginning to appear earlier as the !Kung settle near the pastoral Bantu and abandon their traditional nomadic life and diet.

We can safely assume that there is a biological lower bound for the age of menarche, one we now approximate, as well as an upper limit to mean human height. However, improved living standards have revealed biological potentials of the human organism which, until the recent past, had been masked by the ubiquity of undernourishment. New social conditions do not alter human potential, but they reveal its unsuspected dimensions.

Furthermore, the "new" biology of puberty has its own social consequences. Earlier menarche inevitably implies the earlier establishment of regular ovulatory cycles and enhanced fertility. The potential for earlier fertility, when accompanied, as it is in our day, by the earlier onset of sexual activity and by the failure to use contraception, has resulted in higher rates of pregnancy among young teenagers, pregnancies which carry greater medical hazard for mother and infant as well as serious social risks for both (Berger 1978; Furstenberg 1976). Between 1970 and 1976, the proportion of fifteen- to nineteen-year-old unmarried women who had experienced sexual intercourse grew from 30 percent to 41 percent (Zelnik and Kantner 1977). Now, some 400,000 girls under seventeen become pregnant each year, 30,000 of them fourteen or under (Institute of Medicine 1978).

The very great majority of teenage out-of-wedlock pregnancies are unintended. Thus, about a third of the more than a million abortions in the United States each year are performed on teenagers; among those fourteen and younger, abortions exceed live births. For this population, the Hyde Amendment to the Social Security Act, restricting the use of federal monies for abortion in Medicaid recipients, threatens catastrophic medical and social consequences.

Only six states and the District of Columbia mandate family life education in the public schools. Organized political opposition to a role for the public schools insists that sex education is a parental responsibility, despite the overwhelming evidence, both from teenagers' reports on the source of their sex information and from their actual behavior, that it is one most parents fail to meet. The default of the school and the family in providing teenagers with an informed basis for decision making amplifies the effects of peer-group pressures; the greater the number of young people who engage in sexual experimentation, the more powerful the press on others to comply. Social toleration of child and adolescent experimental sexuality, common to many traditional societies, has few biological consequences so long as menarche is a late event. Precocious sexual activity coupled with the socially induced biological potential for earlier fertility, without information about and motivation for contraception, inevitably generates increasing rates of unwanted pregnancy.

During the very same time period when physical maturation has been accelerated, there has been a marked delay for more and more young people of the age at which full adult social status can be attained. The net effect in the last half of this century has been a remarkable prolongation of adolescence as a developmental stage. In the face of the technological imperative of modern society, the time necessary to education for, and socialization into, adult roles in the managerial classes has been extended to a degree heretofore unknown. Whereas at the turn of the century less than 15 percent of fourteen- to seventeen-year-olds attended high school and only an elite 4 percent of eighteen- to twenty-one-year-olds attended college, today well over 90 percent of American seventeen-year-olds are in high school, about half go on to postsecondary education, and a third of those who enter college go on to graduate school (Coleman 1972). Between 1960 and 1970, the percentage of twenty- to twenty-one-year-old males enrolled in college increased from 26 percent to 43 percent, whereas those in the labor force declined from 68 percent at the beginning of the decade to just over half by its end. In more recent years, the proportion of women entering postsecondary education has increased so rapidly that they now make up just about half of the student population.

Thus American youth, precociously mature in their physical development, experience an enforced delay of the time at which they enter socially productive work. Their families have become far less important units of social cohesion, as more and more of the roles once borne by the family have been taken on by other institutions in society. They are segregated into mass postsecondary educational institutions so large that fifty now enroll in excess of 20,000 students and some as many as 50,000. Sheer numbers ineluctably dictate organizational complexity, proliferation of administrative bureaucracy, and assignment of priority to managerial goals. The value system of the colleges they attend is one in which the student is given the task of improving himself on a competitive basis in which the success of one student is at the expense of another so long as grading is on a distribution curve, and the funnel of opportunities narrows as the student moves from one level to the next. This contrasts sharply with the social function of the young worker who must collaborate with others in producing for society (Coleman 1965). Though each may be motivated by economic gain, he or she can attain it only in a common effort because of the nature of mass production; take-home pay can be increased only by joining with others in collective union activity. If even the adults in contemporary society feel atomized and alienated, how much more must this be true of the student who has no immediate social usefulness and who has had little to say in controlling the destiny of the larger society?

Thus far, of course, I have emphasized the new conditions which apply to that increasing proportion of young people who go on to education beyond high school. If that proportion has increased more than tenfold, it still remains true that half enter—or try to enter—the labor force. In attending to overall statistics, we blind ourselves to the sharp differences in the adolescent experience within population subgroups. Despite gains in the numbers of minority group youth who now complete high school and go on to college, marked differences in the opportunity structure remain. Furthermore, minority adolescents experience a disproportionately high rate of unemployment when they seek work, a rate registered at three- to fourfold higher (even with the use of statistics which are undercounts because those who despair of looking for work are no longer tabulated). Thus one subpopulation experiences delay in achieving independent adult status by virtue of prolonged training; other groups strive for adult work roles but are unable to attain them for lack of occupational opportunities.

Other social and demographic changes have altered the envelope of adolescence. One hundred years ago, the length of the school term was about 130 days per year; now, it is almost 180. Even more striking is the change in days actually attended which, because of higher absenteeism rates, then averaged eighty days and now average 160; a doubling of days in school per year has occurred. The student role has become by far the dominant one among the many roles a young person might have had, and did have, not so very long ago. The student role is one in which young people are set apart in an obligatory dependent state, essentially a passive one, in contrast to the many useful work roles in home and community which once were available. Moreover, the young have been segregated into groups within a narrow age range, clustered first by grade and secondarily into age-grouped elementary, junior high, and senior high schools. This differs markedly from traditional societies in which young and old interact in common work tasks and even from the small schoolhouses in the last century of our own industrial society where children and adolescents mingled in one setting and where older students tutored the younger ones. It is not to deny the formal gains in our school system (more specialized instruction, better equipment, a greater variety of teacher role models) to acknowledge that this has been achieved at a social cost: the losses in more individualized relationships, in mutual caring across age groups, and in sense of community. As Coleman (1972) states, "With every decade, the length of schooling has increased, until a thoughtful person must ask whether society can conceive of no other way for youth to come into adulthood."

Equally decisive have been the demographic changes in our population, changes whose consequences have only begun to become the object of social analysis. Between 1960 and 1970, as the result of the post–World War II baby boom, the subpopulation between fourteen and twenty-four increased by 14 million; during that one decade, we added more adolescents to our population than in all the previous sixty years of this century together! The ratio between those aged fourteen to twenty-four and those from twenty-five to sixty-four rose from 32 percent at the beginning of the decade to 45 percent at its end. The increase in sheer numbers was a major determinant of the youth culture of the 1960s, which the media and manufacturers of consumer goods were quicker to appreciate than most professionals. That cohort of adolescents has become a cohort of young adults in this decade as the tidal wave continues to roll through the age distribution of our population. In its wake lies a reduced cohort resulting from the decline in birthrate in the past generation; we have, at the same time, a smaller number of adolescents in this decade and the one to come and a growing reservoir in the young adult population. A proportion which had reached 45 percent by 1970 will decline to 42 percent by 1980 and 33 percent by 1990. The quiescence of the 1970s in comparison with the activism of the 1960s is not merely a matter of numbers, but as the size of the adolescent constituency continues to decline, it will be unable to muster the recruits once available to it. As another way of putting our nation in perspective: those under fifteen are currently only 25 percent of the U.S. population; in contrast, they constitute 46 percent of the total in Mexico. The age distribution of the Mexican population today is similar to that of the United States at the turn of the century when, in present terminology, we would have been a developing nation (Westoff 1974).

The huge influx of inexperienced workers into the labor market, on one hand, and of young college graduates, on the other, has markedly influenced income possibilities for both groups so that a strictly economic analysis questions the profitability of an investment in college (Freeman 1976). Furthermore, the delayed economic burden for the family of having children closely spaced together has been overlooked in the standard analysis of educational costs. According to government data, family incomes have risen more rapidly than college costs; analysts have therefore concluded that additional student support is not necessary. But this narrow perspective has overlooked the effect of the ''college-age sib squeeze'' (Parke 1979). Whereas fifteen years ago, only about a quarter of the children of an age to enter college had a sibling one or two years older, now (and for the next few years), half will. The average years of double tuition payment rose from 1.8 in 1965 to 2.8 in 1976. This leads to a very different conclusion about the need for a public subsidy of higher education. Although the squeeze will begin to taper by 1980, it will not be until ten years from now that it will fall below the level of 1967.

Welcome as this may be at one level, the demographic transition has been so pervasive in the Western world that several European nations (e.g., France and West Germany) currently have birthrates below those necessary for population replacement, and in both countries pronatalist political movements have arisen. Those of us who have spent restless nights worrying about explosive population growth may find the prospect of its contraction a welcome soporific. However, economic viability depends on the age distribution of each nation's population as well as its aggregate numbers. The developed world has entered a new era, one in which it will be necessary to develop effective long-range social policy to buffer against inordinate swings in birthrate, perturbations whose social consequences do not become fully evident until a generation later.

So much, then, for a cursory survey of the changes over time and place in the biological and social dimensions of adolescence. If these changes were without major impact on psychological development, they would be no more than curious, no doubt interesting, but largely irrelevant matters for psychiatry. The contrary is the case. The more things change, the more rapidly they change. The genetic program that circumscribes human biopsychological capacities evolved over millenia characterized by rates of social change which, despite aperiodic catastrophes caused by pestilence, crop failure, and war, were glacial compared with those of this century. We may be fast approaching a point that will exceed the collective coping capacity of our species. Indeed, the mere enumeration of adolescent health statistics must arouse serious concern.

What stands out is that the major health problems of adolescence are behaviorally mediated (Eisenberg and Eisenberg 1977). Deaths from violence— accidents, homicide, and suicide—account for three-quarters of all deaths between ages twelve and nineteen. Some 60 percent result from accidents, half of them due to automobiles. For nonwhites fifteen to nineteen, both male and female, homicide is the second leading cause of death. For white males, it is suicide. Suicide rates among adolescents have tripled over the last twenty years. However, we know that the recorded rates are underestimates because of social constraints on reporting. Although firm data are hard to come by, there may be as many as 100 attempts for each completed suicide. Deaths from violence in adolescence and young adulthood among males account for the greatest part of the difference in longevity between the United States and Sweden (Fuchs 1974).

Other behavior-linked threats to health—smoking, drug taking, and drinking—are on the increase among American youth, with the earlier age of onset of this self-destructive behavior being the most frightening statistic of all. As Jessor and Jessor (1977) have pointed out, health-compromising behavior represents instrumental efforts to attain a sense of personal satisfaction, a sense of control over the environment, and a sense of autonomy, goals which may be unavailable to the adolescent through other channels. It expresses opposition to conventional society and serves as a way of demonstrating solidarity with peers. Problem behavior tends to co-occur. Thus adolescents who use marijuana are more likely to be sexually active and to drink than are nonusers; such activities have a negative relationship with more conventional attributes such as school achievement and church membership. They are associated with lower expectations of achievement and a high valence on independence and autonomy. Peer behavior, support, and identification are particularly powerful forces in generating deviant behavior. In effect, efforts to prevent behavior that endangers health demand of adolescents that they delay gratifications which are constantly emphasized, widely advertised, and avidly sought by adults. If there is to be any hope of postponing problem behavior, adolescents must have increased access to opportunities to attain the constructive symbols of maturity: the capacity for work, love, and play.

The litany of misfortune is a long one. In major cities, as many as one-third of all juveniles will have a police record by the age of eighteen; violent crimes are increasing. Positive achievement, as measured by an index such as the Scholastic Aptitude Test, has shown a steady decline over the past twenty years, a decline that cannot be explained away by changes in the composition of the group aspiring to college or by changes in the stringency of the examinations which appear, if anything, to be less demanding than they were. And I would add, though this statement is based on clinical impression rather than firm data, that the narcissistic preoccupation with self, so evident in the adult culture of the 1970s, threatens to become a virulent infestation among our youth.

Grim as this may sound, I refuse to accept it as either a necessary or an inevitable Spenglerian account of the decline and fall of the West. On the contrary, if I am right in emphasizing the relativity of adolescence as a set of developmental phenomena which are shaped by what has been up to now blind social change, it follows with equal force that it is within our power as citizens to construct a society in which the potential for healthy growth of personality will be enhanced, just as social conditions have permitted physical maturation to flower.

If we are to do so, it will be necessary to reexamine the prevailing cynicism about the efficacy of social action that has become the received wisdom of our time. For example, the fathers of this republic asserted a faith in public education as a basic instrumentality for creating a citizenry prepared for and committed to democracy. Recall the words Jefferson wrote in defense of his plan for a law on public education:

But of all of the views of this law, none is more important, none more legitimate, than that of rendering the people the safe, as they are the ultimate, guardians of their own liberty. . . . Every government degenerates when trusted to the rulers of the people alone. The people themselves therefore are its only safe depositories. And to render even them safe their minds must be improved to a certain degree. . . . An amendment of our Constitution must here come in aid of the public education. . . . [Jefferson 1783]

Or recall the words of Benjamin Rush: "[Learning] is favorable to liberty. Freedom can exist only in the society of knowledge. Without learning, men are incapable of knowing their rights, and where learning is confined to a few people, liberty can be neither equal nor universal" (Rush 1786).

Yet today, conventional wisdom holds that schooling makes little difference to adolescent achievement. The Coleman study (1966) has been taken to demonstrate few effects attributable to schooling in contrast to the major impact of home circumstance on achievement. Jencks (1972), in his analysis of the Coleman data, reemphasized the importance of social class and cast doubt on the ability of public education to offset social inequality. Educators, already despondent about the difficulty of the task assigned to them, had been provided a weighty rationalization for pessimism. Whereas once cynics about public education reveled in the hereditarian doctrine that IQ determines attainment, we now have the equally deterministic view that social class is all; in either event, there would appear to be little purpose for schooling other than to warehouse the legions of adolescents who must be kept under surveillance and off the streets.

Rutter and his colleagues (1979) at the Institute of Psychiatry in London have reopened the debate by employing a study design that is longitudinal, rather than cross-sectional, so that change over time can be measured; and by employing instruments sufficiently fine grained and appropriate to school-related goals to discern behavioral effects attributable to differences between schools as well as between pupils. They identified twelve comprehensive schools in London whose intake was drawn from a known population. The pupils who were to enter those schools were tested at the age of ten before they entered, again four years later while in attendance, and finally at age sixteen, the minimal school-leaving age. Because the children had been assessed before they enrolled, allowance could be made for the characteristics the children brought with them to the several schools in differentiating those aspects of their later performance which could be attributed to the school experience.

The results are striking. The average level of performance of children in some of the schools was very much better than that in others. Attendance at certain schools was associated with a marked reduction in the frequency of behavior problems and with gains in academic performance; other schools generated a surplus of behavior problems and lower academic gain. Social class remained an important determinant of achievement and was not obliterated by school effects. The successful schools enhanced achievement for both middle- and lower-class children; class differences remained; what is salient is that both groups performed at a higher level. Are we entitled to ask more of public education?

The outcomes measured included academic attainment, attendance, in-school behavior, and delinquency. The independent variables in the school studies included academic emphasis, continuity, teacher activity, rewards and punishment, student conditions, and opportunities for participation.

Academic emphasis (such things as assigning homework and making sure it was completed, the care given to planning courses, the supervision of teachers by department heads, and the like) demonstrated a strong positive relationship with attendance as did high staff morale. Continuity (that is, absence of teacher turnover) did not, somewhat surprisingly, have a major impact. However, the actual time spent teaching was significantly related to both attendance and attainment. Firm discipline, without use of corporal punishment, and liberal reward and encouragement characterized successful schools. Students' feelings that they could approach a teacher were strongly related to positive academic outcome, as was giving students an opportunity to participate in, and responsibility for, planning. An index based on combining the independent variables showed a .8 correlation with behavioral outcomes. Schools do make a difference! Or, at least, schools can make a difference, and a highly positive one, when they are committed to teaching and when they have a representative mix of students.

Schools are, however, not enough. However assiduously cultivated, the talents acquired in school will atrophy without an opportunity for their exercise thereafter. Fairness in school, essential though it is, must be the precursor of fairness in the job market. No youngster will sustain the effort necessary for achievement without reason to believe that achievement will be honored in the world of work. Feedback from recent graduates (and dropouts) will give the lie to the noble principles enunciated in school if they fail to correspond with actuality. Pupils and teachers together can and must

36

engage in uncensored analysis of the real world and participate in the task of making it a better one. Effective educational strategies demand recognition of Frederick Douglass's aphorism: without struggle, there is no progress.

Part of what has led us so badly astray in assessing public education has been a narrow emphasis on the acquisition of prescribed academic content. School is a microcosm of society. Whatever its avowed instrumental intent, it socializes students into the modes of behavior society expects of them. What is learned of human relationships between teacher and student and among peers provides the prototype for human transactions. It is competition or cooperation, hierarchy or equality, reality orientation or denial, social mobility or caste-locked status, that is to be the mode for relations between people? That much we can be certain that students learn, no matter how poorly they perform on formal examinations.

School should nurture the anlage of Erikson's (1950) stage of "generativity." Ties between the extended family have been stretched thin in a mobile society; the lower birthrate and smaller size of the nuclear family had diminished opportunities to learn parenting roles by caring for younger siblings. At the same time, with both parents working, care for infants and toddlers remains an unsolved social problem. Day-care centers and nurseries can and should be situated adjacent to intermediate and secondary schools. Adolescents can not only provide irreplaceable labor but can gain direct experience in parenting as they contribute to the development of the young. Service in tutoring younger children teaches the teacher as well as the taught. In setting classroom goals, emphasis must be placed on group achievement in addition to individual accomplishment; each should feel some responsibility for the success of the other. School and work experience should be interleaved by making time available within the regular program and encouraging experimentation with time out at no loss of right for subsequent reenrollment. Continuous schooling may be an appropriate mode of learning for some, but opportunities for intermittent schooling should be made available to those who can profit from it, at whatever age.

Facile distortions of psychiatric theory have been seized upon to justify the abandonment of firm expectations for prosocial behavior. Pop psychologists regularly recall Freud's (1943) aphorism that "no neurosis [actual neurosis] . . . is present where sexual life is normal" as warrant for indulgence but conveniently overlook his later and more profound comment, "It is impossible to ignore the extent to which civilization is built up on renunciation of instinctual gratifications" (Freud 1930). That freedom is no freedom which is based upon the self alone.

Conclusions

Let me conclude, as I began, by recalling the words of Albert Einstein (1979) in this year of his centennary. Speaking of education he stated,

> Sometimes one sees in the school the instrument for transferring a certain maximum quantity of knowledge to the growing generation. But that is not right. Knowledge is dead; the school, however, serves the living. It should develop in the young individual those qualities and capabilities which are of value for the welfare of the commonwealth. That does not mean that the individual should be destroyed and become a mere tool of the community like a bee or an ant. A community of standardized individuals without personal originality or personal aims would be a poor community without possibilities for development. On the contrary, the aim must be the training of independently acting and thinking individuals who, however, see in the service of the community their highest life problem. [Pp. 315–316]

And further:

> The existence and validity of human rights are not written in the stars. The ideals concerning the conduct of men toward each other and the desirable structure of the community have been conceived and taught by enlightened individuals in the course of history. Those ideals and convictions which resulted from historical experience, from the cravings for beauty and harmony, have been readily accepted in theory by man— and, at all times—have been trampled upon by the same people under the pressure of their animal instincts. A large part of history is therefore replete with the struggle for those human rights, an eternal struggle in which final victory can never be won. But to tire in that struggle would mean the ruin of society. [P. 305]

I can think of no better charter to guide our common effort to reconstruct a social framework to enhance adolescent development.

REFERENCES

Aries, P. 1962. *Centuries of Childhood*. New York: Knopf.
Berger, L. W. 1978. Abortion in America: the effects of restrictive funding. *New England Journal of Medicine* 298:1474–1477.

Coleman, J. S. 1965. *Adolescents and the Schools*. New York: Basic.

Coleman, J. S., et al. 1966. *Equality of Educational Opportunity*. Washington, D.C.: Government Printing Office.

Coleman, J. S., et al. 1972. *Youth: Transition to Adulthood. Report of the Panel on Youth of the President's Science Advisory Committee*. Chicago: University of Chicago Press.

Einstein, A. 1979. In A. P. French, ed. *Einstein: A Centenary Volume*. Cambridge, Mass.: Harvard University Press.

Eisenberg, C., and Eisenberg, L. 1977. On making it at college. Paper presented at the American Academy of Pediatrics. Chicago.

Erikson, E. H. 1950. *Childhood and Society*. New York: Norton.

Freeman, R. B. 1976. *The Overeducated American*. New York: Academic Press.

Freud, S. 1930. Civilization and its discontents. *Standard Edition* 21:64–145. London: Hogarth, 1961.

Freud, S. 1943. *A General Introduction to Psychoanalysis*. Garden City, New York: Doubleday.

Fuchs, V. R. 1974. *Who Shall Live? Health, Economics, and Social Choice*. New York: Basic.

Furstenberg, F. F. 1976. The social consequences of teenage parenthood. *Family Planning Perspectives* 8:148–164.

Institute of Medicine. 1978. *Adolescent Behavior and Health*. Washington, D.C.: National Academy of Sciences.

Jefferson, T. 1783. Notes on Virginia. In R. H. Bremmer, ed. *Children and Youth in America*. Vol. 1. Cambridge, Mass.: Harvard University Press, 1970.

Jencks, C., et al. 1972. *Inequality: A Reassessment of Family and Schooling in America*. New York: Basic.

Jessor, R., and Jessor, S. L. 1977. *Problem Behavior and Psychological Development: A Longitudinal Study of Youth*. New York: Academic Press.

Kenniston, K. 1971. Youth as a stage of life. *Adolescent Psychiatry* 1:161–175.

Levinson, D. 1978. *The Seasons of a Man's Life*. New York: Knopf.

National Center for Health Statistics. 1973a. Age at menarche, United States. *Vital and Health Statistics*, ser. 11, no. 133.

National Center for Health Statistics. 1973b. Height and weight of youths 12–17 years, United States. *Vital and Health Statistics*, ser. 11, no. 124.

Parke, R. 1979. Population changes that affect federal policy: some suggestions for research. *Social Science Research Council Items* 33:3–8.

Rush, B. 1786. A plan for the establishment of public schools and the diffusion of knowledge in Pennsylvania. In D. D. Runes, ed. *The*

Selected Writings of Benjamin Rush. New York: Philosophical Library, 1947.

Rutter, M.; Maugham, B.; Mortimer, P.; and Ouston, J. 1979. *Fifteen Thousand Hours: Secondary Schools and Their Effects on Children*. Cambridge, Mass.: Harvard University Press.

Tanner, J. M. 1962. *Growth at Adolescence*. 2d ed. Oxford: Blackwell Scientific Publications.

Westoff, C. F. 1974. The population of the developed countries. *Scientific American* 231:31–36.

Zelnik, M., and Kantner, J. F. 1977. Sexual and contraceptive practices of young unmarried women in the United States, 1971 and 1976. *Family Planning Perspectives* 9:55–71.

3

TOMORROW'S SELF: HEINZ KOHUT'S
CONTRIBUTION TO ADOLESCENT PSYCHIATRY

ERNEST S. WOLF

Imagine a fourteen-year-old girl who has arranged to watch a procession in the town square from a store which is the place of business of a couple who are friends of the little girl's father. Upon arriving at this place of business the girl found that only the husband was present—he was a man in his forties—and he asked her to wait while he went outside to lower the shutters. When he returned he suddenly clasped the girl to him and pressed a kiss upon her lips.

Now, try to be introspective and empathic with this fourteen-year-old who had never before been approached and ask yourself: What did she experience? Was she startled? Excited? Sexually aroused? Frightened? Embarrassed? Enraged? Erotically stimulated? I have asked a number of people, men and women, this question and the consensus seems to be that the girl probably would be aware of being startled, perhaps of being a little frightened, and perhaps somewhat embarrassed, and, after a short while, she probably would be aware of some anger at the sudden unexpectedness of the attack, an apparent betrayal by a trusted friend of the family.

Most of you who have come with me on this little imaginary journey will by now have recognized this little vignette as the episode of the kiss from Freud's famous case history of Dora. Dora told Freud that she experienced a feeling of disgust. Freud, who usually was a most introspective and empathic analyst, could not or did not really empathize with Dora. He wrote (Freud 1905): "This was surely just a situation to call up a distinct feeling of sexual excitement in a girl of fourteen who had never before been approached." And then he went on to say: "I should without question consider a person

Plenary address on the occasion of the William A. Schonfeld Distinguished Service Award to Heinz Kohut, Chicago, Illinois, May 12, 1979.

hysterical in whom an occasion for sexual excitement elicited feelings that were preponderantly or exclusively unpleasurable."

It is clear that Freud is not thinking of a young girl, of a person, or of a self in a particular situation, a situation which may be experienced as a frightening attack, a humiliating assault, a stimulating intimacy, or perhaps the betrayal of a trust. Freud appears to be thinking only of seeing a nubile sexual apparatus which in proximity to an arousing sexual stimulus failed to respond with sexual excitement. It is as if the girl were merely an appendage to this sexual apparatus, and, therefore, Freud is bound to diagnose the failure to respond with overt conscious sexual excitement as a kind of pathology, as hysteria. In this rare instance Freud has not been empathic with the girl but has put his theory first, the theory which says that the ubiquitous sexual instincts are at the root of most psychopathology. And because he is starting with an a priori theory of the central importance of sexuality, he does not see the girl but sees only the vicissitudes of her sexual responsiveness. In all likelihood Freud was correct in postulating at least a degree of sexual arousal as a result of a kiss, even under the most adverse circumstances. But awareness of such arousal will appear only under favorable conditions. The disgust experienced by Dora had little to do with whatever sexual arousal may or may not have occurred. Her disgust was the appropriate response of an adolescent to the betrayal of trust. Erikson (1963) has discussed this issue, and Freud's countertransference has been noted by others as well. With his usual honest self-examination, Freud admits that he did not succeed in mastering the transference in good time. We may add that it was Freud's countertransference which prevented him from mastering the transference, and we may further add that Freud's countertransference, his passing inability to see the whole girl Dora, was not due to a lack of sensitivity on his part but probably due to his intense commitment to do research and to prove a theory.

All that, however, is peripheral to the fundamental issue of clinical data collection, to theories about clinical observation, that is, to the question of how best to understand clinical material. We all agree that one cannot make observations without some theoretical commitment to guide the selection and the interpretation of data. Classical psychoanalytic theory is a reliable guide for the study of the vicissitudes of sexuality, particularly when distorted sexuality determines the psychopathology, as it does in the psychoneuroses. However, to study the total subjective experience of the person, of the self, requires a shift in focus from being empathic with the drivenness of sexuality to being empathic with the self. I would venture to say that an empathic listener to Dora might have understood her feeling of disgust as an appropriately angry response under the circumstances. Freud's assumption of sexual arousal and his interpretation of the repression, or, to be more specific, the reversal of this arousal into disgust, are not necessarily wrong but are peripheral and irrelevant to the issues at hand, to the girl's main concern, to what had brought her into treatment, to what she wanted from Freud.

It is here that we find Heinz Kohut's first and, perhaps, most important contribution to the understanding of man, including the adolescent variety of our species. My first selection, therefore, among the contributions that Kohut has made, not only to adolescent psychiatry but to psychiatry and psychoanalysis generally, is a shift in the stance of the scientific clinical observer. I am referring, of course, to the seminal paper on empathy (Kohut 1959). Ornstein (in Kohut 1978) has noted that Kohut set in motion a shift in emphasis from the investigation of the external world with one's sense organs to an emphasis on investigating the inner world through introspection and empathy. Empathy, that is, vicarious introspection, had always been implicit as an essential aspect of data collection in psychoanalysis since Freud. Rarely was Freud as unempathic as he was with this young adolescent, Dora. However, Kohut (1959) described the introspective-empathic observational stance explicitly as the one aspect of psychoanalytic observation that defined and differentiated psychoanalysis from other psychologies. Along with interpretations based on empathic data there existed, and in some quarters there still exists, another kind of interpretation which is not based on an empathic grasp of the data but on logical inferences obtained by the application of theory to the data of free association. The theory and the rules derived from it allow interpretations to be made from the sequential flow of associations.

Let me illustrate this usage with another vignette from that adolescent par excellence, Freud's (1905) Dora. Freud, for instance, tells us that Dora remarked on Frau K.'s ill health whenever her husband, Herr K., returned from traveling. "At this point in the discussion Dora suddenly brought in an allusion to her own alternations between good and bad health," and Freud suspected that Dora's states of health were to be regarded as depending on something else in the same way as Frau K.'s. Freud derived this interpretation from a rule which he states: "It is a rule of psychoanalytic technique that an internal connection which is still undisclosed will announce its presence by means of a continuity—a temporal proximity—of association" (p. 39).

Freud's associational rule may well result in correct interpretations much of the time, and, I believe, it was in fact correct in this instance. But I suspect that when interpretations based on logical inference from observational data happen to be correct, they are correct not because of the logic of the inference but because of a hidden empathic component. I believe that when Freud suspected that Dora's state of health was dependent on something else, in the same way as Frau K.'s state of health, Freud had become empathically aware that both women, Dora and Frau K., were sensitive to certain changes in their environment and responded to it with ill health. Interpretations made by logical inferences from extrospective observational data may be correct or incorrect, but they are psychoanalytic only when they also include an introspective-empathic component. It is this component which is responsible for the correctness or incorrectness of the interpretation, and it is this component, that is, the essential aspect of the participation of introspection and empathy, that was first stated explicitly by Kohut and made the center of the analytic method. Making introspection-empathy the basic ingredient of interpretation has resulted in freeing psychoanalytic theory from the restrictions imposed by an a priori assumption that ubiquitous sexuality and conflicts are the all-important and universal motivators of those psychic activities which are significant for potential psychopathological sequelae. Instead of basing psychoanalytic interpretations on a psychoanalytic theory of sexuality and aggression, Kohut (1959) began to base his interpretations on a psychoanalytic theory of observation, namely, the theory which says that all interpretations must be in harmony with introspective-empathic data in order to be psychoanalytic. It is this pivotal step that has had far-reaching consequences for psychoanalytic theory, for psychoanalytic practice, and for our understanding of the human psyche.

As my second step in highlighting the contributions of Heinz Kohut, I will consider those consequences of having put the introspective-empathic method into the center. The most immediate impact was that Kohut began to listen to his patients in a more open and yet at the same time more intense manner. I know this not because he has told me so; and he has not written much about the change in therapeutic posture. But all of us who have followed Heinz Kohut in his clarification of the essence of psychoanalysis have had the experience of listening in a new manner, of hearing the manifestations of psychic constellations that previously escaped our notice. No longer do we quickly dismiss negative responses to our seemingly technically appropriate and correct interpretations as resistance or as negative therapeutic reactions; rather, we have attempted to appreciate empathically what the patient's subjective experience must be like. We took seriously the complaints that we had not really listened, we took seriously the rages, the apathy, or the other numerous negative reactions that our seemingly correct interpretations sometimes evoked so paradoxically. This, I imagine, must have been the impact on Kohut himself when he first shifted from an experience-distant, theoretically determined posture into a more experience-near, empathic analytic posture. In this way he discovered that some patients neither loved nor hated him as the object of their libidinal desires or frustrations but they needed him, sometimes desperately, as a necessary sustaining presence for the coherent functioning of their personalities. These transference-like phenomena, of course, had been noted before by many analysts but had never been fully understood. After an intense inner struggle Kohut finally was forced to recognize that these transference-like phenomena were not the manifestations of unconscious conflicts but the manifestations of a deficiency in psychic structure. In other words, the transference phenomena were an expression of a need to correct the deficiency in structure by filling the gap with functions supplied by the analyst.

Kohut's strenuous and sophisticated efforts to explain his clinical findings within the concepts given by libido theory and ego psychology failed to give an adequate account of the new observations. Inevitably, the introspective-empathic clinical approach put the patient's self at the core of the observed psychic field, and a psychology of the self emerged. Kohut has conceptualized a systematic theory of the self, its development, its vicissitudes, and its treatment.

As the third step in our review of Kohut's contributions we shall proceed to a consideration of specific issues of adolescence.

The importance of adolescence as a period of psychological development and psychological change has only been recognized fully in recent decades. To be sure, there are over one hundred references to puberty in the index volume of the *Standard Edition of the Complete Psychological Works of Sigmund Freud* (Strachey 1974). In contrast, there are only six listings referring to adolescence. Clearly, until recently, psychoanalytic interest was focused primarily on the sexual aspects per se of the adolescent years and not on the adolescent process as a whole. It is also noteworthy to recall that this organization, the American Society for Adolescent Psychiatry, was not founded until twelve years ago, 1967. Those of you who believe that cultural changes are indicated by the many simultaneous parallel changes advancing on a broad front may find some significance in the fact that Kohut's 1966 paper on forms and transformations of narcissism, the first of his publications on narcissism, preceded the founding of our adolescent society here by only one year. These developments have in common an approach that gives the uppermost priority to the study of the whole, in its total context—in the one instance the self, in the other instance the adolescent process.

Furthermore, it seems to me that there is something peculiarly American about the emergence of our interest in adolescence and our interest in the self. It was an American psychologist, G. Stanley Hall, who published in 1904 a huge study, *Adolescence*, which first recognized the particular developmental phase between childhood and adulthood as deserving special attention (Hall 1904). It was the same G. Stanley Hall, a pioneer in American psychology, who recognized the important contribution of psychoanalysis to psychology and who, as president of Clark University, invited Sigmund Freud in 1909 to give the now-famous series of lectures on his only trip to America. I am suggesting that the impact of American culture on the science of psychology led to the proper appreciation of adolescence and that the impact of American culture on psychoanalysis, in the person of Heinz Kohut, led to the proper appreciation of the self. Therefore, it seems quite natural to me that Kohut, from the beginning of his investigations into the self, paid a good deal of attention to the vicissitudes of the self during adolescence.

Thus Kohut (1971), in *The Analysis of the Self*, stressed the importance of adolescence as the time for decisive firming and buttressing of the psyche, especially in the area of the establishment of reliable ideals (1971, p. 43). He also observed—and I must add that his observation here is often overlooked—that much of the sexual activities of adolescents serve primarily narcissistic purposes, that is, even relatively stable adolescents undertake sexual activities mainly in order to enhance self-esteem, particularly when these youngsters have been exposed to the revival of frightening childhood experiences of self-depletion and fragmentation (1971, p. 19n.). The implication is, clearly, of sexual activity not merely as an outcome of pubertal drive pressure but, more important, as an escape from unbearable feelings of self-depletion and deadness. In other words, adolescent sexual activity often is understood to be a secondary manifestation of self-pathology. In retrospect we can see that Kohut already in 1971 recognized that certain kinds of sexual pathology can usefully be conceptualized as a type of self-pathology, a view which he elaborated and expanded more recently in *The Restoration of the Self* (Kohut 1977).

I might interject that it is no accident that Kohut has always been interested in adolescents and particularly in the maturational tasks which confront adolescents, for Kohut was a student and analysand of August Aichhorn, whose uniquely successful work with delinquents is well known. Aichhorn had recognized the need for the creation of an emotional bond between therapist and juvenile delinquent and, through the application of very active techniques, he facilitated the emergence of what we would now call an idealizing transference. Kohut also recognizes the essential importance of narcissistic transferences if one wants to analyze delinquent youths or adults. But, analogous to Freud's abandonment of active hypnosis in favor of free-associational techniques, Kohut rejected the active techniques of Aichhorn in favor of the classic psychoanalytic technique, with, however, the shift in interpretative emphasis toward the introspective-empathic stance.

Kohut described certain types of adolescents or adults who often loudly proclaim their grandiosity because of the embarrassment about the weakness which the underlying preconscious idealizing attitudes seem to imply to them (Kohut 1971, p. 162). "Behind these preconscious fears of social disgrace, however, lies unconscious fear of a traumatic rejection of their idealizing attitude by the idealized object or the anticipation of a traumatic disillusionment with the idealized object—a dread, in other words, of frustration in the narcissistic realm which would lead to intolerable narcissistic tensions and to the painful experience of shame and hypochondria." In discussing the treatment of these adolescent delinquents, and in contrast to Aichhorn, Kohut warned against utilization of any activity for the purpose of bringing about an idealization of the therapist. "We may well heed Freud's relevant warning," Kohut said, "that there exists a temptation for the analyst to play the part of prophet, saviour, and redeemer to the patient, a procedure to which the rules of analysis are diametrically opposed. Yet, while it is analytically deleterious to bring about idealization of the analyst by artificial devices, a spontaneously occurring therapeutic mobilization of the idealized parent imago or of the grandiose self is indeed to be welcomed and must not be interfered with" (Kohut 1971, p. 164). To me this injunction to let transference develop spontaneously is unambiguous and clear, and it remains a puzzle to me that it is so often misunderstood.

As we all know, adolescence is characterized not only by the vicissitudes of miscarried idealization, but also by frequent episodes of irrationality and sometimes even by violence. Hamlet's brooding melancholia and his aggressive outburts of periodic madness are a fair illustration of a not-uncommon turmoil of adolescence and youth. Kohut's analysis of Hamlet's antic disposition shows it to be neither madness nor pretense of madness but a traumatic state of the self which is overburdened by excessive stimuli and therefore cannot contain its fragmenting constituents safely within the boundaries of cohesion. Witness the punning, the recklessly aggressive outbursts, including murder, and the retreat of the depleted self into brooding and melancholia (Kohut 1971, pp. 235–237). It is especially adolescents who are disposed to suffer from this terrible oscillation between the madness of an overstimulated self and the melancholia of a depleted self. Statistically, we know that most crimes of violence are perpetrated by adolescents and by youths who are still adolescent in their psychic organization. Perhaps in some of these cases the overstimulation may also be self-induced as a desperate attempt to escape the unbearable experience of apathy that accompanies depletion of the self. Kohut stated precisely this dynamic connection in the case of other adolescents whose hypervitality, hyperidealism, and overenthusiasm can be understood as attempts to counteract through self-stimulation a feeling of inner deadness and depression. In these adolescents childhood fantasies often become transformed by an intense devotion to romanticize, for example, aesthetic, religious, or political aims. Such hyperidealism may not recede with adulthood but remains but one step removed from the underlying depression (Kohut 1977, pp. 5–6).

In a similar vein Kohut discussed the utilization of sexual excitement. He recognized certain solitary sexual activities and group activities of a sexual nature as an attempt to relieve the lethargy and depression resulting from the unavailablity of a mirroring and of an idealizable self-object. These activities are the forerunners of the frantic sexual activities of some depressed adolescents (Kohut 1977, p. 272).

Kohut's emphasis on the vicissitudes of the cohesion and vigor of the self during adolescence, in addition to the vicissitudes of puberty and resurgent oedipal conflicts, has been elaborated by others. Inspired by Kohut's ideas, Gedo, Terman, and I proposed that the transformation of the self during adolescence was the major task of that developmental phase. We noted the temporary need for substitutive idealization of peer group idols to bridge the gap during the transformation from preadolescent idealized parental imagoes to the postadolescent idealized ethics and values (Wolf, Gedo, and Terman 1972). In a discussion of that paper Kohut stressed that the impact of drive maturation and changing social expectations puts the assertive aspect and the ideals of the self of the early adolescent in jeopardy and reactivates old fears of self-disintegration. He confirmed our stress on the importance of peer relationships, especially the adolescent's "secret society," and elaborated with examples from his own adolescence (Kohut 1978, p. 659).

Let me attempt to bring this rather fragmentary presentation of Kohut's contribution to our understanding of adolescence into some sort of conceptual coherence. Kohut has opened the door to an appreciation of adolescence as an aspect of the unfolding life curve of the self. Life is like a symphony made up of many movements, and, to be sure, the movement which we call adolescence often announces itself with the dissonance of puberty and the recapitulation of oedipal conflicts. And many times we know that adolescence has run its course by the crescendo of what Erikson (1963) has aptly called an identity crisis. But no longer do we fall so easily into the error of mistaking the noisy chords for the symphonic flow. A youngster, whose nuclear self emerged during the second year of life and whose own ambitions and goals were given a familial or tribal cast during the oedipal phase, enters adolescence as a period of potential freedom to throw off what is not genuinely his own and to give his life the direction that is authentic to his individual self.

Historically, in most societies, the glimpse of freedom and the space and time to reconstruct oneself have been brief. The adolescent is prematurely forced to fit himself into the patterns of his forebears. In our society, in contrast—and I hope I am not just blinded by the bias of parochial patriotism—our adolescents are given the time, space, resources, and freedom to transform and consolidate their selves more nearly in harmony with the ambitions and goals of their nuclear self as it emerged in early childhood. Of course, here I am only speaking about those adolescents who come from families above the poverty level. It is only after they have achieved this adolescent transformation of their self that they merge themselves into a social role, an identity, and often they are able to choose an identity that fittingly supports the self—sometimes a very vulnerable self—and allows the self room for expansion and creativity. This adolescent process of firming the self can be very noisy, especially when it requires the exposure of vulnerabilities caused by deficiencies in psychic structure left over from the earliest formative years. The innate flexibility and self-healing potential of the adolescent frequently facilitates significant growth in psychic structure, and, as psychiatrists of adolescents, we are often surprised by the speed with which a seriously disturbed youngster can be restored to healthy functioning.

As you all know, Heinz Kohut had intended to be with us this evening until a severe life-threatening illness put a stop to his plans. For us, his friends and colleagues, it comes as a shock not to see him here with us on the occasion of his being honored. Though Heinz now is convalescing and regaining his strength, we have been painfully reminded how transient is human existence and how difficult it is to accept the human condition. Times like these lie heavy upon our souls and make us look not only backward at past accomplishments but also forward to the future and our hopes for it.

This review of Kohut's contribution to our understanding of adolescents in health and in turmoil indicates that his contributions to adolescent psychiatry are not confined to discussion of specifically adolescent problems. On the contrary and more important, he has discussed the impact of the psychology of the self in altering our theoretical outlook and our therapeutic posture with all patients. I have touched on some of these recent advances, but, inevitably, a comprehensive overview has eluded me. However, as this society prepares to honor this great innovative scientist and devoted healer, I trust that I have given you enough of a glimpse into his achievements so that you may share with me the feeling of pride in our honoring Heinz Kohut here today and also share with me the feeling of being honored by his acceptance of our award to him.

REFERENCES

Erikson, E. 1963. Youth: fidelity and diversity. In E. Erikson, ed. *Youth: Change and Challenge*. New York: Basic.

Freud, S. 1905. Fragment of an analysis of a case of hysteria. *Standard Edition* 7:7–122. London: Hogarth, 1953.

Hall, G. S. 1904. *Adolescence*. New York: Appleton.

Kohut, H. 1959. Introspection, empathy and psychoanalysis. In Kohut 1978.

Kohut, H. 1966. Forms and transformation of narcissism. In Kohut 1978.

Kohut, H. 1971. *The Analysis of the Self*. New York: International Universities Press.

Kohut, H. 1977. *The Restoration of the Self*. New York: International Universities Press.

Kohut H. 1978. *The Search for the Self*. Edited and with an introduction by P. H. Ornstein. New York: International Universities Press.

Strachey, J. 1974. Indexes and bibliographies. *Standard Edition*. Vol. 24. London: Hogarth.

Wolf, E.; Gedo, J.; and Terman, D. 1972. On the adolescent process as a transformation of the self. *Journal of Youth and Adolescence* 1:257–272.

4

REMARKS ON RECEIVING THE WILLIAM A. SCHONFELD DISTINGUISHED SERVICE AWARD

HEINZ KOHUT

The decision of the American Society for Adolescent Psychiatry to bestow the William A. Schonfeld Distinguished Service Award on me pleases me for two reasons. The first and more superficial reason is that any recognition is sustaining to me because, as you know, my work on the self is considered to be highly "controversial," as the euphemism goes, by many of my psychoanalytic colleagues, in particular by those of my own generation. The award pleases me even more, however, for another reason. That you, the members of the American Society for Adolescent Psychiatry decided to honor my work, the work of a psychoanalyst who has all his life treated only adult patients, lends special significance to your approval and constitutes, I believe, an especially important support to the validity of my ideas.

It is always difficult in the psychological field, especially when our findings and theories are culled from experiences obtained in a therapeutic setting, to arrive at a reliable judgment about the validity of a new outlook and of new findings. However conscientiously applied the wholesome skepticism that the researcher brings to bear on his work, however great in particular his caution as he evaluates the improvement of his patients, there remains always the possibility that the inner consistency and explanatory power of the new system of thought are no more than a testimony to the cleverness of a theoretical mind which had been able to arrange a variety of selected data into a cohesive whole. Then the therapeutic efficacy of the new approach is no more than the nonspecific result of the self-righteous conviction of the therapist—however veiled by manifest modesty—who has become the omnipotent, all-healing parent of childhood for the patient. That equally good results may be achieved also by others who are bound to the innovator by transferences and who identify with him will also be open to attack by those who, for rational and irrational reasons of their own, reject the new ideas. All in all, then, it

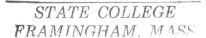

seems that we have to resign ourselves to the fact that, at least in the short run, we will not be able to reach undoubted certainty concerning our new findings and theories and that we must remain vigilant, examine seriously all objections to our explanations, and over and over consider alternatives and improvements.

Still, the situation is not hopeless. With the passage of time the clash between those who are utterly convinced of the validity of the new outlook and those who reject it with equal certainty subsides, and new generations can apply the new viewpoint with dispassion and separate the wheat from the chaff. And, as you have undoubtedly already grasped from the tenor of my earlier remarks, we do not even have to wait for the emergence of dispassionate witnesses in later generations, we have also witnesses in the present time whose testimonial carries special conviction.

What a new system of thought in psychology needs in order to establish the relevance and accuracy of its explanatory approach is not only the concreteness and realism of the innovator and of his close co-workers and friends, but the confirmatory response of workers at a distance from the innovator, of individuals who are not exposed to frequent contact with the teacher figure, and whose views are not influenced by the feelings of loyalty and devotion toward the leader which inevitably arise under these circumstances. The situation that is most favorable in this regard is one in which, not only is there an absence of direct contact, but where we are dealing with individuals who are working in areas that had not been investigated by the primary research.

The fact that explanations obtained in one field—the field originally investigated by the innovator—apply also in other areas I take as a significant confirmation of the essential correctness and relevance of new ideas. I have therefore enthusiastically responded to investigations which examine such other areas from the vantage point of the psychology of the self—for example, investigations concerning the historical process and the traditional applied areas of art and literature—and I have felt reassured by the fact that much is indeed illuminated when seen in the light of the psychology of the self. But here it may still be said that these are areas in which I and some of my friends and collaborators have been deeply interested for many years. Not so, however, with regard to the period of adolescence. Here I must confess that something in me has prevented me from ever dealing in depth with this fascinating period of life. What remarks about adolescence can be found dispersed in my writings were almost always the outgrowth of reflection on my part and not the result of prolonged clinical observation or of empathic immersion into the inner life of my patients, which otherwise have been the near-total empirical basis of my work.

You can see, therefore, that it is not just traditional politeness but the expression of sincere gratification when I thank you for the award which you are giving to me. When I learned of your decision to honor me, I was surprised and delighted that you who work in a field other than my own have found my work to be applicable and helpful with regard to the clinical and theoretical problems that you are confronting in your work.

5 THE MISSING ADOLESCENT

The concept of "adolescence" has become so deeply ingrained within our current thinking that we assume everyone sees what we see and responds to what we respond to when viewing the adolescent. Adolescence has been defined as an adaptive period to pubescence and a developmental stage with special physical, intellectual, emotional, and social characteristics. Adolescents are a visible presence by their numbers, by their behavior, and by our having to deal with them. But do they exist? Perhaps they are nothing but a construction of our thoughts in response to needs.

This and other questions have been raised by comparing current attitudes toward the age group we identify as adolescent with attitudes of other times in history and other cultures. Qualitative differences emerge as the customs and institutions of past civilizations, developing countries, and our own society are examined.

About 3,700 years ago a scribe set forth on Sumerian clay tablets from Ur his admonishment to his son to work diligently and to report home without loitering. He bitterly rebuked his son for his waywardness and expressed deep disappointment at the son's ingratitude. He bemoaned the fact that he had never made his son work behind plough or ox, nor did he ever ask him to bring firewood or to support him as other fathers made their sons do, and yet his son turned out to be less of a man than others. This plaintive cry out of the past can be viewed readily as a comment on the state of affairs between generations. However, the scribe of Ur presented his case in terms of a wayward son becoming less of a man for not having followed the work ethic built into family life. He referred specifically to "family" and to "man" as do most references to the young until the nineteenth and twentieth centuries.

It is only within the last century that the young have achieved an identity of their own. The twentieth century may have become known as the Century of the Child because it was not until then that children acquired a separate

© 1980 by The University of Chicago. 0-226-24053-3/80/0008-3100$01.00

identity through a variety of practices and attitudes which helped set them apart from family. In his historical study, Lawrence Stone (1977) identifies the single major change in the family household in the last 500 years "to be the removal of unmarried agricultural workers and apprentices to lodgings of their own," highlighting the new phenomenon of an independent existence for the young. Practices arising from the industrialization of England and the United States, as well as most of the countries of western Europe, appeared to cause much of this separation of child from family. Child labor in farming had been an accepted practice from time immemorial but had always existed within the context of the family. The early stages of the Industrial Revolution maintained the child within his family with the development of the cottage-industry system. However, with further changes and the introduction of the factory and its accompanying urbanization, children began to live more and more outside of the family of their origin, making the child an individual with a separate identity.

Not only did the children work within the newly developing industrial structure of factory and town, but also many were living apart from their natural families. Examination of some of the practices of child labor and apprenticeship is revealing of how extensive was this movement of the child out of the family. There was a premium placed on the labor of children by the growing need for hands in the mills. Many of these children lived in dormitories associated with the factories. As early as 1654, Edward Johnson praised the people of Rowely, Massachusetts, because they had "built a fulling mill, and caused their little ones to be very diligent in spinning cotton wool" (Bremmer 1971).

The labor of young children was justified by need and sanctified by religious practices. Children were warned that idleness destroyed souls and undermined the social system. The Puritan ethic warned that work was essential to salvation and the mark of good citizenship. It became common for well-to-do parents to bind out their children to other households as servants or apprentices so that they would experience and profit from the discipline of work. A survey of seventeenth-century colonial labor practices suggested the predominance of children among imported servants (Morris 1946). Most were identified as being under nineteen years of age and the average was between fourteen and sixteen. Some were as young as six.

Servitude and apprenticeship were identified as being separate from each other and yet there was considerable overlapping. Apprenticeship obligated the master to teach a specific trade while servitude did not. Apprenticeship was considered both an educational and economic institution while emerging as part of the industrial system. It added to the skilled labor force while producing additional labor. At the same time the practice of binding out poor and orphaned children grew and used apprenticeship as a form of social control and public welfare. Thus two types of apprenticeship affecting children emerged. There was a voluntary system in which the child and his parents entered into the agreement on their own initiative, but there was also a compulsory system in which poor or neglected children were bound out by the authorities. The compulsory apprenticeship resembled servitude. Voluntary apprentices usually served for seven years. Boys were apprenticed between ten and fourteen years of age and usually served until they were twenty-one. Girls served to age eighteen or until married. Compulsory apprentices served until they were twenty-one regardless of their age at the time of indenture. The apprentice lived in the master's household and saw his own family rarely, while many children moved into communal living situations associated with the practice of developing industries.

The tempo and extent of these changes can be seen in the following description of child labor in the United States in the nineteenth century:

Rapid industrialization after the Civil War increased the child labor force, introduced new occupations for children and spread child labor into new parts of the nation, especially the South. By 1900, one-third of the workers in southern mills were children. More than half of them were between ten and thirteen years of age; and many were under ten. In the absence of legislative restrictions the South repeated the experience of New England in its early period of industrialization.

The nation-wide extent of child labor became visible in 1870 when the Census Bureau established a separate category of the gainfully employed who were from ten to fifteen years of age. According to the 1870 census about one out of every eight children was employed. By 1900 approximately 1,750,000 children, or one out of six, were gainfully employed. Sixty percent were agricultural workers; of the 40 percent in industry over half were children of immigrant workers. [Bremmer 1971]

The practices associated with child labor, servitude, and apprenticeship made little distinction between the child and the adolescent, nor did they distinguish the adolescent from the adult. Regardless of age, they placed the children within or outside the family of origin. The master or factory owner acted *in loco parentis,* and all practices and laws reinforced this. Thus, not only were there no adolescents, but the social and economic institutions denied them an existence. It was not until large numbers of children existed outside of their families that the young achieved an identity of their own and could be given distinguishing characteristics.

An amusing but tragic anecdote coming from this lack of specific identity can be found in a report by John Augustus (1852) describing his efforts to keep children out of Boston's jails between 1846 and 1850:

In August, 1850, as I was walking around in Leveret Street jail, I found a small boy who was crying. I asked him why he was there, and he said he did not know. I enquired of the officers and they informed me that he was there on charge of committing a rape; at first, I paid no attention to the reply, thinking of course that the statement was false, but I learned afterwards that such was the fact. He was but seven years old. I proceeded directly to court, and informed his Honor, Judge Hoar, who was then presiding, of the fact. The Judge immediately issued a *capias* and the child was brought into court. By advice, he pleaded not guilty. A jury was impaneled in the case, and though the presumption was that the judgment's instruction to the jury would result in the boy's acquittal, just as the trial was about to proceed, I told the judge that I thought it a shame and a disgrace to all present to proceed with the case; his Honor asked what could be done; I replied, ''let him be sent to his mother and placed in her lap''; I stated that I would bail him, and to this the court readily assented. I bailed him, then moved to have the indictment placed on file, which was done and I carried the child to his home in Chelsea. This is the only case where I became bail when the indictment was laid on file with a plea of not guilty, except when the parties have died. The Grand Jury were not aware that the charge which they investigated was against so young a child. The child upon whom the assault was alleged to have been committed was but ten years old.

I have bailed persons charged with all sorts of crime bailable on the Statute book, but only now and then a case like the above. Some people will insist that I do more harm than good in bailing so many. They say it is of no use to complain of boys or girls, or women, for I manage to get them discharged; that all sorts of crimes, even rape and highway robbery, may be committed with impunity, and I will bail them. But this representation is false. I have indeed bailed a party charged with the crime of rape and also in a case of highway robbery, and as I have related the former, I will briefly give the other.

Sometime during the year 1847, two boys were at play on the Tremont Road, and finally got to quarreling; one seized the other's cap and the other in return took six cents from the first; they then separated. Soon after, the first returned with the cap, and claimed the six cents, but the boy who had taken the money was not disposed to give it up, and a prosecution at the Police Court was the consequence of the refusal.

The boy was arrested on the charge of committing highway robbery, and was confined in jail. His father applied to me to bail him, and I did so; afterwards the parents of the boys by the consent of the court, settled the matter satisfactorily amongst themselves; and here ended the great highway robbery case. One of the boys was nine and the other ten years old. In former times a birch rod would have been law and gospel to them both.

These anecdotes highlight the existence of a body of law and social attitude denying the young a separate identity from their family going back in history for thousands of years. The following quotation comes from the fifth book of the Torah, Deuteronomy:

If a man has a wayward and defiant son, who does not heed his father or mother and does not obey them after they have disciplined him, his father and mother shall take hold of him and bring him out to the elders of his town at the public place of his community. They shall say to the elders of this town, this son of ours is disloyal and defiant; he does not heed us. He is a glutton and a drunkard. Thereupon the men of his town shall stone him to death and thus you will sweep out evil from your midst; all Israel will hear and be afraid.

And from Sir William Blackstone's (1765–1769) comments on English law there is the following: "Under seven years of age indeed an infant cannot be guilty of felony. Also, under fourteen, though an infant shall be *prima facie* adjudged to be *doli incapax* [incapable of michief]; yet if it appears to the court and jury, that he was *doli capax,* and could discern between good and evil, he may be convicted and suffer death."

The need to preserve the significance of the family over the individual was strong and may have been rooted in the transient existence of people of that time. The collective identity offered by the family represented safe harbor and continuity for person, property, and livelihood. The many hazards to life and survival made for a tenuous existence. Infant mortality rates have been reduced only recently to the point of assuring the probability of continued existence to the newborn. High morbidity and mortality rates among the young and their families, coupled with the practices of fostering out children from their home at an early age, made parent-child relations equally tenuous. There were a large number of orphans as well as conditions in which a minority of children had two living parents and were themselves living with their family of origin by the time of their pubescence.

These circumstances may account for the absence of the adolescent in times gone by but also may have changed the nature of being young. The early separation of children from their natural parents may have served to reduce the oedipal conflicts and altered other psychic tensions arising inevitably within the struggle for maturity, independence from parents, and mastery over the problems of budding sexuality. Developmental transition periods may have been accelerated and created a type of very young adult with little or no evidence of an adolescent period. The statement by William Shakespeare (1623) in *Winter's Tale,* "I would there were no age between ten and three-and-twenty, or that youth would sleep out the rest; for there is nothing in the between but getting wenches with child, wronging the ancientry, stealing, fighting," is an unusual statement of age grouping by current values unless we consider the possibility of the existence of a group of very young adults or a very extended period of adolescence which includes children whom we do not ordinarily recognize and identify now with the adolescent period of life. The social and economic practices of the times suggest the creation of a class of youth existing outside of the family whom we would be hard pressed to identify with the adolescent of today. However, with the changing times and the need to control this group of individuals existing both within and outside of the family, the adolescent was born and began to acquire characteristics determined as much by social and economic factors as by biological and psychological ones.

Children were viewed as unfair competitors for jobs within the work force of the budding industrial society. The argument which won passage of the first child-labor law in the United States, restricting the use of the labor of children in our factories, was based on this view. The apprenticeship system was recruited by the guilds to limit the number of children coming into a trade. At the same time the expanding technology of the industrial society produced a greater need for skills requiring education as well as job training. The combination resulted in the expansion of compulsory education and a greater effort directed at its enforcement. The school was made both the training ground for the newly required industrial technician and the warehouse for those young who were judged to be unfair competitors to the growing number of surviving adults. This trend may account for many of the problems we are facing now by harboring our young within an educational system in which a growing number do not care to be. The old work ethic of the family seems in the process of replacement by the ethics of a new system based on sorting, grouping, storing, and distributing our young in a manner which may deprive the individual of essential ingredients contributing to the formation of a concept of the self and the family. This transition appears to be instrumental in the formation of a group of individuals whom we identify now as adolescents with identity crises, family conflicts, borderline or delinquent personalities, and so forth.

The characteristics of adolescence as well as its disturbances appear to be determined more and more by the practices associated with our contemporary society. Not only has the nature of pubescence been identified by technological advances, but its existence has been reinforced by current social practices. Puberty has emerged as the stage of life chosen by society to help the young move out of the family by various rituals and by the sorting and grouping provided by its educational system. This is the period when tracking and departmentalization in the schools are reinforced and broadened to include all children. Many school refusal syndromes, with their link to separation anxiety, appear with both pubescence and movement into the intermediate school system.

Adolescence has emerged also as the stage of life chosen by the educational system to distribute and store children within its secondary schools. This occurs when specialization of educational procedures accelerates the sorting and grouping of the young. It seems to be more than coincidence that the number of school dropouts or school pushouts accelerates at the same time the educator and student become preoccupied with preparatory examinations for higher education. Specialized and vocational high schools have become permanent fixtures in our society at the same time as the truant. Perhaps the peaking of delinquent behavior at the age of seventeen may be linked as much to the discrepancy between the end of compulsory education at the age of sixteen and the acceptance of the young by current industrial practices into the work force at the age of eighteen, as it is to the problems of breakdown of impulse control and acting-out behavior associated with the adolescent period.

Many of our observations and experiences within the developing nations of today's world suggest that their patterns of adolescence are evolving from both the child of the family and from the young of their emerging industrial society. In much of Latin and South America, Asia and Africa, the nations have evolved into a two-tier society—partially agricultural and partially in-dustrial. In many instances the two coexist, and each breeds social values with different attitudes toward the young. Sometimes the adolescent is miss-ing, is present as a young adult, or becomes the symbol and instrument of conflict between the two tiers.

Throughout the developing countries the same statement was made by people coming from the land. "My children are my security. As soon as they are old enough, they will help me in my work. And when my wife and I are too old, they will care for us." Here there is no in between; there is nothing but the child within the family, and there is no transitional stage between childhood and adulthood. There is only the relationship of child to parent and all the attitudes and social institutions that reflect and support this rela-tionship. The concept of "adolescence" has little meaning and no application. Large families are needed and desired because they support the individual and provide a form of social security. High infant mortality rates reinforce the need for higher birthrates in order to assure an appropriate outcome.

In Kenya, a black courier, accompanying us during our travels through East Africa, described in detail his early memories of his childhood in a small agrarian village in the savanna. He described the *manyetta,* the grass hut with earthen floor, of his birth and early childhood. He was able to recall the stories of magic, nature, and strange gods of the land and sky which his mother told him and his many brothers and sisters as they huddled together in a common bed. He talked also of himself and his own family living far away in the new city of Nairobi with more than a million people. He described his difficulties with his formal education at the University of Nairobi, his marriage to a fellow student from another tribe in another part of the country, and their living in an apartment in Nairobi with their two planned children. He talked of his aspirations to advance within the growing tourist industry of his country while he simultaneously offered us vignettes praising the never-changing patterns of existence within the village life of his parents. He took us to a village in the jungle where we were entertained by unmarried pubescent girls doing fertility dances and young boys doing war dances. At the same time he discussed with great concern the high incidence of pregnancy among his country's unwed young and their accompanying high maternal and infant mortality and morbidity rates.

In China, children were presented to us as the symbol of change and a communal effort—the production of their socialist society. Wherever we went they showed us the products of their work—electric motors, farm products, tea, and clothes. Their method of presentation was striking. They would first present us with their commune, its organization, work force, resources, and purpose; then they would show us their techniques of production and, finally, their products of production. Only then would they introduce their children.

We had the following experience within this routine which was followed everywhere. At a farm commune, we were shown chickens in their rectangular chicken house with its central outdoor enclosure, then sows in their rectangular pig houses with their central enclosures, then cattle in their rectangular barns with central enclosures, and, finally, the children in their rectangular nurseries and schools with central enclosures. All had the same order and schedule. All had programs of indoor and outdoor activities. All were part of a plan and organization. It was no wonder that the Chinese could close down all of their universities during their Cultural Revolution. Mao's dictatorship of the peasant needed hands to till the soil and not technicians to serve their poorly developed industries. At that point, the conflict between the two tiers of agriculture and industry was resolved by moving all of the young to the land. There was no need for the university. Now, with China's newly determined goal of a technological society, its young are being moved more quickly than ever into training institutions.

Wherever we went in China we could see the young as the symbol and instrument of conflict between agriculture and industry. The children were presented to us for the most part as individuals produced by but existing outside of the family. Thus we saw no adolescents. We saw children in all kinds of schools being prepared for some role within society. They were orderly. They worked hard. They were not interested in physical sexuality. There was little or no promiscuity. They married late. They had planned and small families. They talked only of their goals for the future. Religion was unimportant and played no role in their lives. The young were visible within ordered groups while we were informed by word only of the strong persistence of the family's meaning in their cultural and moral life.

Conclusions

The agricultural society appears to be linked to the fertility of its land, the variable elements of nature, and a time reference determined by the rising sun with its accompanying seasons. The number of its young seems to be related as much to the fertility and productivity of the land as to human fertility. Children are reared within the biological unit of their origin (family and kin) unrelated to individual ability. There is little need for selection, grouping, or training beyond that offered by the family. If the young survive the tribulations of their childhood, they are integrated immediately into society through their family. Attitudes and thoughts reflect the characteristics of origin by being concrete, task oriented, and devoted to survival and family. Response is to the moment and the here and now. Pubescence brings physical sexuality—fertility, pregnancy, and expanded family. There is preoccupation with the unpredictabilities of life and its changing nature. The unknown is as important as the known. There is belief in magic and the presence of unseen forces. There is no need for movement or distribution other than that determined by the productivity of the land.

The industrial society appears to be linked to its technology, resources, and a time reference determined by its own organization. The number of its young seems to be related to plan and needs. Children are produced, grouped, and trained for specific roles; then they are packaged, distributed, and conditioned to the time frame of the orderly sequencing of industrial technology. Numbers are determined by population planning and birth control. Children are less and less reared within the biological unit of their origin and relegated to nursery, school, and community institutions. The children are subjected to procedures of grouping such as intelligence quotient, ability, and handicap. They are trained specially for a role within the system and moved about according to production needs. If the young survive the tribulations of their childhood, they are warehoused and stored until needed. Attitudes and thoughts reflect the characteristics of the industrial system by being ordered, compartmentalized, and bureaucratized. Pubescence brings frustration and delay to physical sexuality. There is preoccupation with their future and the predictability of its outcome. The known is most important; belief in magic is relegated to the unknown which is to be examined, identified, classified, and recruited by scientific exploration. There is constant need for movement, progress, distribution, redistribution, and growth within the system. The adolescent can no longer be hidden: Adolescence emerges.

It would appear that adolescence as we know it may truly represent a phenomenon of our time. Not only may adolescents' existence be determined by what we do and think, but what they think and do may be determined by our existence.

REFERENCES

Augustus, J. 1852. *A Report of the Labors of John Augustus for the Last Ten Years, in Aid of the Unfortunate.* In R. Bremmer, ed. *Children and Youth in America, Volume I, 1600–1865*. Cambridge, Mass.: Harvard University Press, 1970.

Blackstone, W. 1765–1769. *Commentaries on the Laws of England*. Chicago: University of Chicago Press, 1979.

Bremmer, R. 1971. *Children and Youth in America. Vol. II, 1866–1932*. New York: American Public Health Association.

Morris, R. B. 1946. *Government and Labor in Early America*. New York: Columbia University Press.

Shakespeare, W. 1623. *The Winters Tale*. New Haven, Conn.: Yale University Press, 1918.

Stone, L. 1977. *The Family, Sex and Marriage in England 1500–1800*. New York: Harper & Row.

6 SOCIOCULTURAL FACTORS, LIFE-STYLE, AND ADOLESCENT PSYCHOPATHOLOGY

PETER L. GIOVACCHINI

Both clinicians and sociologists continue to stress the importance of the cultural milieu in determining adaptive patterns, especially during adolescence. The editors of this journal are constantly impressed by the number of manuscripts they receive which question whether adolescence exists as an entity in itself or whether it is the product of a complex rapidly changing technology. Certainly Offer and Offer (1976) as well as Oldham (1978) convincingly demonstrated that the stereotype of a frenetically confused adolescent is not valid for the group of youngsters they have studied. Toffler (1971) has emphasized that, in view of the sweeping changes brought about by our ever-advancing technical innovations, life-styles and cultural orientations have changed.

The adolescent is supposed to be occupied with activities that will prepare him for adulthood. This can hardly be considered a life-style since goals and values are vague. At best, the child, now an adolescent, is entering a phase in which he will discover how he wants to live. Frequently youth fails to construct a framework which will enable him to live comfortably and feel valued and useful, and then we are faced with psychopathology.

Many teenagers insist that the world is in opposition to their struggle to achieve autonomy. They often blame the Establishment for their difficulties, and clinicians are frequently faced with the dilemma of determining whether they are dealing with intrapsychic problems or environmental stress. Of course, every patient can be viewed in terms of both, but the problem is to discover which is the most intense. Freud (1905), when he postulated his concept of complemental series, was involved with a similar question as he noted the reciprocal influences of constitutional vulnerability and external trauma.

The adolescents' need to blame the environment may lead to special technical problems when we attempt to treat them in a psychotherapeutic or psychoanalytic context. They blame their inconstant turbulent surroundings as responsible for their inner agitation. They find themselves in a world in which they find no peace, in which they cannot be soothed. The situation might have been different with previous generations.

The Adolescent's Place in the World

In preindustrial societies, children were valued. Families had to provide for themselves by raising crops for food, chopping wood for cooking and warmth, and weaving their own clothes. Purchasing power was meager, and since mass manufacturing was still unknown they could not avail themselves of ready-made products.

As soon as the male child could walk, he was assigned specific tasks which would increase in quantity and demand increasingly more muscle power. What he had to do and what he had to learn to do were predetermined. Similarly, the girl's development followed an unchanging course. There was never a question as to choice of goals. She would gradually take over more and more of the household chores, and her eventual goal would be to marry and have children. Deviations for both boys and girls were rare and generally frowned upon. Life was characterized by monotonous constancy, but backbreaking labor did not represent a strain on the mind.

No one gave children and adolescents special attention simply because they were children and adolescents. Their childhood status was short-lived. Although the child was still biologically dependent, his helplessness was not as apparent because he had a role to fulfill which contributed to the family's welfare. As he began to experience himself as an adult and as others treated him as if he were one, he felt respected and valued.

As we venture further back in the past, we find that life-styles were increasingly predetermined. Perhaps there are exceptions to this generalization, but these occurred during the unstable times of certain historical periods. The modern era is characterized by instability.

Formerly, the passage from childhood to adulthood was a continuous unbroken progression. Today, discontinuity makes adolescence noticeable, and discontinuity is the product of our vast scientific and sociological achievements. To harmonize with the world, the adolescent must find a role in which he can function effectively and meet his needs in a civilized fashion. There are now countless role choices. Inasmuch as necessity and tradition do not restrict how a person decides to make a living, the adolescent is faced with conflicts in his task of choosing a role—a role which will influence the rest of his life. Although there are limitations as to choice of roles, they are minimal when compared to the past.

Progress has created a stage of life with its own unique features. However, if this phase leads to conflicts that did not previously exist, then we are faced with a paradox. Stated simply, good things lead to bad things. The blatant contradiction of this statement is characteristic of the confusion of today's adolescent and makes it excruciatingly painful to establish a coherent and stable system of values.

Adolescence seemed more stable even as recently as one or two generations ago. Adults were amused by teenage clothing styles and fads, and adolescence did not appear to be a particularly tense or stressful period. Teenagers swallowed goldfish with gusto and no one was the worse off, except the goldfish. Generations were fairly friendly with each other, and youth respected their parents' values and tried to emulate them. At the worst, the adolescent struck the critical adult as childish and frivolous. The adolescent was granted a moratorium in preparation for the somber, more serious commitments of adulthood.

These youths did not trouble themselves with world problems. They had school spirit, a now-outdated loyalty to the extent that some graduates do not even care to attend convocation ceremonies. Youths enthusiastically planned proms, talked incessantly about sex, and drugs were used only by degenerates. The middle-class American did not look beyond the confines of his group.

This brings us to the youth of today who are desperately seeking some meaning to justify their existence. As we trace the journey from childhood through the transition phase of adolescence to final adulthood, we can see the historical progression of the adolescent phase and its markedly different characteristics. Formerly, preindustrial youth possessed a hard and colorless life but felt secure in its monotonous identity. The youth of one or two generations ago were tolerated and found entertaining but not taken seriously. Today, the adolescent's niche is not so easily defined. He must determine his own place in the world.

Emotional Illness and Socioeconomic Background

The phenomena, processes, and goals of adolescence are often profoundly related to emotional illness. Psychopathology has a significant influence upon

67

life-style. Construction of a way of life based upon our personal neuroses is characteristic of our times. Some adults believe that youth is crazy, and it is this craziness that determines how they live. This unwarranted generalization has its effect upon the adolescent. Teenagers who live quiet, unobtrusive lives often view themselves as strange. They perceive their behavior as different from some elusive norm and cannot find the security and self-esteem they need as they relate to the world in a fashion that does not conform to the stereotypic adolescent. This makes the problem of finding a comfortable life-style during a transition period even more difficult.

Some clinicians also consider adolescence a form of psychopathology; I do not agree with such a generalization. Youth has special problems that have to be resolved in a characteristic fashion, as is true of any stage of life. Furthermore, youth's energy, curiosity, and creative exuberance are the antitheses of psychopathology. Although there is considerable psychopathology in the adolescent group, this does not mean that the adolescent phase is a form of emotional illness.

The clinician has a natural tendency to equate the severity of emotional illness, or psychopathology, to the severity of economic circumstances. To some extent, this follows from the combination of material and emotional deprivation commonly encountered in the ghetto. Violence, broken homes, and the lack of constant and stable loving relationships are not exactly favorable conditions for the development of healthy, contented adolescents.

Are ghetto youths really sicker than the affluent? To explore this question I conducted an informal experiment to test the degree of significance of social class on adolescent disturbance. At the time of the experiment, I was a psychiatric consultant to the United Charities, the largest social agency in Chicago. I worked with three branches whose range of clients included poverty levels and lower middle-income status. The social workers who presented their clients for consultation provided me with detailed, comprehensive case histories. I selected several write-ups of adolescent clients belonging to ghetto and lower middle-class groups and several case histories from my own private practice of upper-income groups. I carefully deleted all identifying material revealing social and economic status and described only the symptoms and their development, concentrating solely upon personality make-up and the stresses suffered. I submitted copies of these anonymous patients to social workers, psychologists, psychiatrists, and psychoanalysts who have had considerable experience in treating adolescent patients from all levels of society. I was astonished at their abyssmal failure at guessing the patients' backgrounds. In fact, the relatively wealthy patients from my private practice were judged to be the sickest of all and thereby put in the lowest poverty-level income groups.

Although exposed to flagrant and pathetic cruelty, the ghetto children did not seem as emotionally scarred as the youth from upper-income families. Even more surprising was the fact that, upon rereading the case histories of affluent youth, their backgrounds impressed us as being just as traumatic, if not more so, than those from the slums. Physical fights between parents, broken homes, exhibitionistic sexual activity witnessed by children, cruel beatings, or absolute neglect were frequent findings in the developmental history of these so-called privileged children.

One particularly upsetting example occurred in the childhood of a delinquent adolescent girl who came from a wealthy suburban home. Her past history revealed that at the age of three she stumbled and hit her head on a concrete sidewalk, knocking herself unconscious. The mother saw this happening but did not bother to move one step to help her daughter. The girl lay there for hours until a neighbor carried her into the house. She had fractured her skull, but neither parent showed any concern or remorse.

The manifestations of trauma can be subtle. Physical abuse and gross neglect as occurs in impoverished areas is easily recognizable and often comes to the attention of the authorities and welfare workers. However, situations such as that just described, of the mother and the daughter who fractured her skull, are not as obvious. That mother seemed concerned about her children's welfare, fed them, clothed them, gave them appropriate parties, and generally acted as if she had considerable love for them. Her basic sadism and emotional isolation were grossly revealed in such an incident. Her daily affective assaults and rejections were not readily noticeable, and her damaging influence operated in a covert fashion and was expressed in hidden nuances. Nevertheless, its effects on her children were unmistakable. The daughter, as mentioned, is a severely acting-out delinquent and a son is an institutionalized schizophrenic.

Again, we can formulate the obvious, that is, the environment is a crucial factor in determining whether a child will be emotionally a relatively healthy adolescent or whether he will suffer from psychopathology. Still, as we have repeatedly learned, the important elements that are responsible for either psychic growth or fixation are found in early object relationships. The surrounding world, whether it is the ghetto or affluent suburbia, is important inasmuch as it provides the setting in which, for example, a mother will relate to her child. That setting will have some influence upon how she will function as a mother, but her early life experiences, her own emotional development, outweigh all other factors as determinants to her motherliness.

The Influence of Immigrants on Adolescent Life-Style

The United States is a conglomeration of immigrants who, to this day, have not been completely assimilated into a cohesive unity, nor have they formed a national identity. The adolescent immigrant child, or second-generation child, has been significantly responsible for our orientations and ideologies which, in turn, have spread to other areas of the world. This group has determined practically all of the elements that characterize our culture. Old traditions and our national identity are beginning to crumble in places where they had once been firmly constructed.

We have not had enough time to study the effects of the relatively recent influx of Latinos and Asiatics. I am discussing the wave of immigration that occurred several generations back, that is, from the beginning of the twentieth century to the post–World War I era of the 1920s. The children of these immigrants found methods to achieve specific goals and a comfortable lifestyle. They wanted material success and acceptance by their peer group. They struggled to acquire a self-image which would enhance self-esteem. Sometimes they succeeded. Because of their background and identity problems, they worked and competed in typical fashions. Their method of relating are what we refer to as cultural stereotypes.

No one likes to be classified as a cultural stereotype, and the adolescent in particular strives to free himself from being categorized. Second-generation adolescents could not escape becoming stereotypes. They had to adjust to the new culture in order to maintain their self-respect. In turn, their peers, whose families had been here for many generations, related to personality patterns which threatened the stability of their self-images and disturbed their value systems. This interplay between the children of immigrants and those of established families led to the construction of attitudes and perspectives responsible for the distinctive qualities and unsettling features of our competitive, frenetic society. No other group has so dramatically contributed to a life-style that has had its repercussions on all adolescents.

Boundaries between childhood, adolescence, and adulthood were blurred in the old country. The adolescent had his niche and, within the family system, had a definitive role which commanded respect. His self-representation was relatively secure. Identity problems, in terms of the meaning of life, were scarce. The Europe that immigrants left was a land of hard labor, scarcity, and, sometimes, persecution. With an empty stomach, there is little inclination to deal with what would seem to be lofty philosophical questions. If you are dying of thirst, you do not pause to ponder about the essence of a glass of water.

Immigrants experienced the move to the new world as a precipitous change, a severe cultural shock. The parents and the children who settled here were forced to adapt to an entirely different environment. Their previous adaptations and methods of obtaining self-esteem were not synchronous with the current milieu. They quickly learned that the land of opportunity could supply them with nurture and safety, but how satisfying this would be was another question, and the immigrant used a variety of adaptations. The gifted and enterprising immigrant parent could achieve business success and wealth. He could use his money as the basis for self-esteem and acceptance by the higher social echelons of the new culture. He would seldom succeed, but he might be tolerated—a token acceptance. This generation rarely melted into the surrounding environment.

Consequently, they sought out their own countrymen and maintained the customs and traditions of the old world. The less fortunate immigrant, by far the most common, lived in neighborhoods peopled by fellow nationals and isolated from the main current. Many never learned English and continued to eke out a meager living in sections of the city named after their country of origin, sections that often degenerated into ghettos. Immigrants in the United States voluntarily banded together in these ghettos for safety and security, in much the same manner that European Jews were forced to separate themselves and live apart. When the greenhorn left Ellis Island, he did not have much choice, but his lack of motivation to learn the customs of his adopted country indicated that he was not too eager to break out of his isolation.

The psyche achieves stability and equilibrium when its adaptations and defenses can function efficiently in an environment which supports it. As much as possible, we seek to create such an environment. I have called the process by which this is achieved "externalization" (Giovacchini 1975, 1979), a process which is similar to but still different from projection.

Briefly, the psyche projects instinctual impulses or self and object representations. By contrast, when it externalizes, it seeks to construct an environment patterned after the infantile ambience in which the ego's executive system can adapt. No adaptation can function in a vacuum. An adaptation or a defense requires an ambience in which it can function. For example, the master sergeant who is calm and efficient in dangerous battle conditions, conditions that would terrify most of us, may break down emotionally during peacetime. Imagine what would happen to us if we were suddenly transported into a society in which running and hurling spears were the most esteemed and functional adaptations.

The immigrant parent faced a comparable dilemma when he arrived in the United States. The externalizations that worked in his native country were no longer operative here, at least in the general community. Consequently, he banded together with fellow nationals who also felt threatened by a breakdown of their externalizations. Thus, they created ghettos. The group, as Freud (1921) emphasized, provided these immigrants with an opportunity to identify with each other and with a collective superego patterned after the mores and values of the old country.

The Early Environment and Defensive Adaptations of the Second-Generation Immigrant

The parental home ideally gives the infant child both good nurturing and soothing, in other words, capable, adequate mothering. The child's excitement is contained within the family setting, and he acquires the security that he will be loved and cared for. His adaptations to the infantile environment may be effective and gratifying, and psychic structuralization may optimally occur.

The second-generation child spent infancy nestled in the arms of a woman who hummed, sang, and talked to him in her mother tongue. Mother soothed and comforted him in a language that he would soon recognize as foreign. If the tempo of his rocking maintained a Yiddish, Italian, or Polish cadence, he heard some strange rhythms and sounds when he ventured out into the world beyond the confines of the nursery. The child was literally confronted with uncomfortable noises, sounds that upset a sense of stability and inner harmony. He felt himself out of phase with his surroundings.

Discordance between the outside environment and the one inside the home tremendously affects the later childhood period of assimilation. It is a period in which the child is pulled by opposing forces, although the conflict may be far from apparent on the surface. The parents' viewpoint of the world is clear but different from that of the child's peers. This creates problems. Since many of these children had a good childhood they want to be like their parents, but they feel alienated. They feel guilty because they are led to believe they are abandoning their parents and their traditions, parents who somehow have undergone severe hardships and worked hard to care for their families. The construction of a firm identity sense is not an easy task, and the problem compounds when these children reach adolescence. Second-generation immigrants learn to deal with their conflicting loyalties and idealizations by behaving in fashions which will help them resolve their dilemma.

One such pattern of resolution, a defensive adaptation, is to caricature the parents' orientations and mannerisms, a form of self-stereotyping (Giovacchini 1961). They may tell ethnic jokes which cast ridicule upon themselves. Witness the numerous Jewish, Italian, and Polish jokes frequently told by Jews, Italians, and Poles. This is especially true of Jewish comedians' jokes which make Jews look ridiculous. True, it may be a sign of tolerance and understanding to poke fun at oneself, but much more is involved. By caricaturing their background, these children and adolescents attempt to ingratiate themselves into the peer group. It is a protective device by which they fend off an anticipated attack by attacking themselves first, an example of identification with the aggressor (A. Freud 1946).

Deprecatory caricature also has a subtle manipulative aspect. Although amused, their peers are also uncomfortable. They occasionally feel that something is being put over on them, but they do not know exactly what. Later, during adolescence or early adulthood, it may be apparent that the second-generation adolescent protects himself by disarming others. He has rendered his peers innocuous by diverting their aggression away from him. In the meantime, he works very hard and comes out ahead academically. He is often successful, achieving economic success or a prestigious and financially rewarding profession. This pattern is more typical of boys who feel the pressure of competition keenly and whose thirst for success is immense.

This type of situation may seem extreme, but it is this kind of behavior that determines which patterns of adjustment and life-style will prevail and the price one must pay for them. This adolescent emerged in the threatening, insecure world of the Great Depression. Nothing was really great about the depression, and the second-generation immigrant had to be particularly astute at grabbing every possible opportunity. Being overidentified with the American life-style, he learned to be especially vigilant and developed an exploitive sophistication.

The insecure immigrant parent sought a world of security and opportunity but instead found a crashing economy and unemployment. These immigrants, who were used to deprivation, hard work, and perseverance, could survive in the cataclysmic world of economic depression. More often than not they survived better than those who had been here for generations and knew very little about hardships. Their American-born children developed the same survival instinct. Although they often felt in limbo, they extracted what they could from their teachers. They tried to incorporate the manners and traits of their peers so that they could achieve the success so desperately needed to secure an identity and maintain self-esteem.

Second-generation immigrant adolescents of the depression differed from their siblings born in the old country. The latter had problems of their own, but they were relatively secure in their identity. They suffered conflicts inasmuch as their values and orientations differed from those of the new environment. However, they did not particularly wish to be like their peers; they simply worked to make their self-concept effective, and they were often successful. They exploited their European mannerisms and accent so that their manner of relating could be considered charming rather than intimidating. Whatever turmoil this group suffered, it had none of the frenetic elements of their siblings born on American soil, and their life-style had no particular impact on the general adolescent population.

The effects of the depression on the second-generation immigrant stimulated a competitive struggle for material acquisition. Generally, students worked hard to acquire the skills to enable them to make a good living. The strivings for upward mobility were intense. Still, many adolescents indulged in various frivolities. The immigrant's child, however, usually burned the midnight oil while his fellow students drank beer. They were the tortoises among the hares. They started with all the disadvantages of the neophyte, but they were steady and plodding. They substituted the joys of adolescence for the joys of success. Often their life consisted solely of work and contained no pleasure; work had taken the place of pleasure.

An example of this joyless personality would be someone like Woody Allen, a successful, witty comedian who often pokes fun at his background. He eloquently proclaims that he cannot experience pleasure. He is an exaggeration and the extreme he presents amuses us. Tone down what he displays, however, and we are faced with a person worn out by work, whose pursuit of pleasure impresses us with the toll of hard work. Everything is a relentless struggle, which has become an end in itself. The need to achieve persists and interferes with the pursuit of the aesthetic for its own sake rather than as a status symbol. The capacity for true enjoyment is defective, and this typical picture portrays a depressed personality.

Effects of the Second-Generation Immigrant on all Adolescents

The second-generation immigrant, in order to establish an identity which maintains self-esteem, both idealized and overidentified with the American culture, fully embraced all its standards and mores. Success, an important attribute of our society, became a desperate goal. To support his identification, he had to renounce his background. Many anglicized their names to hide their national origins.

An interesting outcome of the amalgamation of the second-generation immigrant into the host culture is that he, in turn, had a significant influence on his milieu which, of course, had its effects on all adolescents. He created a competitive atmosphere which drew most youth into the arena, at least middle-class teenagers. At the school level, grades became important. The gentleman "C" was no longer acceptable as students struggled for the limited places in professional schools, such as medical and law schools. During the depression, especially, these were among the few occupations which could guarantee a fairly secure income.

In spite of the second-generation immigrant's maneuvers to be accepted by his native peers, he seldom succeeded. In college, he was usually not accepted by fraternities. If he wanted to emulate the nonimmigrant adolescent, he had to form his own group with fellow nationals. This created a paradox because, at one level, he was involved in an activity such as fraternity life which represented an attempt to identify with an aspect of American college culture, a somewhat prestigious organization and, at another level, he was isolating himself by forming a group of his own away from the circle he was seeking to join. This dilemma continues to the present day although to a much lesser degree.

After World War II, there were third- and fourth-generation as well as second-generation immigrants. Many fraternaties disappeared and the immigrant became, more than ever, assimilated into the group. There were and still are exceptions. For example, Jews are still excluded from some organizations, but this is less so than in the past and in some instances they have formed their own institutions and clubs in order to preserve themselves as a group. However, most descendents of the immigrants of the past several decades want to melt into the majority.

The majority, and in this instance that majority which comprises adolescence, has changed in the expected direction of action and counter-action. Though the competitiveness for places in professional schools and colleges in general continues, perhaps even more keenly because more students seek admission to college than in past generations, their shifts in values espouse opposite standards. Success and material acquisition are no longer idealized, or at least they do not rate as high as they once did on priority lists.

Minority Groups, Life-Style, and Psychopathology

With the homogenization of the adolescent group, as distinctions between immigrants and nonimmigrants become increasingly blurred, overt attitudes about minority groups have decidedly changed. Whereas in the past immigrants, blacks, and other minorities were rejected and ridiculed, today we do not approve of such prejudice. Again there is a counteraction of racist attitudes and deriding of certain ethnic groups as evidenced, for example, by the innumerable Polish jokes of the past decade. But, by and large, there is less of this. In fact, as the second-generation immigrant created certain changes in adolescent behavior and attitudes, other minority groups continue to have their effects on society in general and adolescence in particular. These groups, rather than being defined by national origins, skin color, or religious affiliation, are identified by behavioral patterns and ideologies.

Today it is easy to recognize homosexuals because they do not, as a rule, make any effort to conceal themselves. As is now familiar, there has been considerable debate as to whether they represent a form of psychopathology or an alternate life-style. Without becoming involved in this controversy, I simply want to emphasize that what once might have been unquestionably considered to be the symptoms of emotional illness can today be part of a life-style.

For example, cults have been formed by the banding together of persons with similar or complementary delusional systems. Smoking marijuana and taking drugs several decades ago was considered the symptomatic behavior of severely emotionally disturbed persons. With much less acrimony than was present four or five years ago, our youth is still characterized as being part of a drug culture which, to some extent, has spread to adults. Thirty years ago we would invariably diagnose an adolescent with a beard as schizophrenic. The flamboyant and feminine clothing styles of avant-garde male homosexuals have contributed heavily to fashion trends.

Thus, adaptive techniques which once were characteristic of certain types of psychopathology have become incorporated by the general adolescent community. While they have also spread to older age groups, it has usually been the adolescent who has led the way.

Conclusions

The determination as to whether certain constellations of behavior and attitudes are examples of psychopathology has to be placed in a cultural context. Aberrant orientations in some societies might be the norm in other groups or at different times in history.

The second-generation immigrant of several decades ago spent his infancy in an environment that was different from the one he would experience during childhood and adolescence. The methods of being soothed and nurtured and the character adaptations he acquired do not function smoothly in the new world environment. Consequently, the second-generation immigrant constructs special defensive adaptations which are representative of high levels of psychic structure. He may employ the defense of identification with the aggressor which is manifested by ridiculing his group and caricaturing their accent and mannerisms. By contrast, he may identify, even overidentify, with American traditions and values. He struggles to achieve wealth and success in order to gain self-esteem and acceptance by his native peers.

Up until the post–World War II era, the second-generation immigrant had not particularly succeeded in losing his immigrant status and becoming fully amalgamated into the new culture. However, he made his fellow adolescents less complacent and more aware of goals for which they would have to compete. The drive for success of the second-generation immigrant became infectious, and immigrants and nonimmigrants often became fiercely competitive.

With the passage of time and a major war, the second-generation immigrant and his adolescent children were, for the most part, assimilated by the general population. Regarding adolescence, the attitude toward minorities changed from one of scorn and rejection to tolerance and acceptance and, in some instances, to idealization.

Minority groups, including various types of psychopathology, influence life-styles. Now we are faced with an interesting paradox. Whereas formerly individual psychopathology was measured alongside a cultural norm, meaning that the culture determined what constitutes pathology, today the reverse seems to be the dominant theme—that is, psychopathology determines what the cultural norm will be. The attitudes of persons suffering from emotional disorders, their clothing styles and methods of achieving soothing and excitement, such as by the use of drugs, have become incorporated into the behavior and ideologies of many adolescents and have spread to the adult population as well.

REFERENCES

Freud, A. 1946. *The Ego and the Mechanisms of Defense.* New York: International Universities Press.

Freud, S. 1905. Three contributions to the theory of sex. *Standard Edition* 7:123–244. London: Hogarth, 1953.

Freud, S. 1921. Group psychology and the analysis of the ego. *Standard Edition* 18:12–66. London: Hogarth, 1955.

Giovacchini, P. 1961. Ego adaptations and cultural variables. *Archives of General Psychiatry* 5:37–45.

Giovacchini, P. 1975. *Psychoanalysis of Character Disorders.* New York: Aronson.

Giovacchini, P. 1979. *Treatment of Primitive Mental States.* New York: Aronson.

Offer, D., and Offer, J. B. 1976. Three developmental routes through normal adolescence. *Adolescent Psychiatry* 4:121–141.

Oldham, D. G. 1978. Adolescent turmoil: a myth revisited. *Adolescent Psychiatry* 6:267–279.

Toffler, A. 1971. *Future Shock.* New York: Basic.

7 PERSPECTIVE ON FAMILY LIFE AND SOCIAL CHANGE

OTTO POLLAK

The impact of social change on family life has been particularly noticeable over the last few decades although it has been longer in the making. It has found its strongest expression in the structure and function of the spouse relationship and, as a consequence, has influenced child development. The women's movement, the growing economic independence of wives, and the increasing profusion of child-care services, which have released the mother from many demands which child rearing formerly made on her, are only the most recent and most obvious factors that have contributed to this development. Actually, political orientations that have dominated the mental life of the middle classes for the last 200 years have been instrumental in bringing these changes about.

It is amazing how long it took societies with professed democratic ideals to apply these ideals to the position of women vis-à-vis men. Inequality between men and women, the belief in the superiority of males over females, the institutionalized division of labor between the two, and women's lack of the right to vote coexisted for about a century with governmental institutions based on the ideals of equality and liberty. What is probably the oldest inequality among human beings (Tocqueville 1964) was the slowest in being recognized, being made the subject of public debate, and ultimately the object of social reform. As is always true with revolutions, the anger of the suppressed became public only when the reason for the anger had practically disappeared. Brinton (1952) described this phenomenon that explains the anger of the Roundheads under Charles I, the bourgeoisie under Louis XVI, and the workers under Nicholas II. The same explanation appears to be true for women now. Certainly, the women's movement has been instrumental in improving the position of women in America. This improvement, however, is also the result of earlier progress in their social situation, such as educational equality, their attainment of the right to vote, their roles in the labor movement, and their ability to alleviate the manpower shortages during the Second World War.

In consequence of these developments, family life has now to cope with open assertiveness of women where it formerly had to cope with a professed but insincere submissiveness and concealed dissatisfaction with traditional female roles. In some cases, the new assertiveness and self-realization in an occupation or a profession may be social conformity rather than psychological reality. In assessing the consequences of a revolution one must consider that any liberation produces pressures for the acceptance of new styles of behavior. In the present mood of women's liberation it is not easy for a middle-class woman to live nonassertively and to be satisfied with the role of a homemaker. There is little doubt, however, that assertiveness and self-realization have contributed significantly to a social definition of disagreement as a reason for separation and divorce. Disagreement between unequals can be overcome by power or ruses; between equals it can only lead to compromise or separation. In the assertive mood of many young women today, separation will often appear to be preferable to compromise.

As long as men deluded themselves into believing that they had patriarchal powers in family life, and as long as women found it expedient or unavoidable to help men maintain this belief, family constancy, although not family happiness, could be taken as the norm and divorce as the exception. With the destruction of the patriarchal belief, marriage became unavoidably a temporary arrangement bound to be dissolved when it did not seem to provide reciprocal satisfactions. Equals do not stay together if one of them does not like their togetherness. In other words, marriage, instead of being an economic prison for women who had no opportunity to maintain themselves independently, is now one of several options that are available. These other options are: economic independence after divorce, remarriage in search of a better constellation, or adoption of the single life-style. It is perfectly possible that these options are feasible opportunities which were not recognized until long after the conditions for them had come into existence. At any rate, it is becoming more and more difficult to consider divorce a social problem or a personality problem. It is much rather the expression of the temper of our times which requires instant and uninterrupted gratifications from relationships (Pollak 1976). Since the nature of human relationships implies alternating periods of satisfaction and friction, we seem to be approaching a reversal of evaluations of constancy in marriage. Constancy without persistent gratification is about to be considered as pathological and divorce as a result of disagreement and dissatisfaction as remedial.

The entrance of women into the labor force has contributed to this trend by bringing married people into lasting contacts with persons of the other sex. Women, as well as men, meet persons to whom they can attach their fantasies of a better marriage partner at their work.

It should also be noted that the development of the philosophy of existentialism has produced a new morality which drives people into a permanent search for a place or conditions of living which they feel to be right for them (Heidegger 1949). This philosophy has as its central idea the proposition that the existence of every human being expresses only one of several possible alternatives and that this specific existence alternative may frequently not be right for him or her. People are therefore permanently engaged in a search for authenticity, that is, a type of existence which they feel to be right for them. People are not willing to live as dependent variables of conditions into which they were thrown by birth or the decisions of their parents. They demand from their lives a feeling of being right in what they do and with whom they live. In consequence, behavior and life tasks that we ascribed to adolescence, such as deciding on an occupation and the selection of a mate, are now carried on through adulthood. The distinction between adolescent and adult behavior becomes blurred, and general psychiatry should recognize that it has much to learn about modern maturity from the study of adolescence.

The frantic and continuous search for a better life today is probably the result of the loss of the belief of many that one's reward for suffering will come after death. Increasing and widespread loss of faith in a hereafter forces people to search for rewards in the here and now and leads to rebellion against discomfort and unhappiness. Change becomes the remedy of discomfort and the instrument of existentialism. In this context it might be well to point out that the ability to change is certainly better than immobilization and that change is the essence of life (Boszormenyi-Nagy 1965). Still, from the viewpoint of psychiatry, repetitive divorces and remarriages are probably maladaptive because they are likely to lead to many disappointments and to an erosion of ego-strength. They may result in depression after repeated failure and to inappropriate experimentations when there is not enough time left to attain competence in new ways.

At any rate, self-realization has become a virtue and is experienced as being as demanding as maternal nurture used to be. For children, however, this social change implies a noticeable increase in experiences of separation and loss. Child-care centers that were originally planned to make it possible for women in the lower classes to work are now being used by middle-class women for liberation from maternal demands. This has had several results, two of which may be of particular interest to psychiatrists. First, it leads to internal conflict because many women who seek fulfillment in a profession or occupation still feel that their children need them and that they are withholding from their children time which is rightfully theirs. In consequence, these mothers try to compensate by intensified attention when they are with the children and extra effort when they are on the job. No matter whether they are with the children or working, they feel that they should be somewhere else. This leads to conflict which may produce overwork, exhaustion, and anger which will be felt by their family as well as their employer.

This may well be one of the most significant aspects of modern middle-class life. Young mothers want to have jobs and careers but they do not want to give up maternity. They do not even find it easy to give up fully work in the household. Young spouses, of course, share more and more household and child-care tasks. The power of old role assignments, however, is still strong, and even young professional women frequently feel responsible for the running and appearance of the household. They have, therefore, taken on additional responsibility without giving up any substantial part of the workload prescribed by the previous role models. Since the stress and strain of overwork produces feelings of inadequacy and fatigue, it becomes difficult to control one's hostilities. This may be another reason for the increase in our divorce rate, particularly because men are also overworked. Under the impact of inflation and concerns that purchases should be made now rather than later, men assume two jobs where formerly one seemed sufficient. This crosses class barriers: blue-collar workers drive cabs at night and on weekends; college professors become consultants; secretaries take on extra typing; and nobody has time for the other, or even for himself or herself. We can, therefore, conclude this picture by saying that the family of modern times tries to occupy more positions than it can occupy comfortably.

The frequently heralded exchangeability of social roles between marriage partners may also have unexpected consequences for child rearing. The entrance of the father into infant care or nurturing functions for preschoolers may change the traditional experience of children in connecting the expectation of power with femaleness. As long as women were the only child rearers, it was impossible for a male child to grow up without attaching the idea of adult power to the sex of the mother. In cases where fathers assume such functions, female children may now attach the concept of adult power to the male sex. This could well lead to the unexpected result that the daughters of assertive mothers who insist that fathers do their share in child rearing will become submissive wives or—what is probably more likely—conflicted about the assertiveness which social change now demands from women. Males reared essentially by fathers may be as much stimulated in latent homosexuality as girls reared by mothers are stimulated in latent lesbianism. It might be seen as an act of social retribution that the lesbian panic of girls under stress (Blos 1969) may now become paralleled by the homosexual panic of boys under stress.

Conclusions

Although I have presented the changes which I personally feel occur in modern family life from the viewpoint of possible pathology, I would like to conclude my chapter pointing out the advantages that are being derived from these changes. The abolition of inequality between the sexes which we are experiencing now has removed an element of disharmony from our political and social life. One cannot believe comfortably in democracy for 50 percent of the population. The increasing role of child-care institutions in the formative years of the child may actually produce people who will be better able to cope with the endless and repetitive separations of modern life than their parents. Adolescents who go to college away from home will have an easier time if they have learned to cope with separation almost from infancy. Short of the repetition compulsion in the selection of marriage partners, there is at least a statistical chance that the remarriage after divorce may result in a better marriage than the one which was resolved. For people who should opt for the single life-style, there will be the advantage of a far greater experience of autonomy in living than family life permits.

Equality may truly lead to liberty—liberty to change partners and liberty to live alone. Of course such liberty will demand tolerance for loneliness but, here, again, we may find support in the idea that mortality makes separation unavoidable toward the end of life and that people who have been socialized into a tolerance of separation over the whole life cycle will cope better with old age and its unavoidable losses than people who have been socialized into maintaining themselves through the cultivation of relationships.

REFERENCES

Blos, P. 1969. Three typical constellations in female delinquency. In O. Pollak and A. S. Friedman, eds. *Family Dynamics and Female Sexual Delinquency*. Palo Alto, Calif.: Science & Behavior Books.

Boszormenyi-Nagy, I. 1965. The concept of change in conjoint family therapy. In A. S. Friedman et al., eds. *Psychotherapy for the Whole Family*. New York: Springer.

Brinton, C. 1952. *The Anatomy of Revolutions*. New York: Prentice-Hall.

Heidegger, M. 1949. *Existence and Being*. Chicago: Regnery.

Pollak, O. 1976. Group psychotherapy and changing social values. *International Journal of Group Psychotherapy* 24(4): 411–419.

Tocqueville, A. de. 1964. *Souvenirs*. Paris: Gallimard.

VIVIAN M. RAKOFF

While in the past the privileged allowed their male offspring (at least) an extended period of education and development between puberty and the responsibilities of marriage, duty, and career, it was only after World War I, and more notably after World War II, that a lengthy adolescence became a democratized option. Concomitant with the change in social character from aristocratic privilege to an almost universal psychobiological state of the urban middle classes, there developed new ways of being adolescent, with new and characteristic rites of passage. No longer were the choices restricted to the limited career of the young lord expected to choose between one or two ancient universities or being a military cadet; they became extended to the entire domain of leaving home, political action, traveling, finding oneself, and rejecting all notion of context or history in the service of discovering an authentic identity (Aries 1962; Hall 1904; Rakoff 1978).

Of course, I am stating the case paradigmatically. Most young people struggle along through puberty, high school, and college to arrive, with a few ups and downs, at marriage and procreation. But the ordinariness of the process should not obscure the fact that such ordinariness, the creation of an accepted and new form of life career, was the product of revolutionary social changes and social forces that created the massive social discontinuities of the French and American revolutions.

The same historical forces that created the contemporary Western way of being adolescent may also have contributed to the characteristic forms of adolescent distress, anomie, narcissism, complaints of emptiness, loneliness, and existential despair. To the degree that the mass option of extended adolescence may represent an extraordinary social achievement of the Western world during the past 200 years, an understanding of the stresses on the

Based on an article by Dr. Rakoff which appeared in *The Adolescent and Moral Disorders,* ed. H. Golombeck (New York: International Universities Press, 1980).

adolescent may clarify forms of social distress not necessarily confined to adolescents.

To be specific: The notion of the right to individual personality and identity is one of those aristocratic privileges that becomes a democratic option. But whereas aristocratic personality and identity were developed and expressed within the context of clearly defined social relationships and place (old families lived on clearly defined territory and took their names from places, estates, countries, possessions; the landless poor took their names from their crafts or expressed the familial identity in simple patronymics), the democratized right to identity developed from the destruction of historical context.

For most people the historical context of precapitalist, aristocratic, feudal societies was the confining and oppressive expression of those forces that held them from full personhood. In particular, almost all Americans (including Canadians) are the children, grandchildren, and great grandchildren of those who fled the context of a defined past. They fled from kings, emperors, czars, dictators, and religious orthodoxy; in leaving behind the external and usually tyrannical definers of who they were, they extended the opportunity to define themselves, or at least the opportunity that their children might become themselves. Their new myth—the myth that replaced nationhood, class status, language, ancestral landscapes, traditions of cooking, and the graves of the fathers—was that of a pluralist America that offered an open frontier to both the body and the sense of self. The ultimate freedom offered was, in its ideal form, the right to define oneself, to unleash fully one's own energy, and to live, if one wished, dangerously.

While America expressed these ideas most explicitly and consistently, Western society was heir to currents of political development that flowed like a strong, consistent, and broadening stream in England and exploded in continental Europe in the French revolution. The new postrevolutionary capitalist-individual man was released in fantasy from the defined modes of being of the court into the exciting and dangerous territory of what Trilling (1972) labeled, "sincerity and authenticity," a social mode defined by the revolutionary expectation that one not only existed but had the right to express the true self. The task would involve constant conflict. In place of the fixed roles and certainties of the old context, a universe of predictable and more or less certain categories, there would now be the constant labor of perpetual movement and redefinition in the direction of increasing self-consciousness, the Hegelian *Aufheibung,* elevating oneself in stages to an ideal, fully realized, fully conscious personhood (Weisberg 1979).

Those of us who work with adolescents will recognize that these historical injunctions and opportunities offered to all the freed citizens of postrevolutionary Europe and America sound very similar to the task of adolescence defined by Erikson (1963) as establishing a sense of "identity." Its defined opposite and failure were sensed long ago by Nietzsche and Kierkegaard, the one exultantly and the other in despair. The exciting prospect of establishing a true self and of making a personally defined journey through life was accompanied by the twin dangers of social alienation and the loss of a sense of moral significance. Despair clung to hope like a shadow.

Although the emphasis of this chapter will be on history and culture and their possible relationship to clinical pathology, it is not intended to displace our concerns with other important factors of interpersonal and intrapersonal relationships, so clearly significant in the formation of the individual and the capacity of that individual to withstand stress and to relate to others. My concern will be with the problem of how the great ship of history gets into the bottle of the individual psyche. In particular, I will attempt to define some determinants of the psychopathology of a particular group of patients: those who come to us severely depressed, confused about their roles, preoccupied with ethical and moral concerns against a background of poorly defined values, and even some of those who at the extreme we label narcissistic, borderline, or sociopathic personality disorders. Three clinical vignettes may help to focus our concerns.

Case Example 1

Jody, a young woman in her early twenties, was referred to me via a complex pathway by an ex-lover. When she arrived, she had already made up her mind. She was going to carry out her plan to go to India to the center of a major religious organization. She had already bought a one-way ticket and said, "I want to do something drastic about my life."

She told me about her plans using the characteristic language of the seeker after mystical experience. She wanted to discover her true self and live on a plane above the mundane. She did not use the phrase, "the veil of Maya," but when I used it to articulate her concerns, she nodded in vigorous agreement. She felt her life and the lives of people around her were frivolous and nonsignificant. She had an intense conviction that with proper training and with a change in attitude, she would break through to a vivid, meaningful, spiritual experience, which would finally make sense of her life. She said, "I want to renounce everything because there is no meaning to the physical world. . . . I have to find people who are thinking of spiritual things all the time."

She appeared to have no sense that she was one of many, and that her language, preoccupations, and planned solutions were stereotypic. She was in fact surprised that I could supply her with certain phrases to describe both her aspiration and her experience since she had, like many of us, the sense that what she was choosing was totally personal.

She was not psychotic or in any way sociopathic. She had always worked and had used drugs sparingly. During a period with a religious sect in New York she had had some experiences which provided the model for her quest. She described it as a search for "a blissful, detached state, an inner joy."

My inquiry into her family history produced a story which bewildered me as a therapist. Both her parents, she said, were very loving and supportive. "I had a very good childhood, we did lots of things together and we lived in the family." I seized on the phrase, "we lived in the family," and asked her what she meant. She elaborated. "We had to. We never had time to make friends with our neighbors, because we moved every three or four years." She described her various dwellings. Each home had been in a prosperous part of the city. When I asked her about the family's community attachments, such as church, political party, or social networks, she replied, "I can't think of anything. My parents were and are agnostic. They never went to church and I don't think they really were much involved in politics."

Jody comes from an Anglo-Saxon family. She is not underprivileged. Her decision to go to India seems wild were it not for the fact that there are many like her, who either go to India or to some local variant of an India. It would be difficult to place her in any category other than that of an adventure seeker of a curious variety.

Case Example 2

Mark comes from a totally different background. His father spent part of his childhood in a concentration camp. After the war, when the father was fourteen years old, he was sent to Israel alone to live on a kibbutz. Although they had visited him on the kibbutz, he felt that he had lost all connection with his parents. Mark was born in Israel. When he was ten years old the family moved to Canada, where they severed all ties with the past. The children did not receive a Hebrew education, and the family is unrelated to any political or institutionalized, identity-giving organization.

Mark was referred because of behavioral difficulty at school, bad work, and disciplinary problems. From the parents' point of view, the most significant problem was his trouble with the police because of his dealing in marijuana.

Clinical interviews with the family revealed the following. The mother was concerned and appeared genuinely warm. The father was a bit excitable but in no way pathological. It is probably important to note that when he spoke of his work, his comments were flat and direct: "I hate my work. I always say I hate my work. It's a living." The older brother, Michael, who also had behavioral problems in the past, was at the time of the interviews a hyperconformist, model boy.

Mark was sad and lackadaisical. His affect was somewhat flat and he was very casual about his problems. He said his only pleasures came from acting, music, and smoking pot.

Case Example 3

The third picture I would like to present could be contained in a photograph: James's appearance was a display board of the fundamental problem we are trying to address. He dressed in a style reminiscent of the 1960s: a "street crazy" costume striving for individuality but so clearly a fashion of a given time and a given place. He wore a fancy brown fedora hat, not secondhand ("My mother gave it to me for Christmas"). In the hatband there was a razor blade. He had long, unkempt hair, and his jeans were scribbled with obscenities and the names of rock groups. He wore a tie but it was knotted around his neck inside his open shirt collar. The tie pin was a short length of chain pinned with a couple of small, brass safety pins. Attached to his belt was a heavy steel chain fastened to the belt loop with a heavy brass lock. Here and there pinned to his clothing were buttons advertising various rock groups. Among the buttons was a plain blue coat button about the size of a silver dollar—just that, a button, without significance or inscription.

James was not delinquent, stupid, or underprivileged. Why then, I asked myself, was his clothing such a collection of aggressive, ironic references? He was not a punk rocker or a cocaine addict, although he would have liked to look like one. His plain blue button, taken from his mother's sewing box, was as significant to him, it seemed, as those that he wore bearing slogans.

When I asked him about the meaning of his ornaments, chains, and deliberate inversions of conventional dress, he professed not to know what I was talking about. "I do it because I like it." When I pressed him a bit further and asked him if he couldn't see that the chains and the punk-rock safety pins and the dirty words scrawled on his trousers were aggressive signals, he replied, "No, I just do it for fun."

Further discussion showed that he really did not consciously know why he did these things. He has adopted some of the styles of the 1960s without any knowledge or interest in the ideologies of the peace movement, student rebellion, or even the drug culture. He wears the tag ends of fashions and recent mythologies without participating in them.

When I asked him, "Where do you see yourself twenty years from now? . . . What do you want of your life?" he could barely articulate an answer. The most I could get from him was a vague wish to run a rock band. At seventeen, Jim belongs to no church, no political movement, and he has only a couple of friends with whom he is mildly rebellious at his elite private school.

He was born in the West, lived in the East, and has had many moves in Toronto. His family structure is small in its scope. The only consistent figure is his mother, an intelligent, troubled woman, who consciously feels that she has no group of reference. She has recently joined a church of congenial people. For the mother, the friendship she finds in this community is more important than its systems of belief. Her own experience is loneliness and rootlessness.

If one were attempting to understand the origin of James's curious lack of direction, the panoply of ironic signals he does not understand, the loss of any sense of shape to his life, it could be constructed in purely personal, psychopathological terms. His biography contains all the necessary elements. There was no effective father. He and his mother have moved repeatedly, with the result that they have lost all consistent community as well as their extended family. His life is in the most classical sense a recipe for a chaotic superego. But, in fact, in most of his functioning James is not someone without standards of conduct. It is as though he has been deprived of a particular part of his existence which in his behavior and his costuming he tries to satisfy.

If James were alone or even very unusual, he would be interesting enough, but the truth is that like Jody and like Mark, in more or less extreme form, his depression, his lack of direction, his lack of public structure are characteristic of a whole class of adolescents. They appear to be clinical fallout of the great historical forces that bequeathed us many of our most valued freedoms and opportunities.

For purposes of discussion I could have cited the histories of other young people whose families were not notably pathological. Certainly on close examination there were distortions of communication, oddities of personality, some plain nasty bits and pieces of behavior, but none of what I actually saw in these cases seemed to be sufficient cause for the degree of symptomatology shown by the identified patients. These adolescents are depressed, restless, and apathetic. They want creative jobs without first applying themselves to disciplined preparation, study, and so on. They are hungry for authority, meaning, and belief.

I have told you about Jody, Mark, and James as a mnemonic device, not to acquaint you with them in great detail. It will be my thesis that somewhere there is a common thread in their distress. At this stage it is essential to make clear that this is an attempt to unravel only one thread that may contribute to the complex and varied pathologies presented by adolescents. There is no intention to invalidate or ignore other factors of crucial importance in psychiatric disorder: the subtle entanglements of distorted family functioning, the sad tyranny of genetic predisposition or organic diathesis, or the important contribution of economics.

Jody and Mark came from families which seemed to provide everything for human growth, affection, food, education, and money. They came from families that, among other things, encourage their creativity. Jody describes her brother as a very creative person, "into film photography . . . though he hasn't done much yet." And Mark's mother, as she threatens to throw him out of the house, pleads with him to go to a theater school "to develop his great talent as an actor."

They share one other important characteristic. Their families, like the families of thousands of others in our culture, are restless movers, detached from the contexts of place, history, religion, or even similar communal custom. Mark's father was repeatedly detached during his lifetime from country, family, and personal and group history. One of the pieces of information he gave repeatedly is how much he "hates" his work. Jody moved within her language and her city; her disruption is less obvious than Mark's. But her family moved repeatedly and had no group attachments. Perhaps it is also significant that Jody's father is an advertising company president. Jody's very name is cute and fashionable, detached from history and any mythical structure, and reflects only an ephemeral fashion. She, like many others, was named by whim. Her name embodies no history of her family, ethnic group, or ethical community. She was named like actresses are named, or soap is labeled—only to be appealing in the marketplace. She is not like the boys, who have been alienated in other ways, named for figures who were important in the shared myths of society.

While the three adolescents described are representative of our contemporary clinic populations, they are, in their curious social detachment, prefigured in Durkheim's (1951) turn-of-the-century descriptions of anomic individuals. Durkeim's concern with the relationship of anomie to suicide may illuminate some of our concerns. Detachment, alienation, or anomie expressed itself in the most serious form of psychopathology: the desire to kill oneself. The absence of a nurturant community at the level of intimacy or more distant social connectedness may precipitate a psychic "illness unto death."

Some contemporary Canadian suicide data support this observation (Sakinofsky, Robert, and Van Hauten 1975). In Canada it is well known that the lowest suicide rates are in Newfoundland, where people are the poorest in the country and where they move least often. In contrast, the highest suicide rates in Canada are in the big cities and in the western provinces where prosperity is at its highest and physical movement is at its greatest. These provinces and cities attract the rootless and adventurous. But there is another group that must be considered because it confounds some of our assumptions and yet, at the same time, may illuminate the argument. Garfinkle (1979) has drawn our attention to the increased suicide rates of Indian adolescents in Western Ontario. These young people are not alienated from place or community; they exist in reservations within clearly defined community and family context. They are not poorer than their urban counterparts, and curiously their rate of employment is higher than a comparable sample of urban Caucasian adolescents in Ontario. However, they remain alienated in a crucial and significant way that relates them to the anomic figures of Durkheim's description and the white population of British Columbia. They have been alienated not from place or family but from their sense of historical continuity. Their own historical culture has been invalidated by the powerful patterns of the dominant society.

There are, of course, other important factors related to suicide, but the information cited brings into sharp focus the human need for connectedness and for a coherent sense of the self within a culture which we may label, in the broadest sense, as "history." There appears to be an implicit or explicit need for community, for mythology, for—let me make a leap—nonintimate, publicly validated sources of identity, guidance, and personal significance.

The association of the individual with necessary society, a domain of relating within which the family is embedded, is almost universally recognized. But the phenomenon has been expressed within the tradition of modern psychiatry in terms that tend to emphasize the opposition of the individual and society. Beginning with the classical formulations of Freud's (1930) *Civilization and Its Discontents*, the more recent pronouncement of Brown (1959) that "history is the accumulated result of repression" encapsulates the opposition of the individual's oppression by the group and its expression in history. He writes, "Repression transforms the timeless instinctual compulsion to repeat into the forward moving dialectic of neurosis which is history." The universal association of human beings in complex societies has been defined in the language of neurosis and conflict, language echoed by Roheim, Reich, and Marcuse (Robinson 1970).

Fortunately, for our time, Erikson has placed the developing individual within the concentric rings of relationships, each of which is a necessary component of possible achievement or failure during successive stages of human growth. It is now well accepted that there are necessary phases of development, achievements, capacities, and skills which need not be placed within the context of neurosis and conflict. And, in addition, there is a model that may describe a structure which permits the nonconflicted relationship of the individual to a single other—a mechanism permitting association and yet individuation, a mechansim which bridges the symbiotic close-bonded mother-child entity to become the mother and child relationship without destroying the infant's security or basic trust. I am, of course, referring to Winnicott's (1958) concept of the transitional object—the class of things which are not mother or child but which sufficiently contain the mother to be reassurers, talismans of safety, and trust. While they contain the mother, they are also in a psychic sense not only a possession but also part of the child. For our purposes, a further important aspect of these transitional objects should be noted: they exist within a transitional space, a species of psychic territory where one may play and create, and where one is released from emergency and pure necessity. It is the space, Winnicott (1967) suggests, in which culture is elaborated, the source of the essential tradition which must be established before there can be original action. Here transitional phenomena permit the movement of the child from the mother's side to free range within the "ecos," the household, the world of the family, however small or large the household may be in a particular society.

In the culture of the family, the child is loved for itself alone. In positivist rational terms the child does nothing for its keep. It exists, and that existence is sufficient cause for an entire complex of rewards. The essential substrate for this extraordinary altruistic phenomenon is established through the mutual bonding that connects the neotonous, helpless (dirty and noisy) infant to the receiving responsive parent. It is this structure of "being" as the generator of security, bondedness to intimates as opposed to strangers, the notion of family, home, "my parents," "my sisters and brothers," which provides for the needs of intimate man. Ultimately it provides the template for expectation of the self and others in intimate relationships. While it may originate in the parent-child bonded pair, it generates the capacity for affection, erotic intimacy, and transgenerational protectiveness in the fully developed adult.

Beyond the context of the family there is the universal context of a containing society, the world of the clothed and public human being, governed by different expectations from those that operate in the intimate cluster of the family. The bonding in the public context is sustained by a shared membership in a group established through more or less shared belief systems and, crucially and commonly, by a common language. Mere existence is not sufficient to generate reward in this context, which essentially respects and rewards performance. It is in this domain that competence, power, political savvy, courtliness, socially structured politeness, and the playing out of the life career take place. At the most commonplace level membership in such groups, with the use of a common language and respect for the shared assumptions of society, provides an essential component of identity and the sense of self as both subjectively perceived and recognized by others. One is not only John or Jane X, but one is also a Torontonian, an Ontarian, a Canadian, a somebody defined by place and culture as well as by the exigencies of early and intimate experience.

Alienation consists essentially of being detached from a societal structure. It is a central life task to be able to make the transition back and forth from the context of family—the world of the unclothed—to society or public existence—the world of the clothed. There need to be structures which bond the individual to the receiving group, in much the same way that the infant needs to be bonded not only to the initial mothering figure but to the household. The characteristics of such mechanisms would have to be such that they embodied shared perceptions, signaling systems, and common expectations not only of immediate action but of the significance that the individual and society have in time and in relation to ethical concerns.

An examination of transformations of language may illuminate the process of transition from intimate family to public community. In a city such as Toronto there is daily confirmation of the well-known fact that the children of immigrant parents speak in the accent and style of the receiving society, particularly the school, rather than the accent of the parents. The idiosyncratic, fractured language of feeling and the communication of nonperformance needs has to be extended to the language of discourse and social function. The sharing of common social language becomes the basis of communal empathy, much as early bonding relations within the family constitute the basis of personal empathy. Although Kohut (1966) has written, "The capacity for empathy belongs, therefore, to the innate equipment of the human psyche and remains to some extent associated with the primary process," this seems to be too restricted and fails to recognize the empathic sharing of public affective experience, which is the substrate for the powerful emotion of group identity.

Within culture, a common language is a primary vehicle for adults as well as children for the specific bondedness of the nonintimate world. But language is only one of the factors, albeit an early and necessary factor, for the development of "a good enough" (Winnicott 1967) sense of social security. The history of the communal context, which permits the projection of the self into the future because it establishes the continuity with the past; a shared sense of ethical values; and the elaborate compendium of social rituals involving games, art forms, visual symbols such as flags, national colors, group emblems, and badges are all in some way necessary components of the identity of the self within the world.

Winnicott (1967) elaborated his concept of the transitional object as follows:

In favourable circumstances the potential space [between mother and child] becomes filled with the products of the baby's own creative imagination. . . . Given the chance the baby begins to live creatively and to use actual objects to be creative into. If the baby is not given this chance then there is no area in which the baby may have play, or may have cultural experience; then there is no link with the cultural inheritance and there will be no connection with the cultural pool. . . . It is these cultural experiences that provide the continuity in the human race which transcends personal existence. I am assuming that cultural experiences are in direct continuity with play, the play of those who have not yet heard of games.

It is well known that for Winnicott, the transitional object, the thing that is "not me, not mother, but which is between" us signals the potential return of the mother who may have left the child. It is the foundation of security in the personal world.

This concept has been extremely important, and may without difficulty be extended to objects that define our personal space and security in the world. It seems to this writer that the concept, as outlined by Winnicott, may explain further the painful effects of loss of history and the yearning for history which we so commonly encounter in the clinic. However, it will be necessary to take the thought a stage further since, as it stands, it does not carry the concept into the second sphere of human relating beyond the family, the world of "We: not us, not them" which is the great complex of shared experiences between the individual and the other members of his society.

How can one assume that there is indeed a separate sphere of relating that requires a separate set of transitional structures? Why should the maternal child interspace not contain enough potential elaboration to satisfy the object hunger (seeking) of the intimate personal life, as well as the object hunger of the sphere beyond the family? It may be useful once more to consider the mechanism of language. Roheim (1962) reduces language to "the word . . . used to summon the mother when the child is hungry," and Freud (1905) says, "When someone speaks it's as though a light goes on." Language may be these things, but it is another thing as well. The cry may summon the mother, but, as we have said, it also summons the community. The transformations of language into an instrument of intricate social communication, the myth-carrying vehicle for a given society, and the instrument for expressing law, suggest an entire domain of ego necessities specifically developed for nonintimate relating: a genetic anlage for an expected community, analogous to the genetic behavioral structures that anticipate the nurturant mother. These ego necessities can no longer be reduced to the language of infantile need (although they may be contained in primitive form in early needs and interactions) but can, perhaps, be best perceived as essential needs of the psychiatrically neglected public self.

If we accept this hypothetical formulation, the curious yearning for history which takes the form of searching for roots, real or imagined, becomes understandable. It is not a frivolity but is connected with that painful sense of being disconnected that afflicts the cases discussed above. Furthermore, the need for ethical norms, or, at its most elaborate, adherence to a religious community, need no longer be perceived as "comparable to a childhood neurosis" (Freud 1927) but as the expression of a fundamental necessity, the deprivation of which will lead to neurosis. Fortunately, the explication of myth as necessary sense-making structure, the indeed necessary "manifestations of mental functioning" (Goddard 1970), has taken us beyond earlier, excessively simple perceptions of the role of the religious life for the individual.

The development of the secure reality within the context of family appears to be related to maternal function, whereas the movement into the societal context may in human terms be mediated by what Mahler (1975) called "the first stranger," the father or paternal function. In traditional societies, it was principally the male who participated in defense and the preservation of religious continuity and was the political "hero." The loss of paternal authority, commented on by Marcuse (1955) and Lasch (1978), has accompanied the growing failure to recognize the distinction between the domain of intimacy and the domain of public existence. It may also be responsible for what Sennett (1977), perhaps overpolemically, has described as "the tyrannies of intimacy." Sennett specifically regrets the loss of social forms of behavior and the energy people will give to their public demands and requirements when there is a clear distinction between loving and working for what one wants. Furthermore, both he and Lasch have emphasized that the failure to recognize the public arena of action as different from intimate action does not increase a sense of social security but leads, rather, to an increase in (what is now so fashionably labeled) narcissism. This is particularly true in terms of the terror of death, the solipsistic evaluation of events, the vacillation between grandiose omnipotence and the feeling of total weakness, and the incapacity to articulate complex and formal modes of public behavior.

Conclusions

Why do we see so many adolescents whose disorder contains some element of historical or ethical rootlessness? I have suggested that a sense of social connectedness and a sharing of structures of language and history mediated through the paternal function consitute ego needs and are the basis for a sense of security and the development of a realistic career in the working world. Pluralism in democratic societies of North America and Western Europe provided for a long time their own mythology. It was no longer necessary to subscribe narrowly to an identity determined by religion or the nation-states from which the immigrant populations that came to this continent derived. When the myth of American liberalism faltered and all the shared institutions of partriotism and social forms became severely threatened in the postwar years, necessary supports for maintaining one's life were eroded. It is significant that many of those who were such active leaders in the student rebellion and the political movement in the 1960s are now among the most vocal subscribers to almost any new form of belief or therapy that promises rediscovery of the self. The hunger for belief, it seems, will embrace any form where there is vast social absence.

REFERENCES

Aries, P. 1962. *Centuries of Childhood.* New York: Knopf.

Brown, N. O. 1959. *Life against Death: The Psychoanalytical Meaning of History.* Middletown, Conn.: Wesleyan University Press.

Durkheim, É. 1951. *Suicide: A Study in Sociology.* New York: Free Press.

Erikson, E. H. 1963. *Childhood and Society.* 2d ed. New York: Norton.

Freud, S. 1905. Three essays on the theory of sexuality. *Standard Edition* 7:130–243. London: Hogarth, 1953.

Freud, S. 1927. The future of an illusion. *Standard Edition* 21:5–56. London: Hogarth, 1961.

Freud, S. 1930. Civilization and its discontents. *Standard Edition* 21:64–145. London: Hogarth, 1961.

Garfinkle, B. 1979. Completed suicide in Ontario youth. Paper presented to the Canadian Psychiatric Association annual meeting, Toronto, January.

Goddard, D. 1970. Lévi-Strauss and the anthropologists. *Social Research* 37:366–378.

Hall, G. S. 1904. *Adolescence.* New York: Appleton.

Kohut, H. 1966. Forms and transformations of narcissism. *Journal of the American Psychoanalytic Association* 14:243–272.

Lasch, C. 1978. *The Culture of Narcissism.* New York: Norton.

Mahler, M. S.; Pine, F.; and Bergman, A. 1975. *The Psychological Birth of the Human Infant.* New York: Basic.

Marcuse, H. 1955. *Eros and Civilization.* Boston: Beacon.

Rakoff, V. M. 1978. The illusion of detachment. *Adolescent Psychiatry* 6:119–129.

Robinson, P. A. 1970. *The Freudian Left.* New York: Harper.

Roheim, G. 1962. *Magic and Schizophrenia.* Bloomington: Indiana University Press.

Sakinofsky, I.; Roberts, R.; and Van Hauten, A. 1975. The end of the journey: a study of suicide across Canada. Paper presented before the Eighth International Congress on Suicide Prevention, Jerusalem.

Sennett, R. 1977. *The Fall of Public Man.* New York: Knopf.

Trilling, L. 1972. *Sincerity and Authenticity.* Cambridge, Mass.: Harvard University Press.

Weisberg, P. 1979. Adolescence, aufheibung: dream's end and dream's beginning. Presented before the meeting of the American Society for Adolescent Psychiatry, Winnipeg.

Winnicott, D. W. 1958. *Collected Papers: Through Pediatrics to Psychoanalysis*. London: Tavistock.

Winnicott, D. W. 1967. The location of cultural experience. *International Journal of Psycho-Analysis* 48:368–372.

9 CULTURAL DIFFERENCES AND THE WORK ETHIC

PHILIP KATZ

The difficulties encountered by disturbed adolescents trying to function in a work system have not received adequate attention. The behavioral area of work has been seen basically as an extension of the behavioral area of school-ing—with comparisons drawn between responses to teachers and responses to bosses, between relationships with classmates and relationships with work-mates, between attitudes toward academic material and attitudes toward work tasks. The similar organization of educational institutions and industrial in-stitutions has led society to take for granted the structure of the work world, especially its adherence to the clock.

Observations of the conflict between the white work world and some North American Indian tribal work ethics illuminates the vocational difficulties that some adolescents encounter due either to culture or to psychopathology. The rigidities of the work world have, at times, precipitated difficulties with adolescents of all races and cultures. Sometimes these difficulties were due to conflicting personal values, sometimes to cultural differences, and some-times to psychopathological constellations. The result, all too often, was an unemployed adolescent, cut off from the potentially growth-promoting ex-perience of work.

Significance of Work

The significance of participation in the work world can be viewed from several different perspectives. Freud (1930) suggested that work attached the individual to reality and offered a vehicle for the displacement of libidinal components. Holmes (1965) stated his belief that the "dichotomization between the two functions of work appears neither necessary nor fruitful. It would seem that for a given individual work fulfills both functions, to varying degrees. Thus for one individual work may serve primarily as a means of expressing drives and as such will be invested with drive energy, whereas for another individual, work may be invested with neutralized energy and may serve primarily a self-evaluative, planning, and reality-orienting function."

Oseas (1963) looked at the significance of work from a sociological point of view and concluded that "the meaning of work to the individual is the composite of conscious and unconscious attitudes and predispositions toward work learned through the internalization of societal values, identification with significant persons and hypotheses about the self that are generated by direct confrontations with the world of work." Oseas focused on a number of roles that work plays for the individual. He explored its role in fostering self-actualization which is facilitated by providing opportunities for development of the individual's potentials and in encouraging self-identification which is facilitated by society's requiring that the individual find his place in the world of work, resulting in the testing out of ideas about the self. Oseas also looked at the self-enhancement through increases in status, power, and materialistic acquisitions that accrues from work, at the necessary development of social participation that work engenders, and at the opportunities for mastery and security that work offers.

It is evident that work plays a number of extremely important roles in the lives of adolescents by providing the setting for identity formation, development of the self, reality testing, and libidinal and aggressive drive discharge. Failure by society to offer opportunities for work results in a void in the lives of adolescents and may lead, in some, to the establishment of pathological patterns of behavior.

In discussing the role of work in the development of identity during adolescence Erikson (1968) wrote "that adolescence was least stormy in those youths who felt competent in the modern technological world. Those who do not feel so competent become more ideological. If the environment blocks development and integration, the adolescent may become quite savage in his desperate struggle to attain an identity." Smarr and Escoll (1975), looking at the significance of the work ethic in youth, stated that "as youth grow older they make a practical accommodation to the real world. Those who have good ego strength are successful, those who lack ego strength and have a weak identity fail and wind up as patients and/or unemployed."

Culture and Work Behavior

Observations of the effects of traditional cultural values on the vocational behavior of certain North American Indian adolescents help to clarify the difficulties that some disturbed adolescents have in the work world. In the cultures of the Cree and the Saulteaux-Ojibway, the major Indian tribes in the lower three-quarters of the present Province of Manitoba, there are a number of values that are quite different from those of the surrounding white culture. Three of these—attitude toward time, attitude toward property, and attitude toward anger—have significant effects on adolescent attitudes and approaches to the work world (Katz, Carruthers, and Forrest 1979). Parallels to these cultural differences are found in white and other minority-group youngsters, but they are due to psychopathology rather than to cultural upbringing.

ATTITUDE TOWARD TIME

The attitude toward time of the Cree and the Saulteaux-Ojibway originates from a culture that was bountifully nourished by a prairie swarming with buffalo and other game and rich with berry trees and plants. With no concern about food supplies, they developed a here-and-now philosophy that still underlies the thinking of tribal adults and adolescents.

Time is something one uses, not something by which one is controlled. If one visits a friend, there are no set limitations on the visit; it lasts until it reaches its natural ending, whether it be an hour or several days. Whatever one does, one continues doing it until the activity comes to an end; one does not stop to do something else. The something else comes afterward. The white world, with its orientation to the acquisition of property, puts controls on the use of time in order to get more done and to make good use of one's time. These Indian tribes are not similarly orientated. They value their present activities rather than activities aimed at future gain—to be, rather than to become.

Frank (1939) stated that culturally determined attitudes toward time are a significant means whereby a culture affects behavior. The significance of a society's attitude toward time and its relationship to culture and language are described by Whorf (1956): "Just as we conceive our objectified time as extending in the future the same way that it extends in the past, so we set down our estimates of the future in the same shape as our records of the past, producing programs, schedules, budgets. . . . We are of course stimulated to use calendars, clocks and watches, and to try to measure time ever more precisely; this aids science, and science in turn, following these well-worn cultural grooves, gives back to culture an ever-growing store of applications, habits, and values, with which culture again directs science."

Other cultures have different attitudes about time from that of the Western Europeans. Lee (1959) refers to timelessness in the lives of the Trobrianders in the South Pacific as well as their attitudes toward work:

> The Trobrianders are concerned with being, and being alone. Change and becoming are foreign to their thinking. An object or event is grasped and evaluated in terms of itself alone, that is, irrespective of other beings.
>
> Becoming involves temporality, but Trobriand being has no reference to time. With us, change in time is a value, and place in a developmental sequence is necessary for evaluation. We cannot respond with approval or disapproval unless we know that a thing is getting bigger or better or surer.
>
> There is no job, no labor, no drudgery which finds its reward outside the act. All work contains its own satisfaction. . . . The present is not a means to future satisfaction, but good in itself, as the future is also good in itself; neither better nor worse, neither climactic nor anticlimactic, in fact, not lineally connected nor removed.

The compulsive, materialistic coercion of time that has characterized Western European society since the nineteenth century is causing conflicts in many areas of the globe. Lee (1959) writes about modern-day Greeks and their attitudes toward time and work:

> Greeks "pass" the time; they do not save or accumulate or use it. And they are intent on passing the time, not on budgeting it. . . . The clock is not master of the Greek: it does not tell him to get up, to go to the field. . . . Wherever there is no law to the contrary, a man opens his store in due course, not by the clock; however, in the cities he now functions under clocked time because he comes under government and union regulations. . . . To introduce an awareness of time into a meal

is particularly abhorrent to Greeks, though this has to be done where factories set time limits. . . . People are called "Englishmen" when they turn up on the dot at appointments. People often arrive an hour late to an appointment to find that the other person is also just arriving, or, if they find him gone, they usually accept the fact with neither apology nor frustration.

The cultural attitude toward time of the Cree and Saulteaux-Ojibway tribes has major implications for their work ethic. Going to work, day in and day out, five days a week, at a regular time, for a set number of hours, regardless of how one feels, is the basic format of the white urban and industrial work world; it is in stark conflict with the values of these tribes. Those adolescents who want to live outside the reservations, particularly in the urban areas, find themselves in great difficulty. If they are at a party, they feel they should not leave to go to work until the party is finished. If they are not in the mood to work, they do not feel obligated to go. When they have earned some money they wish to stop working and enjoy it. They are not so future oriented, so accumulation oriented, as to go on working and saving their money in order to enjoy more later.

In working psychotherapeutically with these adolescents, one has to help them become consciously aware of the conflict between their traditional value system and the white value system and of the choices available to them. If they wish to live in urban areas, they will have to choose between holding onto their traditional values—with the resultant difficulty in retaining employment and limitation in financial achievements—or accepting the white priorities with the hope of greater financial gain. If they wish to have the material acquisitions of white society, they will have to accept the domination of the clock. Many of the Indian adolescents want material things but find it difficult to think ahead and plan for their purchase.

ATTITUDE TOWARD PROPERTY

Many Indian adolescents find it difficult to save money toward purchases because of tribal attitudes concerning property. The Cree and the Saulteaux-Ojibway, and many other Indian tribes, hold that one cannot own anything. One uses what there is and then leaves it for the next person who comes along. Everything one acquires has to be shared: money, cars, boats, clothes, etc. Chief Dan George (1974) described this attitude thus:

Of all the teachings we receive
this one is most important:
Nothing belongs to you
Of what there is,
Of what you take,
you must share.

This cultural value is very strongly held; native adolescents share far more among themselves than do white adolescents. It makes it difficult to save money since refusal to share money or acquisitions will earn them the open hostility of family and friends. They will be derogated as "apples" (red on the outside, white on the inside) in the current parlance of an emerging Indian-white cultural clash. The incentive to work is destroyed for many youngsters when siblings, cousins, and friends are at home spending their earnings on amusements while they are at work. The alternative is the very painful decision to turn away from the ancestral culture, thereby breaking ties with many relatives and friends, and to attempt to enter the unwelcoming white culture. Refusal to take this painful step usually means a life of comparative poverty.

Clinical example. One patient, who was in a white-run residential treatment center, arrived at an ingenious solution to his desires for some "sharp" clothes, a stereo, and a number of tapes. One day, he suddenly borrowed money from everyone he knew, including this therapist, and bought all that he wanted. Then, in debt, he happily went to work, arranging with the staff that they receive his paycheck and allocate most of the money to pay off his debts. He did not mind sharing his tapes or clothes with the other residents, but he had not wanted to see his money go for parties.

ATTITUDE TOWARD ANGER

In the traditional Cree and Saulteaux-Ojibway cultures, anger is not expressed openly except when drunk. It is therefore very difficult for a youngster to object to the way a relative or friend uses the money and things he has acquired by working.

Clinical example. One seventeen-year-old Cree patient was well settled into a job and small apartment when a good friend, the friend's brother, and a friend of the brother moved in with him and began living on his income. He found it hard to leave them and the parties to go to work. He knew that

105

he would have no rent money at the end of the month but felt helpless to do anything. He therefore stopped going to work and gave up his apartment. After the others left, he secured another job and apartment.

To the adolescent who tries to work in the white world, prohibition of the expression of anger presents other problems as well. It becomes difficult to deal with racial discrimination since failure to react angrily to racist comments often invites more of them. Suppression of their anger interferes with normal emotional interplay with workmates and cuts them off from many positive experiences such as establishing an identification with other workers. This cultural value, the suppression of anger, is weakening rapidly. The urban-reared Indian youngsters are much more open with their anger.

These three traditional cultural values—attitude toward time as open-ended and present oriented; attitude toward property as something which cannot be owned and must be shared; and attitude toward anger as an emotion that must not be expressed in the sober state—make it virtually impossible for many of the Indian boys and girls to succeed. The only work that is available to them—the urban, white, work world—creates parallel psychopathological findings of a disturbed sense of time, inability to accept material rewards, and excessive repression of anger which severely handicap disturbed adolescents in their attempts to obtain or hold a job.

WORKING MODELS

The significance of the working model can be seen in many of the Cree and Saulteaux-Ojibway reservations, particularly in the southern part of the province, where work is very scarce. For many decades, Indian boys growing up on the reserve had no opportunity to see Indian men in working roles. Boys coming from these reserves do not have fantasies of themselves working at anything, and when asked about their future plans state that they will "go back to the reserve."

Castellano (1970), an Indian social worker, pointed out that "for the middle-class urban child the range of role fantasies is almost limitless. But if the child is poor and rural and Indian and perhaps even fatherless, the basis for identification with varied roles shrinks into virtual non-existence." On the other hand, Indian youngsters from the more northern reserves, whose fathers still hunt, fish, and log, or those who have been in foster homes where they have had good relationships with foster fathers, tend to have fantasies about good jobs and lots of money.

The girls also have difficulty identifying with working models even though the mothers cooked and looked after the home. The mothering roles were seriously derailed by removing the children from their homes into residential schools. Here they could not experience mothering, which resulted in a generation of unparented children who did not know how to parent (Katz, Carruthers, and Forrest 1979).

VOCATIONAL IDENTITY

Duke Redbird (1970), an Indian poet, wrote:

I am the Redman
Son of the tree, hill and stream
What use have I of china and crystal
What use have I of diamonds and gold
What use have I of money
Think you these from heaven sent
That I should be eager to accept.

The polarization between what is seen as the white man's materialistic world and the Indian's spiritual world makes the choice of a vocational identity very difficult for Indian adolescents. The Indian culture stresses personal development and spiritual values, especially naturalistic ones, over the future acquisition of material goods. Chief Smohalla (1971) said, "My young men shall never work. Men who work cannot dream; and wisdom comes to us in dreams." By its subtle and not-so-subtle demeaning of their race and culture and by its insensitivity to cultural differences, the educational system, which was supposed to prepare adolescents for the work world, so antagonized Indian adolescents that many of them felt that to subscribe to the values taught by this educational system was to accept the dishonoring of their race. To choose a vocational identity among those that were available to them meant the surrendering of their Indian identity. Castellano (1970) described this situation: "For the majority of mature Indians, education has negative connotations because it is equated with the schooling which they have found destructive of their self-esteem and irrelevant to their practical needs. They regard the informal transmission of skills and wisdom which

107

goes on continuously in their associations with one another as something quite different. So long as this myth survives, that education is distinct from living, young Indians will continue to be pulled by family and community to plump for identity rather than vocation.'' She points out that this conflict between vocational identity and cultural identity is occurring amid a widespread clash between an educational system that is geared to meet the requirements of an industrial machine that, in itself, is undergoing rapid change and a society that is demanding that more attention be paid to developing human potential.

Havighurst and Gottleib (1975) describe their findings in many middle-class college youth:

> There appears to be an emerging work ethic which places a much greater demand upon work. The expectation is that work can and should be of greater significance to the individual and of greater value to the society. . . . Work, for many of these youth, is not seen as an activity which should be separate or isolated from one's family or private life. . . . Work is not considered to be a means to an end, but rather as a potential source for enhancing self-sufficiency and family relationships. At the same time, work and career needs are not expected to take priority over family relationships. Occupational mobility will be sacrificed if it must come at the expense of family needs and desires.

Differing cultural values and differing life situations lead to many minority-group adolescents and lower-socioeconomic-class and some middle-class adolescents establishing vocational identities and work ethics that do not fit into the general structure of the work world, particularly into the structure of the urban industrialized work world, which for many of them is the major source of employment opportunities.

Psychopathology and Work Behavior

Many adolescents are unable to establish themselves in the work world because of psychopathological difficulties. These difficulties parallel the cultural factors that block the minority-group adolescent from succeeding vocationally.

Disturbances in the sense of time, often seen in an adolescent psychiatric practice, are the psychopathological parallels to the Cree and Saulteaux-Ojibway attitude toward time. Greenacre (1945) described disturbances of time perspective in severe personality disorders. Schlosberg (1969) and Seeman (1976) reported on time disturbances in schizophrenics.

Hartocollis (1972) stated that "schizophrenia or borderline conditions are characterized frequently by boredom and a sense of depersonalization. Both of these affects are dominated by the sense of time—time as present. Psychotic depression and morbid anxiety also are dominated by a sense of time that is specific to these conditions—the sense of an irrevocable past and a dreadful future." In another study on time (Hartocollis 1975), he said that one's awareness of time is normally unconscious but that in schizophrenia and borderline states time tends to dominate consciousness.

Erikson (1959) discussed disturbances of time as time diffusion, when the ego's functions of maintaining perspective and expectancy were lost. These adolescents seemed to manifest a mistrust of time, believing delays, waits, and expectations to be indications of trouble.

Chambers (1961) found disturbed concepts of time in children who had experienced a major degree of maternal deprivation.

These disturbances of the sense of time, while found in the psychopathology of many different diagnostic entities, may become manifest clinically in the work area in a variety of ways. Difficulties in getting to work on time may occur because of the patient's poor judgment in budgeting his time for the previous night's activities and sleep, or his poor judgment in planning the timing of his preparatory activities prior to leaving for work, or because of the meaninglessness to the patient of the set time at which he is supposed to be at work. Difficulties in tolerating an eight-hour day may occur because the patient finds eight hours to be tortuously long. The patient may function poorly in those jobs that require good time judgment. For all adolescents who have difficulties with time, whether it be due to cultural upbringing or psychopathology, our rigidly clock-oriented work world looms as an almost immovable obstacle to their further development.

The impact of no ownership of property on the vocational behavior of the Cree and Saulteaux-Ojibway indicates the significance to the work ethic of a system of ongoing rewards. Many disturbed adolescents do not have a sense of ownership and do not seem to value what are considered to be their possessions, such as clothes, records, books, furniture, etc. While very interested in being gifted with these objects, they do not take care of them, suggesting that it is the symbolic indications of being loved rather than the wish to possess these objects that motivate their requests. At a residential treatment center for adolescent boys, it is a frequent experience to have a youngster plead for a shirt or a record only to find it, within a few days, lying on the floor or thrown in a corner. It is difficult for those adolescents who, as Laufer (1968) observes, feel that they do not even own their own body to envision owning anything else.

This inability to experience tangible rewards causes some disturbed adolescents to have difficulty motivating themselves to work. The whole routine of getting up every morning and going to work seems meaningless and burdensome, reducing the likelihood of their succeeding in the work world.

The suppression of anger in the Indian culture has its parallel in the excessive repression of anger found in some psychiatric patients, which results in a lack of aggressiveness and often an overall passivity that hampers the patient's functioning in the work situation. Concomitant with a severe repression of anger, there is often an inhibited emotionality which interferes with the patient's relationships with workmates. The accumulation of anger and frustration sometimes results in an outburst which may cost the patient his job, but more often he quits his job in fear of such outbursts occurring.

Just as in their cultural equivalents, these three psychopathological constellations—disturbances of the sense of time, inability to experience tangible rewards, and excessive repression of anger—cause severe difficulties in obtaining and retaining jobs and in establishing a vocational identity.

Discussion

While for many adolescents a job is a catalyst to emotional maturation, for some it is an anvil against which their psychopathology hammers them. Disorders of the sense of time are widespread throughout the psychopathologies of adolescence resulting in major difficulties in work attendance, punctuality, performance, and often in the loss of the job. Other difficulties, such as repression of anger, poor object relations, and restricted capacity for abstraction, also seriously interfere with job performance, especially if cooperation with workmates is involved.

To be unable to hold a job, to be repeatedly fired, is a destructive situation for the adolescent. Unless culturally reinforced to believe that a job is unimportant, the patient who has no job at all feels a constant corroding sense of failure and has an awareness of himself as a target for society's abuse.

It is evident that the therapist who works with these adolescents needs to be oriented to the various causes of work disorder and how the different structural components of work are affected by different psychopathologies.

110

He has to be particularly cognizant of the difficulties with time, be prepared to explore them, make the patient aware of them, and try to resolve some of their underlying causes. It is necessary to educate the patient about time and to assist the patient in learning to cope with time.

However, for many severely disturbed patients, psychotherapy will not be enough. They will not develop further without the growth experience of working. Just as some patients need special education facilities, so do these patients need special work facilities.

The provision of these special work facilities and programs would require government funding. The alternative is that they and their future families will spend endless years on the welfare lists—at far greater cost to the government. In addition, their talents and abilities will not have been put to use. The failure of our society to provide such facilities and programs up to now has resulted in a tremendous wastage of human resources.

Conclusions

Cree and Saulteaux-Ojibway adolescents have difficulties in the work world that are caused by such cultural values as different attitudes toward time, toward ownership of property, and around the expression of anger. Similar difficulties are found in emotionally disturbed adolescents due to psychopathology rather than to cultural differences. Disturbances of the sense of time are widespread among adolescent psychopathologies. The Indian adolescents share with many lower-socioeconomic-class adolescents difficulties in finding working models with whom to identify. They share with many troubled adolescents of all classes and races a set of values that clash with those of the industrial work world, leading to a conflict between their personal identity and their vocational identity.

These difficulties may be instrumental in their failure to obtain or retain work, with the resultant formation or strengthening of pathological behavior patterns. There is a need for special work facilities and special work programs.

REFERENCES

Castellano, M. B. 1970. Vocation or identity: the dilemma of Indian youth. In Waubageshig, ed. *The Only Good Indian.* Toronto: New Press.

Chambers, J. 1961. Maternal deprivation and the concept of time in children. *American Journal of Orthopsychiatry* 31:406–416.

Erikson, E. H. 1959. *Identity and the Life Cycle. Psychological Issues* 1. New York: International Universities Press.

Erikson, E. H. 1968. *Identity Youth and Crisis.* New York: Norton.

Frank, L. 1939. Time perspectives. *Journal of the Philadelphia Psychoanalytic Society* 4:293–312.

Freud, S. 1930. Civilization and its discontents. *Standard Edition* 21:59–145. London: Hogarth, 1961.

George, Chief Dan. 1974. *My Heart Soars.* Saanichton, B.C.: Hancock House.

Greenacre, P. 1945. Conscience in the psychopath. In *Trauma, Growth, and Personality.* New York: Norton, 1952.

Hartocollis, P. 1972. Time as a dimension of affects. *Journal of the American Psychoanalytic Association* 20:92–108.

Hartocollis, P. 1975. Time and affect in psychopathology. *Journal of the American Psychoanalytic Association* 23:383–396.

Havighurst, R., and Gottleib, D. 1975. Youth and the meaning of work. *Youth* 74:145–160.

Holmes, D. 1965. A contribution to a psychoanalytic theory of work. *Psychoanalytic Study of the Child* 20:384–393.

Katz, P.; Carruthers, H.; and Forrest, T. 1979. Adolescent Saulteaux-Ojibway girls: the adolescent process amidst a clash of cultures. In M. Sugar, ed. *Female Adolescent Development.* New York: Brunner/Mazel.

Laufer, M. 1968. The body image, the function of masturbation, and adolescence. *Psychoanalytic Study of the Child* 23:114–137.

Lee, D. 1959. *Freedom and Culture.* New York: Prentice-Hall.

Oseas, L. 1963. Work requirements and ego defects. *Psychiatric Quarterly* 37:105–122.

Redbird, D. 1970. I am the redman. In Waubageslig, ed. *The Only Good Indian.* Toronto: New Press.

Schlosberg, A. 1969. Time perspectives in schizophrenics. *Psychiatric Quarterly* 43:22–34.

Seeman, M. 1976. Time and schizophrenia. *Psychiatry* 39:189–194.

Smarr, E., and Escoll, P. 1975. The work ethic, the work personality, and humanistic values. *Adolescent Psychiatry* 4:163–173.

Smohalla, 1971. *Touch the Earth.* Compiled by T. C. McLuhan. New York: Simon & Schuster.

Whorf, B. 1956. *Language, Thought, and Reality.* Cambridge, Mass.: M.I.T. Press.

10 THE CULT PHENOMENON:
TRANSITION, REPRESSION, AND REGRESSION

SHERMAN C. FEINSTEIN

Among the vicissitudes of adolescence and young adulthood, with their problems of transition, a new dilemma with ancient roots has become of great interest. In the past decade the emergence of a surprisingly large number of fringe religious groups or exotic cults using modern, psychologically oriented recruitment practices, which some people believe is a form of thought control, have enlisted a large number of middle-class educated youth. Between the ages of seventeen and thirty, these youth are attracted by promises of making the world a better place, finding God, or living in an ideal society.

Lifton (1963) described ideological totalism as a thought reform with a psychological momentum of its own resulting from the union of excessive character traits and a grandiose ideology. This ideology, consisting of emotionally charged convictions about man and his relationships, may be propelled in an all-or-nothing direction and develop into an exclusive cult with absolute philosophical and emotional assumptions. Lifton further noted that a cult manifests several characteristics: milieu control of communication leading to disruption of balance between self and outside world; mystical manipulation with a sense of higher purpose; demand for purity with emphasis on simplistic splitting into good and bad; an obsession with confession as a vehicle for personal purification and self-surrender; an aura of sacredness as evidenced by prohibitions against questioning basic assumptions; the development of an esoteric language which produces individual constriction; the subordination of human experience to the claims of a doctrine; and, finally, the creation of the right to dispense existence to those who are worthy.

Psychiatry is a newcomer to the phenomenon of young people joining fringe religious groups in large numbers. The small amount of research available and my own personal experiences indicate that these youths are representative of a cross section of the adolescent population and do not represent any particular cluster of psychopathology. A large percentage of those who have been evaluated before, during, and after a cult experience does not show evidence of serious mental disorder although a larger percentage than the normal population has psychopathology.

Because of the obvious unavailability of cult members, there are very few scientific studies of them as a group. There have been, however, two studies made of cult members with the cooperation of their leaders.

Levine and Salter (1976) were able to examine 106 followers in nine religious groups in Toronto and Boston. Galanter, Rabkin, Rabkin, and Deutsch (1979) examined 237 native-born Americans who were full-time members of the Unification Church and living in residences in a metropolitan area. Demographically both groups were similar: largely unmarried, white, and in their early twenties; a slight majority were males, but there was a preponderance of girls in the younger age groups (Levine and Salter 1976). The majority had at least some university education and virtually all had completed high school. In the Galanter et al. study, 42 percent attended school at least half-time before joining the church. Although members tended to leave school after joining, the dropping-out process had begun somewhat before entering the cult. The few professionals among the sample were not working at their chosen field. Most did odd jobs, part-time or occasional work, or worked within the structure.

Their religious backgrounds formed a pattern. Galanter et al. reported that 67 percent were only moderately committed to their family's religion before age fifteen. The Levine study found little religious involvement, but the members of Catholic and Jewish origin tended toward religions of oriental derivation. Those with Protestant backgrounds tended to be interested in similarly oriented religious groups. There was little uniformity among previous attitudes toward religion. None of the cult members were heavily committed to any religion before their conversion, nor was there any correlation between strictness or laxity of childhood religious training and subsequent religious involvement.

Seventy percent of the group studied by Levine and Salter came from relatively large families with three or more children; 10 percent were only children, 20 percent were the firstborn. Most came from intact families; only 25 percent came from divorced homes and 10 percent had suffered a parent loss through death. Almost all of those examined claimed to have an average to good relationship with their parents prior to joining. Only 40 percent felt determined to get away from the parental environment, and almost all reported that their parents felt negative about their conversions.

114

The parental reaction to conversion was one of great intensity. Parents viewed it as a severe loss and responded with strong mourning reactions. Impulsivity, anger, and desperation predominated and frequently complicated the radical change the relationship was undergoing.

In one example the mother visited her son's cult residence and stayed for a recruitment session. She decided to confront the speaker and argued vociferously about the irrationality of their beliefs. She reported that each statement she made was greeted with "knowing smiles" by the various cult members. She later discovered that her son had been warned that since his mother was "possessed by the devil" she would make certain comments which clearly revealed she was under demoniac control. Of course her attempt to question the cult's principles confirmed exactly the predictions of the members about her attitude.

Previous history of psychological difficulties was reported in a significant number of followers but was by no means ubiquitous. In the Galanter study 39 percent reported "serious" emotional difficulties: about seventy had had psychiatric treatment and fourteen had been hospitalized. This incidence is at least twice as high as the 10–15 percent reported in the normal adolescent population but is very far from describing all members of the group as having emotional difficulties. Most respondents indicated marked relief from anxiety after joining a cult, with 35–45 percent reporting transcendental experiences of "a special unfamiliar feeling in my body," "the presence of someone important to me," or "time passing slower or faster than usual."

About half of the interviewees in the Levine study reported active sexual lives before joining cults. Those more active seemed to join the oriental groups, while the less sexually involved were attracted to quasi-Christian or Western groups. A similar distribution was found in prior drug usage. Alcohol was the most frequently used; some used hard drugs (amphetamines and heroin); those that used hallucinogens (marijuana, hashish, LSD) tended to be in the oriental groups.

Reasons for Joining

Levine reported a variety of reasons for joining. The most common were: feeling lonely, rejected, sad, and alienated; life seemed to have no meaning; they were influenced by members who were proselytizing and seemed happy in their personal lives; running away from unpleasant personal or family crisis; searching for a religious experience; drugs and/or yoga gave them a heightened spiritual awareness and demonstrated a void in their lives; and an idealistic desire to help society or humanity.

Both study groups reported considerable and sustained relief from neurotic distress following conversion. The members offered clearly spiritual, transcendental, or mystical rationales less frequently than intrapsychic or interpersonal reasons. The followers reported feeling calmer, healthier, happier, having achieved self-actualization and personal growth. A majority felt great improvement in interpersonal relationships with more and better friendships since joining. In fact, most former cult members recall this element for a long period after leaving the groups. Many mention that in spite of rejecting the whole concept of their conversion and subsequent exploitation, they remember with great fondness the intensity and closeness of the relationships they formed.

This attachment is exploited by cult leaders in an attempt to frustrate leaving the group. For example, during a deprogramming procedure cult members often attempt to find and break into the place the deprogramee is being held. Chanting, singing familiar songs, shouting, and attempting to talk to the former member and emphasize the closeness of the relationship along with an offer to return, the group members attempt to arouse the bonding aspects of the relationship.

Galanter et al. (1979) felt the average convert was in emotional distress prior to joining a cult and that continued membership appeared to support a certain stability in psychological status. Levine's study pointed out that while no overtly psychotic individuals were seen, a significant number of the members could have been described as neurotically anxious or depressed prior to conversion. A small number were difficult to interview, resorting to ritual chanting, gross intellectualization, and denial to avoid any sort of self-examination or affect. These few resembled the popular version of a brainwashed individual. While it can be said that many followers were unhappy before their conversion and a disproportionate number were manifesting symptoms, psychiatric diagnoses could not be applied to the majority of cases. Most might be described as "homoclites," a description of average, follower-type personalities, without any particular charismatic qualities (Grinker, Grinker, and Timberlake 1971). Ungerleider and Wellisch (1979) studied two deprogramees who returned to their group after escaping. Evaluation again revealed no serious psychopathology but rather evidence of some ego defect with marked interfamily conflict. The authors concluded that these dependent, immature young people received the external controls, interpersonal constancy, and approval they needed from the group and were competent to make an informed decision to join a cult. Deutsch and Miller (1979) studied, in depth, a twenty-seven-year-old woman who had been a cult member for four years. They found her repressed and inhibited and characterized her defensive style as one of benevolent transformation. The authors believe that some of her psychological conflicts and character trends appeared to influence her conversion to a religious cult.

Developmental and Psychosocial Issues

The particular young people attracted to conversion to fringe religions are a young, white, well-educated, predominantly middle-class group. They come from stable backgrounds, and their emotional, drug, and sexual histories do not seem remarkable. Those attracted to the religions having an oriental flavor tend to be older, better educated, more experienced sexually and chemically, and more interested in mysticism and altered states of consciousness.

Young people seemed to be motivated to join religious groups by two factors: (1) a dissatisfaction with their status quo, and (2) slow resolution of their identity crises. The clinical picture of acute identity crisis is recognized in young people who are unable to utilize the usual social or intrapsychic moratoria provided by society and are struggling unsuccessfully with adolescent demands for simultaneous commitment to physical intimacy, competition, and psychosocial definition. The resulting transitory regression is manifested by: being unable to make decisions, a sense of isolation and inner emptiness, an inability to achieve relationships and sexual intimacy, a distorted time perspective resulting in a sense of great urgency as well as a loss of consideration for time as a dimension of living, an acute inability to work, and at times the choosing of a negative identity, a hostile parody of the usual roles in one's family or community (Feinstein 1975).

I do not believe, however, that this is a particularly pathological group. The religious cult may have made its presence felt at a crucial moment in the lives of these young people and, using highly developed recruitment techniques, extracted a yield of vulnerable members. On the other hand, this group has much to offer a cult in the way of energy, education, and social skills. They are a relatively inexpensive group regarding health care and nutritional needs. They are capable of working long hours with great intensity.

The research findings indicate that the conversion resulted in considerable and sustained relief from neurotic distress. Continued membership in the group provided a stability in psychological status (Galanter et al. 1979). Levine and Salter (1976) report similar results but have some reservations owing to the suddenness and sharpness of the change.

This steady state of psychological health may be actually a pathological resolution of the existential anxiety with which these young people are struggling prior to conversion. Anna Freud (1958) warned of the danger to adolescents who showed no outer evidence of inner unrest. Wrapped up in family relationships, considerate, submissive, and in accord with the ideas and ideals of their background, these young people have built up repressive defenses against drive activities and become crippled by the barriers against the normal developmental process.

Shortly after conversion, the follower frequently breaks off relationships with the family. The parents are seen as being demonically possessed. The new cult member is described as "glazed" and operating in an automatic fashion. Meditation, chanting, or ritualistic observations are adopted. One adolescent when encouraged by his parents to join them for dinner or an outing would explain that he was "busy and had many things to do." Over the weeks and months this became a slogan which allowed him to avoid much contact with his family and kept him away from their attempts to influence him to leave his group.

After leaving the cult, usually by drastic means, the former member of the group is in a fragile emotional condition. I have had an opportunity to examine several youths shortly after deprogramming and found that they resembled a state seen following a psychotic alteration of consciousness. This period, called a postpsychotic regressive state, is manifested by fragility of ego controls with a constant danger of regression from almost any stress (Feinstein and Miller 1979). In the cult refugee, during and immediately after deprogramming, a stage of "floating" is described which is characterized by an episodic drifting into fantasy or panic. The deprogramming team must interpret this drift and encourage concentration and contact with the rehabilitation staff.

A dramatic experience may occur if cult members find the site of the deprogramming. Intrusion into the quarters may result in a major regression. In some cases the deprogramee will leave with the cult members or run away. The reason for regression may be the hearing of familiar voices, a song on a radio, or a passage from the Bible resulting in a return of old, dependent, symbiotic attachments to the cult group.

This violent reaction to removal from the cult environment is a marked exaggeration of the transitional problems usually seen in developmental change. The intense separation anxiety has a psychotic quality and gives credence to the idea that adaptations had taken place influenced by powerful suggestions. One former member of the Children of God told me that she and 150 others lived in a bare loft in New York. Although she had beautiful clothes to wear to her job as a secretary, she lived on a starvation diet and was kept up very late at night to listen to repetitive lectures by the leader. Still, she ran away from her first deprogramming and participated in a kidnapping lawsuit against her parents and the deprogrammer (resulting in his conviction). Her second deprogramming was successful, although she was still in a vulnerable state six months after leaving the cult.

Singer (1979) described her experiences with ex-cult members and also pointed out the monumental failures most professionals have in giving assistance to the recent cult departees because of their unfamiliarity with cult ethos and the tendency to see cult membership as a psychopathological expression. Following leaving a cult, a period of deprogramming or meeting with reentry counselors, ''an intense period of information giving,'' is advised. A period as long as eighteen months may then be necessary to recreate a sense of cohesiveness and personal competence. During this period group therapy with leaders familiar with psychosocial aspects of cults aids in the slowly developing integration. Postcult emotional difficulties include: mental blocking and inefficiencies, a ''floating'' phenomenon including drifting into altered states of consciousness, identity diffusion, and a ''fishbowl effect'' from ideas of reference.

Discussion

How should one view this seemingly irrational, uncritical adulation and total abandonment of the ethics and protection of a middle-class background? A cult is a group with a living leader who makes absolute claims to divinity, omniscience, and infallibility. The follower must have complete acceptance, loyalty, and allegiance to this mysterious, proselytizing totalistic group (Levine 1979).

In a fundamental sense, conversion (Hall 1904) is a natural, universal process at a stage when life pivots from an egocentric preoccupation with self- and object-related structures to the synthesis of an identity. An identity requires the persistence of a self-sameness and an ability to share. It is manifested behaviorally by physical intimacy, occupational choice, energetic competition, and psychosocial self-definition. An inability to make use of the transitional structures of society (school, dating, working, and other psychosocial moratoria) creates anxiety and diffusion of identity.

Kierkegaard treats the psychology of sin and conversion as resting essentially on the feeling of anxiety. Historically, epidemics of conversion have occurred before. In 1802, one-third of the students at Yale University abandoned their studies to go off with a charismatic revivalist minister. Other examples abound (Hall 1904).

The fringe religions attract and hold young people's attention because of their vulnerability and also because the inherent structure of the belief fulfills needs not being met elsewhere. An intense belief is extremely comforting to an individual. Everything that is confusing becomes comprehensible and no longer threatening. Unfortunately anything which provides such simplistic resolution may be anti-intellectual, pseudoscientific, incomprehensible, and probably dangerous.

For example, in *A Season in Heaven*, Gibson (1974) describes the vedantic philosophy behind Transcendental Meditation. There are sixteen strata of consciousness in the cosmos. In the highest state of consciousness "all decisions are spontaneously right." The words of the guru, from his level, are only fragmentally understood by the ordinary person. The real world is only relative; that which is not real is absolute (boundless, timeless, spaceless, omnipresent, changeless, and eternal). Meditation together with right action refines the nervous system as a channel to the absolute. The fourth or transcendental state is considered a crucial act of faith—perception of boundaries is relative and absolute. In the fifth state the mind is restful in the midst of activity and reveals finer values. In the sixth state one can see electrons—a state of glorified consciousness. In the seventh state limitations of the individual ego are left behind, knowledge is no longer imperfect, decisions are "spontaneously" right (there is not only a hope for heaven but a certainty).

Individuals who feel they are drifting aimlessly are often pleased when structure is given to their lives. It is paradoxical that in the swinging seventies these religions espouse a rigid puritanism with strict prohibition of drugs, alcohol, and sexual activity. Marriages take place by arrangement with followers obeying without questioning the decisions of their leaders.

There are elaborate repetitive rituals that must be followed which add to the mystery and cult aspect as well as making sense in religious terms. Rituals have been shown to be important components of all societies (Milgrim 1971), and their diminishing role in our society may be felt by our youth, who renounce rituals in traditional society but recreate them in their own subculture.

Another theme is communality; a sense of belonging to a like-minded group and sharing values, feelings, and experiences. It is this aspect of the group process that at first attracts lonely young people. The introduction to the cult is frequently via a "love bombing." When a young person leaves a group, the memories of the closeness and attachment continues. One ex-moonie said: "Leaving the group was a very difficult period. After three or four weeks one is set about being out, but I still think about them. I dream about them every night and it's been almost two years. I dream I am still in the movement. I wake up and say, 'Oh my God, maybe I slipped back.' "

Conclusions

These findings give rather clear evidence that most of the group of young people attracted to cults are not fundamentally ill psychologically but are, rather, in a vulnerable state developmentally. It is, in my opinion, incorrect to conclude that only the emotionally disturbed would be susceptible to a charismatic conversion experience.

As Levine (1979) points out, the all-encompassing nature of the belief and the uncritical adulation should lead to skepticism—who can take fanatics seriously? Nevertheless, thousands of intelligent middle-class youth are regularly indoctrinated into a wide variety of fringe religions and believe they are improving their lives. It is important to know which young people are most susceptible to these influences and for what reasons. But it is also important to know where our society is failing and how these groups fill voids in the lives of their members. If we feel these groups are less than desirable, it is our responsibility to encourage and provide alternatives for our young people.

The role of the psychiatrist should be to provide counsel at every step of the way for both the parents and the cult member, if available. An understanding of the processes involved and the emotional needs of the cult member before, during, and following separation from a cult will allow the experience to be used as a growth experience rather than a traumatic, destructive episode.

REFERENCES

Deutsch, A., and Miller, M. J. 1979. Conflict, character, and conversion: study of a "new religion" member. *Adolescent Psychiatry* 7:257–268.

Feinstein, S. C. 1975. Adjustment reaction of adolescence. In A. M. Freedman, H. I. Kaplan, and B. J. Sadock, eds. *Comprehensive Textbook of Psychiatry/II*. Baltimore: Williams & Wilkins.

Feinstein, S., and Miller, D. 1979. Psychoses of adolescence. In J. D. Noshpitz, ed. *Basic Handbook of Child Psychiatry*. Vol. 2. New York: Basic.

Freud, A. 1958. Adolescence. *Psychoanalytic Study of the Child* 13:255–278.

Galanter, M.; Rabkin, R.; Rabkin, J.; and Deutsch, A. 1979. The "moonies": a psychological study of conversion and membership in a contemporary religious sect. *American Journal of Psychiatry* 136(2): 165–170.

Gibson, W. 1974. *A Season in Heaven*. New York: Atheneum.

Grinker, R. R., Sr.; Grinker, R. R., Jr.; and Timberlake, J. 1971. "Mentally healthy" young males: homoclites. *Adolescent Psychiatry* 1:176–255.

Hall, G. S. 1904. *Adolescence*. New York: Appleton.

Levine, S., and Salter, N. 1976. Youth and contemporary religious movements: psychosocial findings. *Canadian Psychiatric Association Journal* 21(6): 411–420.

Levine, S. V. 1979. Adolescents, believing and belonging. *Adolescent Psychiatry* 7:41–53.

Lifton, R. J. 1963. *Thought Reform and the Psychology of Totalism*. New York: Norton.

Milgrim, A. E. 1971. *Jewish Worship*. Philadelphia: Jewish Publication Society.

Singer, M. T. 1979. Therapy with ex-cult members. *National Association of Private Psychiatric Hospitals Journal* 9(4): 15–18.

Ungerleider, J. T., and Wellisch, D. K. 1979. Cultism, thought control and deprogramming: observations on a phenomenon. *Psychiatric Opinion* (January), pp. 10–15.

11   THE ROLE OF PSYCHIATRY IN THE PHENOMENON OF CULTS

SAUL V. LEVINE

Recent tragic events in Guyana have precipitated a renewed public outcry demanding investigation of, and legislation controlling, the various fringe religious cults in North America. These cults are variously seen or depicted by many as dangerous, exploitative, sinister, or destructive. Conversely, there are some who defend them on civil libertarian grounds—in the context of the history of all religious persecution—or even in laudatory terms.

I have, in the course of one major study (Levine 1978; Levine and Salter 1976), subsequent research, and considerble clinical work in this area, interviewed well over 200 cult members, worked psychotherapeutically with about fifty members, usually after their leaving their respective groups, and seen upward of 150 parents of adolescents and young adults in religious groups who were very concerned about the fate of their offspring. Approximately twenty-five different cults have been involved in this total sample.

On the basis of this work, a variety of theoretical and practical issues, both clinical and social, have been derived. These may prove helpful to those psychiatrists called on either to offer elucidation of this complex area or to work with families of members or with the members themselves.

Cults and Cultists

A cult has been defined as having the following characteristics. It is a group which follows a dominant leader, often living, who may make absolute claims that he is divine, God incarnate, the messiah, or God's emissary, and

Reprinted with permission from *Canadian Journal of Psychiatry* 24 (1979): 593–603. © 1979 by the Canadian Pyschiatric Association.

that he is omniscient and infallible. Membership is contingent on complete and literal acceptance of the leader's claims and acceptance of his doctrines and dogma. Complete, unquestioning loyalty and allegiance are demanded together with a total willingness to obey the cult leader's commands without question—which may include a unique way of viewing the world, of acting, of dressing, or of thinking.

It is important to note that cults need not be religious; they can be political or even therapeutic. All cults should not be seen as intrinsically evil or dangerous any more than they should be praised indiscriminately. Cults have been in existence in North America for at least a hundred years (Noyes 1966; Wallace 1961), and contemporary established religions were once seen as dangerous and were persecuted. During times of uncertainty, "cults of unreason" offering solutions or special salvation have been particularly attractive (Cohn 1957; Evans 1972). But never have these movements been so popular and open; never has there been such a concerted search for a new consciousness and life-style (Bourguinon 1974; Nicholi 1973; Roszak 1969, 1972); never have there been so many social philosophers offering rationales and encouragement to these movements (Dass 1974; Leary 1970; Needleman, Bierman, and Gould 1973; Roszak 1969; Watts 1966); and, finally, never have so many of our youth experienced religious awakening with such obvious personal involvement (Farnaro 1973; Romm 1974; Zaretsky and Leone 1974). I have worked with members from many groups, but the majority have come from the Hare Krishna, Unification Church, Divine Light Mission, Children of God, Jesus People, Scientology, Process and Foundation churches, plus a number from twenty others.

All the members I have studied and worked with were Caucasian, middle-class, Canadian- or American-born youth or young adults ranging in age from fourteen to thirty. Both sexes have been equally represented. Most have come from intact families and have been fairly well educated (Levine 1978; Levine and Salter 1976). There is little doubt that they joined the cult movement because of personal dissatisfaction with their lot. This, however, was owing to the fact that the religious group made itself available at a psychological correlate of a critical period in their lives. If not for that fortuitous happenstance, the young person might have gone an entirely different route, not necessarily religious in nature.

Young people have always been more susceptible to ideologies, belief systems, and mass movements (Adelson 1976; Braungart 1976; Toch 1965). Alienated, demoralized youth, with a poor sense of self, are especially receptive to "easy answers" (Levine and Salter 1976). We have found that these young people feel alienated from their peers, families, and society before they join (Levine 1978). In Seaman's terms (1959), feelings of norm-lessness, powerlessness, futility, and leaderlessness abound. They are search-ing. In Frank's (1973) conceptualization they would be seen as "demoral-ized" and potentially good candidates for psychotherapy. Although some have friends, many report a sense of "aloneness," with a poor sense of self. Susceptibility to beliefs and indoctrination is increased in youth with low self-esteem (Rosenberg 1976). This is not to say, however, that these represent a particularly disturbed group of young people; many of our youth harbor these feelings (Keniston 1965; Masterson 1967; Pasamanick 1959).

Joining the religion gives them two powerful reinforcing forces, which in turn enhance a third (Levine 1979). First, a strong belief system is engendered, a raison d'être, a seemingly coherent system of ideas and values. Second, and perhaps more important, is the rapid development of a sense of belonging, of communality, of being an integral part of a group which shares the mem-bers' feelings and aspirations. These two experiences—believing and be-longing—serve to produce a significant increase in the individual's self-es-teem. What we have then is an individual with a strong sense of identity, with good feelings about himself or herself, with a powerfully supportive group and a shared ideology, affect, and catharsis. Alienation, demoraliza-tion, and low self-esteem are at least temporarily, but unequivocally, alle-viated or eradicated; their needs have been fulfilled.

What has struck me about the various groups examined is that for all their proclaimed uniqueness of theology and deliverance of salvation, the com-monalities far outweigh the differences. All are charismatic in nature—that is, via an intense emotional appeal, they engender devotion and inspiration in their followers. This may involve a charismatic individual at the top (for example, Jim Jones, L. Ron Hubbard, Reverend Sun Myung Moon, etc.), but by no means is this an absolute necessity (for example, Maharaj-ji). They all have rituals, mystical pretensions, a quasi-intellectual theological tome, rigid hierarchy and rules, relative asceticism, high-powered fund-raising tech-niques or tithes, and houses of worship. They all promise some degree of personal salvation. They vary in their flirtations with violence (zero to con-siderable), their total obeisance to an individual, their bizarre aspects, their relative prominence, their sense of persecution, their use of dishonest pros-elytizing techniques, and their use of funds. What becomes clear, however, is that the particular content of the theology is never as important as the trappings, and certainly not nearly as significant as believing, belonging, and the increase in self-esteem. Bombay could be Jerusalem, or San Fransisco Moonies could be Children of God or Hare Krishna. The members could be called Premis or novitiates or devotees. But all groups give simple answers

125

to the complexities of modern life; there are no longer any existential dilemmas; life becomes secure, comfortable.

Scenario—Joining the Cult

When one listens to the stories of hundreds of parents, one hears sequences of experiences that seem almost identical and interchangeable between families. There is a progression of events that represents a gradual—sometimes rapid—escalation of confrontation. A typical scenario is as follows: At first the young person (let us say, a son) expresses tentative interest in the cult to his parents. Their initial reactions vary from bemusement and confidence that "he'll come to his senses" to being concerned or even aghast. As their son becomes more enmeshed in the ritual and the worship, the parents almost invariably become frightened, angry, and appalled. Discussion and reasoning soon give way to overt anger and demands. Some parents try to "understand," to learn as much as they can about the particular religion in question. Their sensitive, empathetic attitude often leads nowhere and gives way in fairly short order to restrictive demands or punishments (grounding, withdrawal of privileges, cutting allowance, etc.), or attempts at "deals" ("If you do your homework, eat with the family, maintain your friends, we'll let you go to the Ashram one night a week").

The family feels the inexorable ebbing away of their hold on their son. They fear the worst, that they are losing their offspring. They call friends, relatives, their minister or rabbi, their family doctor, all to no avail. There is no reaching their child. They become panic-stricken and preoccupied with the cult. Altercations become frequent, intense, vociferous, and painful—there are threats, recriminations, epithets, tears, ultimatums. Occasionally, there is violence—a slap in utterly frustrated anger, a push in bitter helplessness and confusion. Finally, there may be a schism, estrangement for a short or prolonged period. The family goes through a period of grieving and mourning not dissimilar from that experienced after the loss by death of a young loved one.

And what of the cult member? He regrets the altercations with his family, but he recognizes that they cannot begin to understand; they are still entrenched in the morass of their decadent or destructive life-styles. They are so blind, so misguided, so to be pitied. He feels morally and spiritually uplifted, released, even euphoric. He senses that he is on the verge of a great period in his life, perhaps even in the life of the world.

126

He is a true believer. He has overwhelming faith in the righteousness of his cause, in the clarity of the religious writings. He feels totally secure, satisfied, filled with warmth and joy. He is closed to conflicting ideas. He has some contempt for ersatz religions, copies of the real truth (his). The others are seen to be exploitative, superficial, or dishonest. Only his religion provides real answers to life's dilemmas.

He manifests varying degrees of egocentrism. At times he can be benevolently tolerant of his parents' fears and concerns. More often, however, there is bemused derision of one's parents and old friends, or angry impatience with their confusion and sinful or misguided ways. Icy hostility is not unusual.

There is a singular lack of genuine sensitivity, of emotional empathy. If it is there at all, the empathy is a combination of pity and cognitive or intellectualized caring. The converted young person develops a closed-mindedness to conflicting ideas and arguments, often seeing them as ridiculous or even sinister. A garrison mentality develops, which is engendered and encouraged by the group. He is now well-nigh unreachable.

Role of Psychiatrists

Psychiatrists can be called—most often by the parents—at any time during the period that the cult has any degree of influence on a young person. This can be before their son or daughter has officially committed to the religious group, during the period of total involvement with the cult, toward the end of that time, or for a considerable interval after having left the religion. We shall deal with each of these very different situations individually. There is, however, an important and general caveat which must be emphasized. Not all fringe religions are harmful. Some are actually helpful; not all individuals suffer, and some are actually helped. Further, it should not be assumed that all members are by definition disturbed individuals—there is no evidence for this. Blanket condemnation or, conversely, total praise is usually not indicated. In an earlier report, it was shown that the phenomenon is too complex for glib opinion or simplistic judgments (Noyes 1966). Some members were in difficult physical and emotional straits prior to joining their cults, and in a very short time thereafter they looked, felt, and acted better. Some had voluntarily seen mental health professionals during their earlier period of personal deterioration, to no avail.

Before any kind of constructive discussion can take place or any decisions made a number of questions must be answered. The clinician should note who is doing the reporting or complaining, their previous and present relationship, their reliability, as well as their history.

PRIOR TO THE CONVERSION

In my experience, this is the least likely time that a psychiatrist would be called by a family. This is in large part due to the variations in a sequence of escalating confrontations and a seeking or grasping at other kinds of help. For a period of time, the parents know nothing of their son's or daughter's new haven and friends. And when they first find out, they may either dismiss it as temporary or try other means of dissuasion. The family attempts discussions, cajoling, demands, and ultimatums; the young person is highly attracted to the religious group and becomes even more so. The antiprohibition aspect of the experience adds to the mystery and excitement of the cult.

If a psychiatrist does gain access to the family and especially to the young person at this crucial time, and he is convinced that there is potential harm to that individual, then it is a critical time to act. Action entails utilizing all the resources at one's disposal. It involves considerably more activity than most psychiatrists are accustomed to. It might mean interviews in the home, direct confrontation, longer or irregular hours, and appealing to both intellect and emotions. Close friends and authority figures, with whom the young person is particularly close (uncle, teacher, doctor, etc.), might have to be mobilized. The potential convert is confused and vulnerable. He is more open at this point than he will be for a considerable time to come if he should become heavily committed to the religion.

An attempt at a mental-status exam is indicated. If the clinician happens to be dealing with a psychotic decompensation (uncommon), for example, hospitalization may be indicated. Other diagnoses might determine indicated specific courses of action, but, more importantly, would tell the clinician the degree of disturbance, if any, he is working with, and the opportunities of reaching the individual. The procedure also serves the important function of setting some kind of baseline status for the young person. This may be important in future involvement. Similarly it is likely that the psychiatrist will be involved with the family for a considerable period of time; he will learn about the family dynamics, stresses, and relationships, and will determine how best to be of help to them.

128

COMMITTED TO THE CULT

During the period that the young person is an active member of a cult, it is not at all unusual for the family to call a psychiatrist. Very often his work is restricted to information exchange (if he is knowledgeable) and support for the parents in a time of extreme crisis. It is not a time for uncovering insight into neurotic conflicts or attaching responsibility. The families are preoccupied with the loss of their child—they are in a period of grief. They are also angry, confused, and guilt ridden—"Where did *we* go wrong?" is a common question. They are totally frustrated by their own impotence and the seeming unwillingness or inability of anyone—police, lawyers, doctors, etc.—to help them. They are often considering radical, even violent alternatives.

Aside from any definitive plans that might be made regarding their son or daughter, the parents will often benefit from ongoing supportive psychotherapy, either on a regular or on an ad hoc basis. At times the intensity of the preoccupation with the religious groups and the apparent loss of their child becomes an omnipresent obsession. They eat, sleep, drink the ruminations—they get no respite and neither does anyone who lives with them. They become countercult proselytizers, every bit as rabid and intolerant as those they fear and detest.

Mothers and fathers in this situation need as much valid information as possible regarding other people's experience with this particular cult. They have to know what the possible alternative outcomes are, and what kinds of expectations they can have. They also have to be encouraged to carry on with other aspects of their own lives and those of their other children. As with so many other types of crises, obtaining support from other parents who have gone through or are at present undergoing the same type of experience can be extremely helpful.

Getting the cult member to see the psychiatrist at this time is often a difficult task. If the parents are estranged from their child, there is obviously no possibility of seeing him. The parents, however, will still need the clinician's help. The young person may adamantly refuse to cooperate for a variety of reasons; there is then little gained in belaboring the point. Psychiatrists are often perceived by the religious group as dangerous, destructive, or sinister, and this is conveyed explicitly to the young member. If the member, however, is willing to please his parents, or avoid deprogramming, the psychiatrist can expect a number of possible reactions: (1) *Open hostility—*

the young person makes it quite clear that he is there only as a favor to his parents, that he mistrusts and either fears or loathes you. (2) *Bemused tolerance*—in these situations, the member is smug and arrogant. He appears to be listening to you, but this is a sham: he is obviously closed-minded. (3) *Ritualistic*—at times the individual will begin chanting and praying overtly to close his sensorium to any kind of verbal overtures that you might make. (4) *Proselytizing*—I have seen young members "too eager" to come in, and my suspicions have been justified. There is an overt attempt to preach, convert, sell books. (5) *Guarded openness*—at times there is a serious open interchange; the young person is committed to his course, is not about to be dissuaded. He listens, he thinks, he argues.

Often the referred member will be in the constant company of an "elder" of the religion and will only speak to the clinician in the presence of that individual. In my experience, there are very few inroads that the clinician can make with the young people at this particular point. One positive effect of these meetings is that the clinician, if he has been well received, might serve as a facilitator, or a conduit of communication between parents and child. One other possible occurrence is the implantation of seeds of doubt; these may well be reaped at a later date.

The members seen at this point do not all fit the popular depiction of brainwashed individuals—wide-eyed; programmed; and spouting rote, verbal productions. While such converts are certainly seen, the majority appear well adjusted, and psychiatric labels cannot be readily applied. At times we do find a curious happiness that is paradoxically devoid of affect; the smiles, gestures, and words are all appropriately there, but one gets a distinctly uncomfortable feeling with this bliss.

SEEDS OF DOUBT—IDENTITY CRISIS

There is one circumstance during the young person's involvement with the cult which provides the best chance for success in attempts to convince him to leave. This is usually not due to an outsider's influence, but rather comes from within, and resembles an adolescent identity crisis. The individual begins to doubt his commitment. He sees hypocrisies, dishonesty, inconsistencies, lies, and outright exploitation, and he begins to question his blind faith. When this happens, he often becomes frightened and confused. If he confides in his religious leaders, they can relatively easily, via pressure, shame, support, love, threats, etc., bring him into line rather quickly. If, however, he shares these feelings with his family or outside friends, they are in a good position to act, if they can get him away from the cult, alone, for a period of days.

This is not an uncommon occurrence—I have seen more than a dozen individuals in similar circumstances. The process we are discussing here involves a member who is already amenable to the possibility of leaving. This is the kind of work that Daphne Greene and her associates in California do, and which they call deprogramming.[1] It most emphatically is not deprogramming. There is no kidnapping or violence. There is no hyperstimulation, deprivation, browbeating, threats, or locked doors. This is an approach that many psychiatrists can use and involves sensitive interviewing—getting the individual to open up in order to be in touch with his fears and anxieties. It involves uncovering and the use of cathartic techniques. The clinician concentrates on the doubts already raised by the individual; he brings the hypocrisies or deceptions (if they are there) into the conversation. Because of the nature of the work, long hours on an emergency or an ad hoc basis may be indicated. Considerable activity on the part of the clinician is indicated, and again, the utilization of close friends or family is often desirable at this point.

The results of this particular kind of work are impressive. But this is not an end point; it is in fact only a beginning. The real process of psychotherapy only commences when the individual finally wrenches himself away and returns to his family or a semblance of his former life.

AFTER THE CULT

Whether the individual comes out on his own or is helped, as described, most are in dire need of rehabilitation and psychotherapy. There is inevitable culture shock. There are difficulties with relationships which have ended or changed markedly. There are insecurities about the future, about fitting in to old activities, about resuming career tracks or school. These are all realistic concerns which are almost invariable and inevitable. Superimposed on these is the young person's unique personality, his irrational thoughts and actions, and his neurotic needs and conflicts.

Many of the ex-cultists are beset with guilt and shame. They may feel that they have sinned—they have contravened their belief system and have committed sacrilege. They may believe that they have let down or, worse, deserted their friends within the group—they have contravened their belonging. And just as an individual's self-esteem rises with believing and belonging, so conversely does it fall when these basic needs are disrupted. Low self-esteem, doubts, self-recriminations are extremely common.

Another common affect experienced by the ex-cultists is fear. This is not free-floating neurotic anxiety but a real fear which may take one of two forms: it is either impersonal (spiritual or religious) or personal (physical) in nature. The former has to do with breaking the precepts of the religion, or sinning; it implies vague but powerful punishment from the deity or his incarnation on earth. The latter represents fear of retribution at the hands of cultists who have been betrayed. This fear occasionally prevents ex-members from sharing any information about their former religious groups. This fear is usually irrationally based, but certainly has validity in some situations and, if there is any possible basis in fact, it should be investigated and the individual protected.

Often the ex-cult member will show depressive affect and mood. There is no doubt that a loss has been sustained, and it takes time and a process of working through to handle the depression. Related to this are regretful thoughts, and at times obsessive ruminations about his departure. At times the guilt is highly complex and dichotomous, because there are equally powerful feelings expressed that they have wronged or made their families suffer needlessly. Ambivalence is often seen; the individual asks himself if he did the right thing. He answers affirmatively, tentatively, qualifies it, and then, answers negatively; his confusion is apparent.

An experience somewhat akin to "flashbacks" among psychedelic chemical users occurs occasionally to ex-cultists. There is a sudden feeling of having been carried back against their will to an intense emotional state or even to an altered state of consciousness. The individual tells you that he experiences "being there" in the cult; he can "hear" the liturgy or chants, songs, and sermons. This is followed immediately by intense fear and confusion.

The clinician will see many or all of these affects and thoughts in the same patient. He may at times use tranquilizers if the personal discomfort becomes too difficult for the individual to cope with, or if the flashbacks become too frequent or real. I have found that at least six months of once-weekly psychotherapy sessions are necessary to enable the ex-cultist to feel liberated from his group.

Deprogramming

For our purposes, we are using the term deprogramming to involve: (1) coercion—utilizing subterfuge, false pretenses, or force to lure the unwilling cult member to a private location; (2) detention—locked or guarded room or setting; (3) numbers—invariably more than one, often more than two deprogrammers; (4) hyperstimulation—confrontation, browbeating, constant input, and unidirectional; (5) wearing down—little or no letup; surprise or random breaks and resumptions; and (6) substitution—of a better belief system.

Others may disagree with this definition, but it comes closest to my personal experiences with this process. It is an issue reft with philosophical, ethical, legal, civil libertarian, and psychological concerns. The very nature of the term pejoratively describes the process by which young people go into the fringe religions. We are not impressed with the whole area—the process, the people who do it, or the results. I have heard of quite a few, but have only seen one successful deprogramming, that is, the avoidance of the religious group for longer than a year after deprogramming and the maintenance of a normal, symptom-free life outside the cult. I have seen the results of numerous failed deprogrammings: total estrangement from families, return to the group, popular appearance of being brainwashed, and emotional decompensation.

Without impugning the motives of the deprogrammers or casting aspersions on their expertise, they fail to impress me with their sensitivity, intelligence, and efficacy. This is an unpleasant, dangerous, and avowedly illegal procedure. If means to an end excuses the process, we should at least have confidence in the ends—unfortunately, this is not always the case.

But anyone who has worked extensively with cultists and their families can easily see how parents are driven to this alternative. It is very difficult for a mother and father to see their child, after years of upbringing, shared joys and pains, love and aspirations, enter a way of life which they consider to be sinister or dangerous. It is a frustrating and poignant situation. I cannot, in good conscience, support the procedure, but neither can I censure it in all circumstances. For example, if a child of fifteen years of age is in a cult, deprogramming might be considered, if all other methods have failed (e.g., conservatorship). Like so many other clinical issues, this does not lend itself to easy answers.

Conclusion

It is incumbent upon our profession to learn more about this entire phenomenon. As an important beginning, I recommend reading recent publications to get an overview of the major cults, in addition to familiarity with some of the dilemmas facing the families (Adelson 1976; Cox 1977; Levine 1978). There have been a number of reports which usually take an entirely negative view of the cults (Bugliosi and Gentry 1974; Jewish Community

Relations Council of Greater Philadelphia 1979; Lefkowitz 1974; National Ad Hoc Committee for a Day of Affirmation and Protest 1976; Terrorist Information Project 1977). There are also a few classic books which can serve to educate, in depth, regarding the areas of brainwashing, deprogramming, and coercive persuasion, on the one hand (Lifton 1961; Sargent 1971), and true believers, on the other (Hoffer 1951; Koestler 1952).

In our experience, most young people in these groups do come out on their own or with some general encouragement. It is incumbent on those who work with these families to encourage the maintenance of channels of communication. I have never seen the situation of wholehearted support on the part of the parents, but usually there is a tenuous rapprochement, whereby there is an agreement to disagree. Not uncommonly there is complete estrangement—a tragic consequence in families that a few months or years earlier may have been warm and cohesive. This might be obviated if a third party could serve the role of a mediator, facilitator, or a liaison between the young person and his family, as well as being a strong support to the parents.

While Jonestown was a horrible aberration, there is no doubt that the control exerted over many young people by the cults is overwhelming. The members' ideology, fervor, and energy is dedicated to the satisfaction of the wishes of the religion. I have sat through too many rallies of one or other of the cults and observed the universal bliss (again, not infectious) and total adulation directed at the leader. This is real power that can obviously be abused, as with the People's Temple or the Manson cult (Bugliosi and Gentry 1974). Again, it is important to note that not all fringe religions (or other fringes—political parties, or social movements, or therapeutic groups) are inherently dangerous.

If one accepts the still controversial premise that psychiatrists and other mental health professionals have a role to play in this area—without getting into controversial civil libertarian issues—we can summarize various roles that the psychiatrist might assume.

He (she) can be a facilitator, helping to maintain avenues of communication between the cult member and his family and friends. He can function as an advisor to families, presenting and considering with them alternative paths to follow. He might be an educator, removing the mystery from both the group and the pattern of reaction of the young cultist. He can function as a consultant to institutions, groups, authorities in his community, regarding specific approaches to the phenomenon.

These are worthy activities and must be pursued. But the major role of the psychiatrist will be in ways with which he is most comfortable and has the most expertise—psychotherapy. The specific psychotherapeutic approach will differ with the individual patient, his personality, and the time he is being seen. Crisis intervention, directive psychotherapy, supportive work, and transactional therapy, and even insight-oriented, uncovering psychotherapy can be used with different patients or even with the same patient at different stages. Similarly, work with the family of the patient may entail a variety of individual and conjoint family techniques.

Finally, a novel role for the psychiatrist, and yet vital, in this area, is as an "exploiter" of seeds of doubt manifesting themselves in the cult member. This involves availability, flexibility, sensitivity, directive and yet gentle prodding of the young man or woman. Considerable activity on the part of the therapist, and the mobilization of friends and family is occasionally indicated.

There is no doubt in my mind that psychiatrists have a vital role to play in this area. What is most telling, in addition to the various functions we can play, is the effectiveness of our efforts. This is gratifying work.

NOTE

1. Regarding Daphne Greene and associates, plus Rabbi Davis's technique, see Stoner and Parke (1977).

REFERENCES

Adelson, J. 1976. The development of ideology in adolescents. In S. Dragastin and G. Elder, eds. *Adolescence in the Life Cycle*. New York: Wiley.

Bourguinon, E. 1974. *Religion, Altered States of Consciousness, and Social Change*. Columbus: Ohio State University Press.

Braungart, R. 1976. Youth and social movements. In S. Dragastin and G. Elder, eds. *Adolescence in the Life Cycle*. New York: Wiley.

Bugliosi, V., and Gentry, C. 1974. *Helter Skelter*. New York: Norton.

Cohn, N. 1957. *The Pursuit of the Millennium*. New York: Essential Books.

Cox, H. 1977. *Turning East*. New York: Simon & Schuster.

Dass, R. 1974. *Spiritual Community Guide*. San Rafael, Calif.: San Rafael Publications.

Evans, C. 1972. *Cults of Unreason*. England: Harrop.

Farnaro, R. J. 1973. Neo-Hinduism and acculturation: alternative to instant chemical religion. Paper presented before the International Symposium on Anthropology and Ethnology, Chicago.

Frank, J. 1973. The demoralized mind. *Psychology Today* 6(11): 22–28.

Hoffer, E. 1951. *The True Believer*. New York: Harper & Row.

Jewish Community Relations Council of Greater Philadelphia. 1978. The challenge of the cults. Report. January.

Keniston, K. 1965. *The Uncommitted: Alienated Youth in America*. New York: Dell.

Koestler, A. 1952. *The God That Failed*. New York: Bantam.

Leary, T. 1970. *The Politics of Ecstacy*. London: Paladin.

Lefkowitz, L. 1974. *Attorney-General's Report on the Children of God*. Albany: State of New York.

Levine, S. 1978. Youth and religious cults: a societal and clinical dilemma. *Adolescent Psychiatry* 6:75–89.

Levine, S. 1979. Adolescents, believing and belonging. *Adolescent Psychiatry* 7:41–53.

Levine, S., and Salter, N. 1976. Youth and contemporary religious movements: psychosocial findings. *Canadian Journal of Psychiatry* 21:411–420.

Lifton, R. 1961. *Thought Reform and the Psychology of Totalism*. New York: Norton.

Masterson, J. F. 1967. *The Psychiatric Dilemma of Adolescence*. Boston: Little, Brown.

National Ad Hoc Committee for a Day of Affirmation and Protest. 1976. *The Unification Church: Its Activities and Practices*. Arlington, Tex.: N.p.

Needleman, J.; Bierman, A. K.; and Gould, J. A. 1973. *Religion for a New Generation*. New York: Macmillan.

Nicholi, A. M. 1973. Youth and religious renaissance. Paper presented before the American Psychiatric Association, Hawaii, May.

Noyes, J. H. 1966. *Strange Cults and Utopias of Nineteenth-Century America*. New York: Dover.

Pasamanick, B. 1959. A survey of mental disease in an urban population. In B. Pasamanick, ed. *Epidemiology of Mental Disorder*. New York: American Association for Advancement of Science.

Romm, E. G. 1974. The yinning of America. American religion: from cosmos to chaos. *Humanist* 34(5): 31–33.

Rosenberg, M. 1976. The dissonant context and the adolescent self-concept. In S. Dragastin and G. Elder, eds. *Adolescence in the Life Cycle*. New York: Wiley.

Roszak, T. 1969. *The making of a Counterculture*. New York: Doubleday.

Sargant, W. 1971. *Battle for the Mind*. New York: Harper & Row.

Seaman, M. 1959. On the meaning of alienation. *American Sociological Review* 24(6): 783–789.

Stoner, C., and Parke, J. A. 1977. *All God's Children*. Radnor, Pa.: Chilton.

Terrorist Information Project. 1977. Brownshirts of the seventies: a report on the national caucus of labor committees. Arlington, Va.: N.p.

Toch, H. 1965. *The Social Psychology of Social Movements*. New York: Bobbs-Merrill.

Wallace, A. 1961. Religious revitalization—a study of religion in human history. Paper presented at the Eighth Institute of Religions in an Age of Science, New Hampshire.

Watts, A. 1966. *The Book on the Taboo against Knowing Who You Are*. New York: Vintage.

Zaretsky, I., and Leone, M. 1974. *Religious Movements in Contemporary America*. Princeton, N.J.: Princeton University Press.

12 RURAL COMMUNES AND RELIGIOUS CULTS: REFUGES FOR MIDDLE-CLASS YOUTH

EDWARD M. LEVINE

When future historians begin to describe and analyze the 1960s, they will have an unusual wealth of material to examine and sort out. This decade, perhaps more than any preceding it, spawned a number of novel and seemingly unfathomable social changes, many of them generated by adolescents and young adults. The purpose of this chapter is to single out two among the host of social experiments that emerged during this period—the formation of noncreedal rural communes and the joining of religious cults, both phenomena of white middle-class youth—in order to ascertain their significance from a social-psychiatric perspective. Despite striking differences between the life-styles of communards and cultists, it is suggested that they share certain personality characteristics which shed more light on their motives for joining these movements (Levine 1978).

Background

Only a short time after rock-and-roll had become the dominant music of the youth culture, adolescents and young adults created another original cultural trend which was as mystifying as it was wholly unanticipated. Quite suddenly, growing numbers began an exodus from the cities to form noncreedal rural communes. As Berger, Hackett, and Millar (1974) have noted, these communes were substantially different from the urban religious groups, such as the Unification Church, Hare Krishna, Children of God, and others,

This chapter is an extended and revised version of a previous study, "Middle-Class Urbanites in Rural Communes: A Social-Psychiatric Analysis" (Levine 1978).

in that they did not subscribe to or share a doctrine that infused and dominated most of their daily activities and way of life. While the noncreedal rural communes had no doctrines, certain of their basic beliefs played a key role in their formation. Furthermore, they also differed from the many urban communes whose members shared a common domicile but kept their jobs. Few rural communards were gainfully employed as a matter of choice. Furthermore, they deliberately severed many but not all of their ties to urban life.

While no reliable statistics are available, various authors have estimated that approximately 3,000 communes, mostly rural, were formed between 1960 and 1970. Though such data are based on impressionistic evidence and speculation, the number of those who joined probably ranged from 40,000 to 80,000. Studies do indicate that this group consisted almost entirely of white middle-class and upper-middle-class individuals whose ages ranged from the late teens to the early thirties (Berger et al. 1974; Kanter 1972; Otto 1971). For the most part they had had at least some college education. Numbers of them left well-paying, attractive occupations; others had only briefly ventured into the business world. In addition, there were "floaters," persons who apparently were unable to stabilize their lives and become productive, and numbers of divorced or separated young women, often with one or more children.

Rural Communes: Quest for an Ideal Life-Style

EQUALITY AND INDIVIDUALITY: THE CONFLICT BETWEEN BELIEF AND REALITY

Because comparatively few communes have been studied, the findings in the literature are limited in scope. Nevertheless, a common theme does much to explain why so many were drawn to communes. In essence, communards shared a deep conviction that only rural life, uncluttered by the trappings and demands of urban living, could bring about the complete equalization of all important social relationships—the true goal of social life whose realization had been thwarted by urban society. They also shared the conviction that those truly committed to this belief would be able to achieve individuality much more completely in communal life than they could in urban settings. Another goal of nearly equal importance was to have living arrangements which provided them with ongoing, close, highly personalized relationships with others, and the openness and caring that they found so lacking in city living.

Berger and Hackett (1974) have described their belief in equality as follows:

> By "equalitarian ethos" we refer not to a sharply defined creed, but to the reluctance, even resistance, of many communards to being defined in terms of almost any kind of standard which indicates differentiation even remotely conceivable as exploitative or binding or restrictive of one's broadly human characteristics . . . so also young people (or "small persons" as they are sometimes deliberately, perhaps preciously, called) are not regarded as primarily members of an autonomous category of "children," but as persons, members of the communal family just like anyone else—not necessarily less wise, perhaps less competent, but recognized primarily by lowering one's line of vision rather then one's level of discourse.

The communards' dedication to equality and to the fulfillment of individuality stood in marked contrast to certain fundamental characteristics of urban-industrial society in which competition (for jobs and sales), hierarchically ordered relationships (in the family, educational and religious institutions, the professional and business worlds, etc.), and the necessity of implementing occupational directives which are set by others govern much behavior. Indeed, rural communards regarded these values, standards, and social arrangements as the primary causes of much that is fundamentally wrong with urban life because, in their judgment, their pervasive influence precludes self-actualization and harmonious, cooperative working arrangements in attending to the humanistic needs in life.

However, the realities of rural communal living sooner or later revealed that the goal of social equality as it was understood by the communards could not be achieved. It also gradually became evident to them that equality and individuality, both so fundamentally important to the meaning and existence of commune life, were often mutually exclusive and in conflict with each other, thereby threatening and at times destroying the fragile consensus upon which the survival of communes depended.

These dilemmas first became apparent when communards attempted to determine the specific purposes that they wished communal living to serve, and their endeavors to resolve such issues ordinarily involved three crucial problems. The first is related to the structure of authority. Thus, while there was general agreement that all (at least major) decisions should be made unanimously, this did not actually happen. Those with dominant personalities frequently initiated and advocated ideas, made decisions arbitrarily, or settled disagreements (Berger et al. 1974; Rothchild and Wolf 1976). Some communards, of course, agreed to decisions because of passive personalities, newcomer status, or indifference. Thus, while complete social equality remained the ideal in decision making, it frequently was not realized in practice. The outcome of this was the emergence of informal power structures, even if some did not recognize them as such, denied their existence, or considered them morally wrong. At any rate, decision-making authority was not equally exercised in practice (as is true in all societies), which sooner or later weakened the appeal of communes for numbers of those who joined them in their quest for egalitarianism.

Even when there were no extended and demanding discussions and debates about what greater ends communal living should or might serve (e.g., ecology, peace, etc.), certain practical decisions had to be reached concerning basic requirements of group living. At this point, the idealized vision of group living began to tarnish as it lost the utopian character the communards believed was a realistic alternative to urban values and life. The originally undefined and ambiguous meaning of group living and social equality, which each member was able to define or interpret as he wished, became modified as detailed, practical decisions had to be made. The criteria for admitting new members, how many the commune should have, and where the communards were to derive their sources of income for fundamental needs are basic survival concerns which practicality alone, rather than enthusiasm and ideology, can resolve. In such ways the demands of survival dulled the glow of the ideological incentives and the eager search for a better way of life.

THE CONFLICT BETWEEN EQUALITY AND INDIVIDUALITY

The communards were unavoidably confronted with another difficulty when disagreements and disputes arose in the course of attempting to resolve group problems, particularly those involving the assignment of chores. Conflicting interests and preferences (not to mention personalities) frequently made it impossible to reach decisions. Personal desires at times conflicted with the decisions of the group. As this occurred, the ideals of equality and individuality began to lose their force as incentives for remaining in the commune.

After all, such tasks as caring for vegetable plots, cooking, cleaning, and repairing buildings and automobiles, and supervising and educating children were scarcely what drew members to communes in the first place. There is ample evidence that the centrifugal force of individual preferences became dominant in most living arrangements (Kanter 1972; Otto 1971; Rothchild and Wolf 1976), with the result that the once-shared hope of attaining an idealized future for a group of like-minded individuals faded as members began to leave.

The problems invariably generated by attempts to define group goals, the unwillingness to attend to routine but important tasks, and the tendency to pursue personal preferences and whims all helped to weaken the cohesiveness of the communes. Disinterest and dissatisfaction with commune living became increasingly prevalent, with the result that communards themselves said that communes succeeded if they lasted as long as one or two years.

WERE COMMUNES A REALISTIC RURAL ALTERNATIVE?

For all their commitment, inspiration, and impressive efforts to establish and maintain a communal way of life, the communes were not genuinely rural. In some instances, one or more individuals purchased or rented homes in which others lived and contributed what they could or wished and many lived rent free. Others built crude, makeshift domiciles. But in various ways they were visibly dependent on urban-industrial society for food stamps, welfare and unemployment checks, doles from parents, loans from friends, and income from a few who continued to work in nearby cities. Cities alone provided them with medical and dental services, books, hardware items, records, radio and television programs, appliances, fuel, and numerous other goods and services they could not produce themselves. Thus, their independence from urban life was illusory. However, as Kanter (1972) has shown, their belief in the moral superiority of communal over urban living was crucial in enabling communards to achieve that degree of solidarity without which their communes would have floundered and dissolved even more quickly than was the case.

Nor was their conception of or dedication to personal growth a rural value or pursuit. The self-development of most individuals is a continuing process experienced during the course of socialization and education and, later, in work and professions. These activities are supplemented by avocational interests, involvement in community organizations, politics, and by starting families. In contrast, communards devoted most of their time to discussions, personal criticisms in group encounters, observing Eastern or other mystical rituals, and frequently to the use of drugs and alcohol. They spent time casually, attending to personal and group chores, hosting friends who visited periodically, and intermittently looking after their children. But they involved themselves in little else.

While some may have gained a clearer understanding of themselves and of the meaning and purpose of life through such experiences, there was little to indicate that they then used such knowledge to improve important aspects of their lives. For example, apart from the few rural communes that were efficiently organized (largely as a result of the charismatic leader who was also the symbolic head of a secular religion), communes usually were settings for self-indulgent living. The members' time orientation was entirely in the present, each person involved in little else than a largely self-centered, impulse-gratifying existence. The emphasis given to the fulfillment of their individuality, as well as their belief that this could be achieved only in communal living, involved a great deal of self-deception.

That their ardent and unremitting involvement in such utopian pursuits and a self-serving life-style went untempered by the realities of their precommune years, and even by much that they experienced in communal life, strongly suggests that they were primarily and intently in search of meaningful values to fill an anomic void in their lives. These emphases, coupled with their propensity to indulge themselves in sentient pastimes, their desultory lives, and their depreciation of urban living, all suggest that their impulse life was far more dominant in guiding their quest than is generally realized. With sounder and stronger ego and superego development, it is likely that they would have had more thoughtful visions of and prudent concern about their longer-run future and that of their communes and that they would have been reasonably involved in and methodical about working to attain these objectives.

Keniston (1960) found similar characteristics among middle- and upper-middle-class college youth in whom emotional problems and the paucity of meaningful values in their lives impaired their ability to commit themselves to productive work and to establish sound object relationships with members of the opposite sex. Fitzgerald (1971), upon cataloging the disappointments of disillusioned ex-commune members, said, "it certainly should not surprise us that communes can easily become escapes from personal social difficulties."

If their joining of and involvement in communes had been less a reactive quest for meaning in life and less prompted by their impulse needs, communards would have realized that such unorthodox ventures in living as communes require numbers of people to support the standard of living they took for granted. The basic health, safety, welfare, educational, and convenience needs of a truly viable commune sizable enough and with sufficient means to support its inhabitants would actually defeat the original objective communards shared, since this would be a small, urbanized community with many of the amenities and characteristics they found so displeasing in the cities they abandoned.

COMMUNARDS' CHILD-REARING VALUES AND PRACTICES

The most vivid illustration of how greatly the communards' impulse life influenced their lives—their proneness toward impulse gratification, self-centered dispositions and ways, and a present-orientation—may be found in their child-rearing values and practices. Residentially isolated in settings in which they were the elders, they were free to favor and use those values and socialization practices that they considered best suited for their children's day-to-day needs and development.

To an extent unknown among children of middle-class urbanites, commune children acted much as they wished because of parental default, indifference, disinterest, or approval (Fairfield 1972; Rothchild and Wolf 1976). While studies of communes range from autobiographical sagas to perceptive descriptions to scholarly analyses, they almost uniformly convey the impression that children received extremely little parental guidance or supervision. They spent their time much as they pleased and were seldom given tasks by their parents, who were largely unconcerned with what the children did or whether they were liked by their age mates. The fundamental tasks of child socialization and ego and superego development were largely neglected or ignored, with the result that children adopted values, attitudes, and behavior—mainly hedonistic ones—from observing and being with their peers, older children, parents, and adults.

There was little that was constructive about their parents' lives which would have necessitated the children's thoughtful examination and emulation in order to internalize and incorporate such examples. Consequently, their way of life became very much like that of adults: one primarily given to impulse gratification, self-centered pursuits, and living in and for the present. It is no exaggeration to say that such rural communes were prototypical, miniature, anomic cultures.

Parental indulgence and indifference to the needs of their children's socialization and ego and superego development stemmed from their own aimlessness, a life in which much discussion and time were devoted to sentience and self-exploration. However, the grossly deficient socialization of children, as well as their inadequate ego and superego development, also resulted from their status—of the way they were regarded and dealt with by adults. That is, given the prevailing view that children were essentially smaller equals, and the preference that children address parents and other adults by their first names, children lacked experience with both the symbols and exercise of parental (and adult) authority in their daily lives. They seldom encountered or were instructed to respect parental authority, since parents neither accepted nor fulfilled their tutelary responsibilities.

Children often were allowed to smoke marijuana among themselves and invited to smoke with adults during communal gatherings, rather than learning why it was sensible not to indulge themselves in impulse-freeing pastimes. Gratifying their impulses—a primary-process existence—became their reality, and the latitude of this hedonistic, self-centered life extended beyond these meandering margins, for numbers of parents of preadolescent and adolescent children believed it was proper for them to engage in sexual intercourse. Their rationale for this was a belief that sex is a natural aspect of life that is far too often encumbered with inhibiting traditions and guilt-instilling moral sanctions that diminish individual fulfillment (Berger et al. 1974).

Thus, the penchant of parents and adults for present gratifications and self-centered living and a disregard for the future resulted in their abdicating their responsibility to help their children develop the ego and superego strengths necessary for controlling their impulses effectively. In their later years, therefore, we can hypothesize that such youngsters will very likely be even more impulse ridden and unconcerned about others, with faint interest in and commitment to the future. Their lives appear to be the ideal breeding grounds for severe characterological defects.

Further illustrative of the communards' inattentiveness to and unconcern about their children's present and future needs is that most communes could not provide any education except by sending children to schools in nearby towns. Most accounts indicate that such attendance was not regular and that the children's educational achievements did not keep pace with those of their school-age mates. Getting them up, fed, and to the school bus or driving them to school were often insurmountable chores for their parents (in many cases a divorced or separated mother). Educational underperformance was compounded by grossly inadequate or no tutoring at home. Rarely, if at all, did communes provide adequate facilities and qualified individuals for their children's education (Rothchild and Wolf 1976). More often than not, adults felt that a formal education was not really necessary or that somehow children would learn what they needed to know when they were ready to do so.

From the foregoing it is evident that the carefree, desultory lives of adults made them poor models for children to emulate. Least of all did they exemplify for their children the value—and the practical advantages—of education. As a result, the communard children were victimized by being unprepared to function in and adopt either a truly rural (farming) way of life or to return to urban living with the values, habits, skills, and commitments prerequisite for their being able to adapt to its demands. Yet this was the inevitable outcome of their parents' conviction that children should be free to grow without adult interference, direction, and guidance. It seems not an exaggeration to say that these children were the real emotional and social casualties of the communards' search for meaning and community in this self-deceiving, illusory alternative to urban living.

Of the adults whose dissatisfactions with communes finally prompted them to return to the cities, many will have lost time that could have been devoted to completing an education, gaining job experience and income, or embarking on marriage and family. For some, of course, spending a year on a commune was not much more than a refreshing contrast with or change of pace from urban-industrial society, but they are probably the well-adjusted exceptions.

In retrospect, the middle-class urbanites in rural communes appear to have been more quixotic than realistic in their efforts to translate their understanding of equality and individuality into the realities of daily life. They found themselves alienated by the social fragmentation and anomie that pervade the lives of so many people in urban-industrial society. They were, after all, utopians in quest of *gemeinschaft*, aware that a comfortable material existence and advanced education do not compensate for or counteract the disturbing effects of anomie and anonymity so prevalent in life today.

Religious Cults: The Middle-Class Escape from Freedom

If those who joined rural communes perplexed and angered their parents and adults by their blatant renunciation of the latters' basic values and lifestyle, the growing numbers of individuals who have joined religious cults since the mid-1960s (e.g., the Hare Krishna, the Unification Church, Jews for Jesus, Meher Baba, the Divine Light Mission, Scientology, the Children of God, etc.) have equally mystified and often incensed their families and the public. These cultists, like the communards, are preponderantly white, middle-class youth and young adults. The appeal of religious cults—their inducements to those who join them—can be more adequately understood if they are regarded as the antithesis of those that led people to join rural communes. That is, while the communes appeared to provide the opportunities to maximize one's freedom, the cults provide those who join them with escape from freedom. It may be that those cults which impose the most stringent limitations on the daily lives of their members attract unusually dependent individuals who are least capable of coping with the responsibilities and demands of freedom of choice. The focus of what follows is limited to those cults about which more reliable information is available and to those which most regulate the daily lives of their most dedicated members. In addition, it will deal primarily with the kinds of incentives that lead individuals to join them.

Religious cults attract their members with a variety of strongly appealing incentives. First, their leaders are charismatic personalities who exude a deep, unshakable conviction in themselves and in their religious views. Because of this, cult members readily gravitate toward and identify with them. Next, the religious beliefs espoused by these leaders are advanced as being both ideal and practical means of dispelling and resolving the confusion over and anxieties about the identities and beliefs of those whom they attract. In addition, certain religious cults (and nonreligious cults such as Synanon) establish stringent regulations that govern major aspects of the daily lives of their members. Thus, members are given what appear to them to be basic, clear-cut answers and explanations about the meaning of life and equally specific and inflexible standards as guides for their interpersonal behavior, both of which provide an alternative of substance to the anomic culture from which they seek to escape. Furthermore, the cultists find comradeship and the feeling of being appreciated and worthy. They have close, ongoing relationships with like-minded others who, both during and subsequent to the recruitment process, bolster the self-image of those who are drawn to the cults.

The doctrines and standards of these cults are presented dogmatically, with consummate conviction and steadfastness, however subtly and indirectly this may be done. Recruits and members are told and accept basic distinctions between what is right and wrong. Thus, they are relieved of the need and opportunity rationally to evaluate and choose their newly adopted set of beliefs and standards. Their acceptance of them is in large measure due to the indoctrination and reinforcement of the peers with whom they first come into contact. Most cults turn their members against the outside world, including their parents' and their beliefs and ways of life, which are depicted as evil and threatening to the cult and its religion. While dividing the moral cult from the evil outside may function to maintain cults, it is also a technique used to convince newcomers that they have found a far better religion and group of people than those they have known. Numbers of individuals find that religious cults meet their compelling needs so that, subsequent to their conversion, many of them experience appreciably less emotional distress and discontinue acting out.

Discussion

There are those who continue to believe that the most significant characteristic of the rural communes and religious cults has been that they offered numbers of youth and young adults new and personally more meaningful beliefs and ways of life than were available to them in mainstream society. Some argue that religious cults are actually beneficial since they are able to introduce order, meaning, and stability into the lives of numbers of young people who have been drifting and involved in drugs.

The view advanced here is substantially different. The evidence more than suggests that those who opted for the all but unlimited freedom of rural communes little understood the limits and meaning of freedom and responsibility, and that much of their lives was given to indulging themselves in gratifying infantile needs. Indeed, their directionless, anomic existence was partly responsible for the inability of communes to endure. The insistence on pursuing individual interests at the expense of group needs led to the demise of communes, just as it has been a central factor in the growing rate of divorces. The incentives of equality and individuality cannot supersede group needs if groups are to continue to exist.

From today's perspective, rural communes seem to be an archaic subcultural offshoot. The cultural pendulum has swung from one extreme to the other, as the appetite for maximizing freedom and minimizing responsibilities to others has yielded to the desire to abandon freedom to authoritative, persuasive figures who will determine for their followers what they should believe and how they should live—a seeming paradox in a democratic society whose dominant values wholly oppose such a posture. Yet the question remains of why so many white middle-class youth and young adults have personality and value needs that are met by charismatic religious figures and

148

their cults. Why, for example, have their traditional religions and families not sufficed? Why have they turned against their parents and their religions?

The answers to such questions, in my judgment, are found in the character of the families and society in which such persons have grown up. The nuclear family, the most prevalent form of family life in urban-industrial society, is clearly floundering due to various strains which undermine its ability to perform its basic responsibilities for the ego and superego development and socialization of children. Having lost or abandoned their traditions, with weak or atrophied identification with religion and with tenuous, if any, ties to kin, nuclear family parents have fewer and feebler standards than ever to instill, by precept and example, in children during their formative years.

In this anomic society, the standards that are ascendant today, especially among the middle and upper middle classes, are those which emphasize impulse gratification, self-centeredness, and a disregard for the future in contrast with those favoring impulse control, regard for others, and a future orientation. The former set of standards has become increasingly prevalent because of the dominance and isolation of the nuclear family. This has occurred largely because of assimilation, residential mobility, higher levels of educational achievement, and affluence—all the inevitable, pervasive results of urbanization, industrialization, and a society that gives precedence to the values of equality, independence, and individual fulfillment, highly valued ends that are also forces leading to the erosion of family cohesiveness and stability, as well as the decline in parental authority (Levine and Shaiova 1971, 1974, 1977).

More than half a century ago, Aichhorn (1925) described a type of delinquency which he attributed to what he termed an "excess of love." He noted that this type was "found disproportionately often in middle-class homes and is the source of great sorrow and despair." It is clear from his description that excess of love is really permissive parenting that stems from the inability of adults to use their authority with assurance and assertiveness. It results in an excessive devotion to the wishes of children (impulse gratification). It fails to assist children effectively to adopt and use values and standards that have practical use in their lives and which are central to the development of sound egos and superegos.

A concomitant of the decline of parental authority is that children grow up with fewer and weaker internalized standards that are prerequisite for their ego and superego development and are, therefore, much more subject to the dominance of their impulse life. They appear to be persons who have developed character disorders and are much more susceptible to the influence of their peers whose values and standards tend to favor impulse gratification, self-centeredness, and living in and for the present. Thus, those who have joined religious cults are also the victims of an anomic society.

In keeping with the importance of the incentives that cults provide those who join them, it is hypothesized that those persons who undergo the most complete identity transformation adopt the most rigid and demanding standards in their daily lives and lead group-isolated lives. They tend to do so, in my opinion, because they are burdened with intense emotional problems which are alleviated by conversion and joining the cult. Their transmuted personal identity and life of self-abnegation within their cloistered community suggest extreme dependency needs that they cannot resolve independently or in their social relationships in the outer society. However, only further research comparing the personality traits of the members of different religious cults can determine whether there are significant differences in the emotional disturbances and the need for direction and clarity in life among the members of the various religious cults (Galanter and Buckley 1978; Galanter, Rabkin, Rabkin, and Deutsch 1979; Judah 1977; Lofland and Stark 1965; Patrick and Dulack 1976; Singer 1979; West and Delgado 1978).

In sharp contrast to an anomic society whose values are weak, ambiguous, and in a state of flux, in religious cults absolute values and standards are presented by individuals who are their determined, committed advocates. A normless society is difficult enough for most adults to cope with competently, even for those not troubled by emotional disturbances. But it is apparently overly exacting and worrisome for numbers of white, middle-class youth and young adults, for whom religious cults appear to be their only alternative to resolve their behavioral problems and anxieties about the uncertainty of life today. Grasping for persons and standards to give meaning and direction to their lives, they are reminiscent of the masochistic persons Fromm (1941) described, who are plagued with feelings of "inferiority, powerlessness, and individual insignificance."

In this age of disbelief, when virtually all fundamental values have been thrown into question or dismissed as irrelevant by young people (and increasingly by adolescents and preadolescents), an effort must be made to attempt to indicate the practical disadvantages for the lives of those who join religious cults. What first comes to mind is that their serious dependency needs may, in time, again flare out and disrupt their lives during their adult years and middle age.

For those who become sufficiently disenchanted or dissatisfied with their cult's religion, emphases, and way of life, leaving it may be quite difficult if the only alternative is to cope once again with anomie, anonymity, and

150

anxiety. Carving out a new existence without the psychosocial supports they had in their associations and life in a religious cult could be emotionally taxing. Then, too, it is likely that they will lack economic security unless their religious cult permitted or encouraged them to have savings accounts, pension plans, social security funds, and health and life insurance. Yet unknown numbers will not have these provisions because of the nature of their community life or because the bulk of their income was taken by their religious cult. It will be a grim challenge for those who leave cults to start life anew with sparse resources to cope with emergencies, provide themselves with housing, pay for their children's education, and support themselves during their years of retirement.

It cannot be said whether or not religious cults will increase their membership significantly in the years ahead. Current estimates are that religious cults have approximately 50,000 members. It may be that they have run the course of their popularity, or that the massacre in Guyana may dissuade numbers of individuals from joining religious cults who might otherwise have done so. However, it is not the cults themselves that are the issue, for it is not imaginable that the tremendous variety of purposes and interests could be united in order to exert some baneful influence on the rest of society.

Conclusions

Cults are symptomatic of certain disturbing conditions of our times, effects rather than influences. It is evident that there are persons from lower income levels as well as the middle class who are easily captivated by the promises and claims of an authoritative, charismatic figure. The widespread interest in both religious and secular cults suggests that this society has produced growing numbers of persons who have significant unresolved dependency needs (emotional and creedal) which are the result of an increase in narcissistic character disorders. Lacking such basic traditional social institutions as the family and religion to which they can turn with assurance, and finding that considerable numbers of young people have been involved in secular (and religious) cults of one kind or another, such persons may be even more susceptible to the beguiling personalities and deceptive promises of demagogues who may appear on the political scene if they sense a growing need to meet crises of belief or the unrest stirred up by a more general social malaise.

151

REFERENCES

Aichhorn, A. 1925. *Wayward Youth*. New York: Viking, 1973.

Berger, B., and Hackett, B. 1974. On the decline of age grading in rural hippie communities. *Journal of Social Issues* 30(2): 163–186.

Berger, B.; Hackett, B.; and Millar, R. 1974. Child rearing practices in the communal family. In J. Skolnick and A. Skolnick, eds. *Intimacy, Family, and Society*. Boston: Little, Brown.

Fairfield, R. 1972. *Communes USA: A Personal Tour*. Baltimore: Penguin.

Fitzgerald, G. 1971. *Communes: Their Goals, Hopes, Problems*. New York: Paulist.

Fromm, E. 1941. *Escape from Freedom*. New York: Rinehart.

Galanter, M., and Buckley, P. 1978. Evangelical religion and meditation: psychotherapeutic effects. *Journal of Nervous and Mental Disease* 166(10): 685–691.

Galanter, M.; Rabkin, R.; Rabkin, J.; and Deutsch, A. 1979. The "moonies": a psychological study of conversion and membership in a contemporary religious sect. *American Journal of Psychiatry* 136(2): 165–170.

Judah, J. 1977. Attitudinal changes among members of the Unification Church. Paper presented at the meeting of the American Association for the Advancement of Science, Denver, January.

Kanter, R. 1972. Getting it all together: some group issues in communes. *American Journal of Orthopsychiatry* 42(4): 632–643.

Keniston, K. 1960. *The Uncommitted*. New York: Dell.

Levine, E. M. 1978. Middle class urbanites in rural communes: a social-psychiatric analysis. *American Journal of Psychoanalysis* 38(4): 327–344.

Levine, E., and Shaiova, C. 1971. Equality and rationality v. child social-ization: a conflict of interests. *Israel Annals of Psychiatry and Related Disciplines* 9(2): 107–116.

Levine, E. M., and Shaiova, C. 1974. Biology, personality, and culture: a theoretical comment on etiology of character disorders in industrial society. *Israel Annals of Psychiatry and Related Disciplines* 12(1): 10–28.

Levine, E. M., and Shaiova, C. 1977. Anomie: its influence on impulse-ridden youth and their self-destructive behavior. *Adolescent Psychiatry* 5: 73–81.

Lofland, J., and Stark, R. 1965. Becoming a world-saver: a theory of con-version to a deviant perspective. *American Sociological Review* 30: 862–875.

Otto, H. 1971. Communes: the alternative life-style. *Saturday Review* (April 24), pp. 16–21.

Patrick, T., and Dulack, T. 1976. *Let Our Children Go*. New York: Ballantine.

Rothchild, J., and Wolf, S. 1976. *The Children of the Counter-Culture*. New York: Doubleday.

Singer, M. 1979. Coming out of the cults. *Psychology Today* (January), pp. 72–81.

West, L., and Delgado, R. 1978. Psyching out the cults' collective. *Los Angeles Times* (November 25).

PART II

DEVELOPMENTAL RESEARCH AND ADOLESCENT PROCESS

EDITORS' INTRODUCTION

The growth patterns of adolescents have been studied in depth for many years, yet we find ourselves in the infantile stages of investigative analysis and attempts at understanding. Recent studies in narcissism and the psychology of the self have forced us to reexamine such basic concepts as adolescent rebellion, emancipation, and individuation. It is often difficult to differentiate the normal adolescent process from psychopathological states. The only certainty is the end product: a young adult who is, or is not, prepared to make his way in the world through successful vocational choice or academic adjustment and an ability to form meaningful intimate relationships.

Robert L. Arnstein describes the concerns of student mental health professionals in helping students with emotional problems that interfere with academic performance and furthering development toward full potential. He reviews the maturational process literature and discusses the key concept of emancipation from the family of origin as an experimental process of a conscious nature deeply affected by sociocultural factors. He concludes that the element of choice underlies the process of becoming an adult. The university experience strengthens the individual's identity in terms of career choice, exposes the student to a world of others and to intense peer relationships, and encourages development of individual coping behavior.

Richard C. Marohn in his studies of delinquent adolescents examines the intrapsychic determinants of adolescent rebellion. He believes that parental ties cannot be described solely in terms of libidinal attachments and must be seen also in relation to the narcissistic line of development. He traces the transformations of the self through the adolescent defensive processes and sees rebellious behavior, that may be viewed as defiance, as an attempt to repair the deficits precipitated by adolescent differentiation.

Mark J. Blotcky and John G. Looney review the literature on adolescent development in both males and females and stress fairly typical sex-defined differences. They conclude that adolescence is a period of regression, recapitulation of earlier stages of development, and movement toward autonomy. Comparing clinical and empirical studies of normal adolescents, they find adolescence to be an orderly, modulated process, with ego strength rather than psychotic-like regression emphasized, and serious loss of control and severe control conflicts with parents not usually evident. Research-based studies indicate that most teenagers perceive their parents as supportive and reasonable. Sexuality is troublesome to the adolescent but much more manageable than expected, resulting in a steady progression toward intimacy in late adolescence. The emancipation process proceeds with some difficulty but is characterized by reasonable order and is not torn by excessive rebellion. Persistent delinquent acts or extreme emotional upheaval suggest disturbance. Blotcky and Looney stress the need for expanded research especially in the areas of psychophysiology and psychosociology.

Jeffrey R. Mitchell evaluates the effects of past and present understanding of adolescence on opposing groups: those who view turmoil as normative for adolescents and others who believe that continuity with earlier and later phases outweighs discontinuity. He believes that clinicians who view normal adolescence as a long period of discontinuity and disorganization are not likely to look beyond the symptoms of a disturbed adolescent. Others who view normal adolescence as continuous with earlier stages will not confuse serious pathology with transient disturbances and will emphasize the need for continued contact and evaluation.

Sidney Weissman and Peter Barglow review recent contributions to the theory of female adolescent psychological development and their impact on psychoanalytic theory. They examine contemporary neurophysiological research and conclude that the quality of the libido is different in children and adults. Weissman and Barglow raise doubts about the validity of the classical view of libido: behavioral differences between boys and girls may reflect a biological basis, not solely a psychological one based on early identifications; developmental differentials of the growth of thought processes may affect transformations of narcissistic thinking during adolescence; and self-psychological development in adolescence is especially helpful to comprehending female developmental issues since biological and cultural factors provide structure to women's self-expressive needs.

Irving N. Berlin writes that the physiological and psychological stresses of adolescence foster a regressive plasticity which results in a capacity for new solutions to previous failures in adaptation. Berlin believes that parents should provide support in those areas where judgment is not sufficient. In pathological development, family therapy techniques can be utilized to trace the history of dysfunctional alliances and correct the consequential effects on development.

John Toews approaches the developmental challenges of marriage in young people as the need to share intimately while at the same time maintaining and enhancing individual autonomy. Successful completion of adolescence is required to facilitate the relationship. Failure to achieve completion may result in a derailment of the relationship with resulting sadomasochistic interactions. Treatment is planned to help the couple view the conflict from a developmental perspective, to understand themselves at their own particular stage of the life cycle, and to avoid the therapeutic pessimism reflected in their behavior.

Ronald M. Benson considers the fate of narcissism during adolescence and the transformations undertaken on the way toward the establishment of a cohesive sense of self. His studies suggest a series of normative aids present at the various levels of development which serve as narcissistic guardians and allow the transitions to take place in a continuous rather than stormy fashion. These guardians, transitional objects, imaginary companions, and the career fantasies of adolescence represent a self-object in the transitional zone of experience and are important in self-esteem regulation.

13 THE STUDENT, THE FAMILY, THE UNIVERSITY, AND TRANSITION TO ADULTHOOD

ROBERT L. ARNSTEIN

The majority of students when they enter the university are still immersed emotionally, psychologically, geographically, and usually financially in their family of origin. By the time of graduation from the university, many, if not most, will have achieved a measure of independence, and are or will be on the road to establishing a family of their own. In the interim in some semimysterious fashion the individual will become an adult in society's view, although the definition of this state is left rather vague. In doing so the student's relation to his or her family of origin will inevitably change, and both student and family will have to adjust to this development.

Historically, mental health professionals working with students have always had two concerns: (1) helping students with emotional problems that interfered with their academic performance, and (2) furthering students' psychological development so that their full potential would be realized. The methods by which these goals are accomplished are not always very clear, but the intention is enthusiastic. A full development into a gratifying adulthood is also a covert aim of the university, for although its primary purpose is to offer the matriculant an education, the term "education" in the United States is commonly expanded to include not only intellectual accomplishment but also the rather diffuse process frequently referred to as personal development or maturing.

A modified version of this paper was initially given at the Triennial Conference of the Australian and New Zealand Student Services Association, University of Canterbury, Christchurch, New Zealand, January 22, 1979. This work was supported in part by NIMH-Psychiatry Branch grant 5 TO1 MHO6536-22.

Adulthood

Maturity or adulthood is a state often referred to with the implication that a relatively clear concept is being communicated. Webster's dictionary (1971) defines *mature* as "having attained the normal peak of natural growth and development" and *adult* as "fully developed (as in size, strength or intellectual capacity)."

In human growth and development, however, the "normal peak" is not clearly agreed upon, and the standard against which maturity is measured is both multiplex and variable because the human has a series of abilities and biological systems that reach peaks and also begin gradual involution at different times.

In measuring maturity one can use a standard of physical development, psychological or emotional development, intellectual development, so-called sociocultural development, or some combination of the four. The biological and physical, of course, would include the changes that occur at puberty and make the individual capable of reproduction. Many societies have defined maturity or the adult state in relation to these changes. Beyond the age at which genital sexual behavior and reproduction can occur, bodily growth continues so that one could also use as an endpoint that age at which growth in height stops, weight reaches a relatively stable state, and various physiological measures are at a maximum (Timiras 1978). Intellectual development can be measured by various tests, although certain mental abilities may not have easily defined zeniths and such capacities as judgment may be almost impossible to determine. The sociocultural standard is the most variable and will differ from one society to another and even among different groups in one society. Anthropological studies demonstrate that there are widely different ages and customs to designate admission to adult status. In Western society, which displays some consistency in attitudes toward maturing, there are variations at least partially determined by educational systems, for one measure is the ability to be relatively self-supporting and to take responsibility for an adult work role appropriate to society. This usually implies having graduated from student status.

Prelinger (1974) has stated that adolescence is a culturally created stage in the life cycle between physical maturation and the sociocultural definition of adulthood. If this is true, then as culture changes, there are changes in the state of adolescence. One of the sociocultural changes that we all are currently struggling with is the gradual increase, for some groups at least, in the length of adolescence that has occurred during this century. This probably has been partly caused by the increasing complexity and technology of modern society but may also have been influenced by the increase in life expectancy and economic factors having to do with the need, or lack of need, for workers. Needless to say, sociocultural factors have also affected the function of the family and its place in the scheme of the maturing individual. Specifically, there has been a change in attitudes toward family formation. Where once full adulthood would have included assuming responsibility for a family and include procreation and assumption of care for the next generation, in our current era of varied life-styles and concern about overpopulation this may no longer be considered an important measure. Furthermore, the development of relatively foolproof methods of contraception has made the issue of pregnancy more controllable and, consequently, affected attitudes toward sexual behavior and family size.

When one comes to the emotional and psychological, however, the definition of the standard becomes most difficult. Should it be measured by one's internal psychological state or by one's external behavior, in which case it would appear to be difficult to separate from the sociocultural standard? Maturity as defined by Stone and Church (1957) encompasses a wide range of qualities. The individual must be capable of: continued change, self-determination, wisdom, humor, good reality-testing, adequate self-esteem, accepting the importance of human relationships, concern with social problems, tolerating solitude, commitment to a democratic code of ethics, assessing and repudiating if necessary ready-made values, and possessing consciousness of one's own mortality. This definition may posit an impossible ideal, but it delineates the complexity of any attempt at a comprehensive description.

Erikson (1950) has outlined a series of tasks which he has related to specific phases in the life cycle, and one can infer from these tasks a definition of maturity if one uses the biological standard to determine the age at which a person should at least approach maturity. Erikson stresses the concept of identity with the implication that one has reached adulthood if one can consolidate an identity which includes the capacity to work and to achieve intimacy with another individual. He states:

Young people must become whole people in their own right, and this during a developmental state characterized by a diversity of changes in physical growth, genital maturation, and social awareness. The wholeness to be achieved at this stage I have called a sense of inner identity. The young person, in order to experience wholeness, must feel a progressive continuity between that which he has come to be during the long years of childhood and that which he promises to become in the anticipated future; between that which he conceives himself to be and that which he perceives others to see in him and to expect of him. [Erikson 1968]

An important aspect of Erikson's theory involves periods of "crisis" which he looks on as turning points rather than times of potential catastrophe. Marcia (1966) interprets Eriksonian periods of crisis to mean periods of experimentation, and periods of commitment to mean periods in which identity elements are decided upon. Four states are described: "moratorium," during which the individual is in crisis; "achievement," in which commitment has occurred following a period of crisis; "foreclosed," in which the individual has assimilated the parental values without a period of crisis; and "diffusion," in which commitment has not been achieved but the individual is not actively experimenting as in a crisis period.

In research done on middle-aged males, Levinson, Darrow, Klein, Levinson, and McKee (1978) constructed a stepwise progression into and through adulthood with each major phase introduced by a transition period. They described the transition into early adulthood as occurring between the ages of seventeen and twenty-two. This is followed by a consolidation phase that they labeled "early adulthood." The transition phase is described as having the twin tasks of terminating preadulthood and beginning early adulthood. The former involves questioning the nature of the preadult world and one's place in it; modifying or terminating existing relationships with important persons, groups, and institutions; and reappraising and changing the self that formed in it. The second task involves exploring the possibilities of the adult world, imagining oneself in it, consolidating an initial adult identity, and making and testing some preliminary choices for adult living. The individual is on the boundary between adolescence and adulthood, and the transition ends when the boundary is crossed and a life is created within the adult world.

What then is the process of maturing that the individual must go through to proceed from adolescence to adulthood? A key concept in many of these theoretical formulations is emancipation from the family of origin. This clearly means emotional or psychological emancipation, not necessarily geographical, although physical separation often seems to further the process or to highlight conflicts if the process is not going smoothly. Levinson et al. (1978) describe leaving the preadult world as separating from the family of origin along many lines, including possibly moving out of the familial home, becoming financially less dependent, and entering new roles and living arrangements in which one is more autonomous and responsible. They state that internally it involves "an increasing differentiation between self and parents, greater psychological distance from the family, and reduced emotional dependency on parental support and authority."

Offer and Offer (1976) in their study of normal adolescent males using interview, rating-scale, and projective-test techniques describe three major types of growth patterns: continuous, surgent, and tumultuous. The continuous group moved smoothly through adolescence and were characterized by an intact family that encouraged independence, no serious clash of values, good peer relationships with appropriate progress toward heterosexual intimacy, and a sense of contentment. The surgent group functioned equally well but experienced greater emotional conflict, more difficulty in peer relationships, more concern about control of sexual impulses, and some conflict over values. The tumultuous group showed considerable inner turmoil and some overt behavioral problems with family conflict and general discord, although the group was as successful academically and vocationally as the other two groups. Offer and Offer conclude that "there is more than one normal developmental process from childhood to adulthood" but do not suggest an explanation as to why an individual took one path rather than another.

Fry and Rostow (1942) wrote about this period: "Detachment from the family is a necessary step toward the emotional maturity of an individual; it is a prerequisite to the smooth development of other growth processes." Similarly, Lidz (1968) states: "The transition from adolescent to adult behavior involves becoming a person in one's own right, not simply someone's son or daughter, and one who is recognized by the community in such terms. . . . It is concerned not simply with inner organization but also with how that organization permits the individual to move properly into the social roles permitted an adult and expected of him in a given society and its subsystems." Blos (1967) refers to the "shedding of family dependencies, the loosening of infantile object ties in order to become a member of society at large or, simply, of the adult world," events that he labels the second individuation process of adolescence.

To backtrack for a moment, one of the consequences of the development of psychoanalysis, with its emphasis on tracing the impact of earlier events on the individual, was a repeated demonstration of how often in the most surprising and unexpected ways earlier relationships within the family influence subsequent relationships. The refrain "I want a girl just like the girl that married dear old dad" frequently turns out to be an accurate account of our romantic involvements even when we think we are choosing someone with precisely opposite characteristics. Freud (1905) felt this to be so true

164

that he felt the individual never totally relinquished early attachments to parents, but he felt that some detachment was essential. He wrote that "one of the most painful psychical achievements of the pubertal period is . . . detachment from parental authority, a process that alone makes possible the opposition, which is so important for the progress of civilization, between the new generation and the old. At every stage in the course of development through which all human beings ought by rights to pass, a certain number are held back; so there are some who have never got over their parents' authority and have withdrawn their affection from them either very incompletely or not at all." In commenting on this passage, Schafer (1973) expands on the view that much of the tie to parents really involves unconscious fantasies extending back to childhood. He points out that the adolescent attempts to eradicate the influence of the parents as they actually are in the individual's adolescence. Schafer states that the unconscious situation makes it impossible for the adolescent to solve developmental problems by avoiding or overwhelming the actual parents, though in some respects such moves may be necessary and beneficial; but what is needed most urgently is the transformation of the so-called inner world, particularly the "archaic infantile world." Schafer feels this transformation will necessarily be "slow, subtle, ambivalent, limited, and fluctuating," but he is not certain how it occurs.

Schafer's point about eradicating parental influence is often seen clinically. A student, when his father was brought up as a possible source of difficulty, said, "There is no need to discuss my father. He has never had any influence on me whatsoever. I have never done anything he wanted me to do." If one accepts the validity of family influence (and I do not really see how one can deny it), questions arise of how the family influences the transition to adulthood. Are the theorists correct, and must one achieve some emancipation from the family to become adult? If having one's own identity is essential to being an adult, how is this achieved? And how does the university experience affect the process?

I believe that some consolidation of one's own identity, which involves some measure of psychological independence from the family, is important if not essential for those living in the United States. This feeling is based on the assumption that individuals will have some freedom of choice in career or life pattern and in choice of mate and/or friends. Prelinger (1974) states that, if we lived in a society that expected children to follow the career and life pattern of their parents and to participate in an arranged marriage and predetermined social relationships, it is less clear that separate identity and independence are so necessary. Levinson et al. (1978) agree, stating that in a relatively stable, undifferentiated society a young man's choices are highly limited, but that "in a technologically advanced, fragmented and changing society such as the United States, he has the advantages and the burdens of greater choice. More options are available in his environment. He is encouraged to seek his own way rather than to follow literally in his father's footsteps."

Does a psychological process go on inwardly which makes someone adult even when the outward manifestations are minimal? In a sense this question harks back to the psychoanalysts, who clearly feel that adulthood is only attained psychologically by overcoming or modifying unconscious fantasies related to erotized early attachments to parents. Anna Freud (1958) feels that, although this is essentially an unconscious process, its conscious manifestation is a kind of turmoil that is a necessary concomitant to the process. She seems, however, to be discussing mid adolescence, so it is possible that the process is usually completed by the time of entrance to college. Schafer (1973) writes that negativism toward parents, though it can be an aspect of the late adolescent to early adult period, is not really the significant process. He is, however, forthright enough to say he does not know how the significant process occurs. I think that in addition to whatever may be going on unconsciously in the adolescent-adult transition, there is considerable experimentation of a conscious nature, although it is not clear that the individual involved thinks of it as experimentation. The process may be summarized: The child establishes that "I am I," the adolescent asks "Who am I," and the adult is the "who" the late adolescent has consciously chosen to be within the limits unconsciously set up in childhood, and as those limits are affected by sociocultural factors (Arnstein 1979).

The element of choice, then, is perhaps the key factor underlying the process of becoming adult. As I have already suggested, in fixed, stable societies elements of choice may not exist, and the process of development may be quite different. In mobile societies, however, choice becomes a predominant factor because it suggests that the individual has the opportunity to select his or her own identity, life pattern, value system, and code of behavior. Given this opportunity, there seems to be considerable proclivity to experiment and establish a combination which is individual and distinguishes one in some way from one's family. The choices involve occupation, type of relationships, life-style, and a code of behavior and may extend to religion, politics, and morality. It is important to recognize, however, that choice has a negative aspect. If one makes a particular choice, it almost inevitably means giving up other possibilities. The ability to accept limitations may be as significant a part of the maturing process as the ability to commit oneself, and, clearly, some individuals find this to be the most difficult part of the process. Seymour Sarason has suggested (personal communication,

1974) that symbolically this limitation may be unconsciously equated with the final closing off of death, and therefore the individual for the first time must face the fact of mortality. For whatever reason, it seems to be a prominent feature in those individuals who are having particular difficulty with the transition.

The Role of the University

It is apparent that the very fact of applying to and entering a college or university has almost by definition forced choice on the individual, for occupation will be greatly or totally determined by the curriculum chosen. Furthermore, the university inevitably opens a new world of experience as a result of meeting new people, being exposed to new ideas often deliberately skeptical, and hearing challenges, both direct and indirect, to the value system with which one enters. Although higher education is seen as a *desideratum* by most parents, and parents are very proud when their son or daughter is accepted by a college or university, they are often quite disapproving of, if not shocked by, the actual impact the experience has on their child. "We're not sending you to college to become an atheist or a Marxist or an intellectual snob" is a not-so-infrequent protest of parents. If the student asks what they *are* sending him or her to college for, the parents might either be at a loss or have some general answer ("to get an education") or a specific answer ("to become a lawyer"). "To learn to think for yourself" is not a response that many parents would be likely to give, although that is exactly what the university faculty would probably say. In the last decade many parents did become accustomed to the idea that their sons or daughters needed to "find themselves," although that particular pursuit was usually advanced by students as a reason not to be in college and as a justification for why their parents should support them in growing organic vegetables or in studying esoteric religions.

How does the university experience contribute to the maturing process? First of all, it strengthens the individual's identity in terms of career choice. Although this is a rather conscious aspect of identity, it seems to have an important influence on one's sense of self. Second, the university exposes the individual to a world of others, many of whom will have had difficult earlier experiences and often will espouse different values. This may help the individual to see his or her own family in better perspective and, by demonstrating that others can survive with different values, help the individual to attain greater autonomy. Third, the individual frequently experiences during these years the first serious emotional relationship with a peer. It may or may not include overt sexual experience, but if it does, it may help to consolidate a sexual identity and to provide a period of experimentation, which gives the individual a clearer sense of what will be fulfilling in the way of an intimate relationship. Fourth, the individual today is often separated from the family and living in a dormitory or an apartment off campus. This gives the individual some opportunity to try out taking care of oneself in everyday practical matters, such as providing food, doing laundry, regulating study and sleeping habits, etc. Although these activities probably do not make specifically for maturity, the psychological ability to cope with such demands without undue anxiety or disruptive upset is probably an aspect of the maturing process.

The idea that education is apt to foster and promote differentiation from the family is only dimly perceived, I believe, by most families. I am not even sure that it is very clearly perceived by the entering student. The university may be approached with a sense of excitement and a readiness for new experiences, but I rather doubt that the student consciously anticipates the forming of a new identity or even necessarily a changed relationship with the family. If the student is to live in a dormitory and the university is at a distance from the family, he or she will recognize that there will be superficial changes in how details of living will be managed. But the student does not necessarily see this as altering the fundamental relationship, good or bad, with parents. If the student continues to live at home and commutes to college, the anticipation of change may be even less, which, if change occurs, may make the impact even greater. It must be remembered, however, that change does not mean cutting off the relationship completely. Levinson et al. (1978), in making this point about relationships that have had great meaning to the individual, cite the young adult in the process of separating from parents as an example and state: "His developmental task is not to end the relationship altogether, rather, he has to reject certain aspects . . . to sustain other aspects, and to build in new qualities such as mutual respect between distinctive individuals who have separate as well as shared interests. Neither the young adult nor his parents find this an easy task."

The Transitional Process

The transitional process is not easy for the student because very often independence and adult status are frightening as well as desired. There is some evidence to suggest that those individuals who have especially stormy relations with the family during the transition are really fighting with their own dependent feelings. In other words, they are so threatened by their own wish to stay dependent on the family that the only way they can disentangle is by wrenching maneuvers. These frequently consist of viewing the parents as totally unsympathetic, authoritarian, and probably stupid, so that there seems to be justification in denying parental authority, influence, and sometimes even existence.

From the family's standpoint there also may be considerable anxiety, if not actual distress, at the process. First of all, as I have already noted, the student views the period as an opportunity for experimentation. It takes a family with considerable fortitude to absorb with equanimity some of the experiments. Although parents may console themselves with the thought that "it's only a phase," it is difficult not at least to consider what the future would be like if it were not a phase. Furthermore, some parents may be relatively relaxed about almost any experiment that occurs within a certain age period, but their view of when that age period should end may differ from the student's view, a concept Sternschein (1973) refers to as a "social clock." And if the student is really in a struggle with the family, he or she may be astute enough to prolong the period of experimentation so that the family eventually becomes unrelaxed.

Second, parents may be attempting to deal with their own problems at the same time that the student is seeking emancipation. Most parents of university students will be in middle life, and the student's problems may inadvertently exacerbate conflicts that the parents are having either as individuals or as a couple. These problems, in turn, may have a reciprocal effect on the student. At this moment in the United States many young women are being affected by their observations of their mothers' dissatisfaction at not having pursued a definite career. The student's problems may also reactivate conflicts that the parents had during their own adolescence, as Kernberg (1974) points out, and consequently the parents may overidentify with the student and encourage solutions that they found viable or inveigh against solutions that they found unsatisfactory.

Third, the process of letting go may be difficult for certain parents. This may be because they want to protect their children from the mistakes that they think are being made, because they are genuinely alarmed at the choices that they see being made, or, more problematically, because the dependent state of the child is important to the psychic economy of the parents, most often the mother but occasionally the father. Siggins (1973) has pointed out that the family's attitudes may differ if the student is female rather than male. The family may value a girl's academic work in elementary and secondary

169

school but look on college as an opportunity for her to meet eligible men for the purpose of marriage; they may even consider academic excellence as a handicap in the mating process on the theory that men are threatened by women who are too smart. Whereas a male student will be praised and encouraged in his academic work as an important step in his career progress, family response to a female student's similar accomplishment may be ambivalent if not disapproving.

Mistakes have been mentioned, and this is a complicated issue. First, what parents feel are mistakes may be viewed very differently by the student. Second, one cannot really talk about experimentation without accepting the possibility or even probability that many of the experiments will be found to be unsatisfactory. It is difficult to know, however, that this interest or friend or style of living is not the right one unless one has tried it. Parents who attempt to spare the student disappointment, pain, or wasted motion are essentially indulging in a contradiction in terms; if one has not experimented and evaluated an experience for oneself, it does not contribute to an independent identity. Although the fact of making mistakes in late adolescence does not guarantee a smooth and satisfactory adulthood, it does seem that individuals who effect the transition with no side trips or uncertainties often later experience conflict about the choices made.

Various factors having to do with the college or university, the family, and the times will also influence the process. If there is a wide discrepancy between the socioeconomic position of the family and the climate of the specific university a student attends, the necessary adjustments by both student and family may be considerably greater than if the family milieu is culturally consonant with the university. Thus, if the student feels the parents are lacking in education or in sophistication, which is not infrequent in a mobile society, he or she may feel inferior in the university setting and, in an attempt to deal with this feeling, adopt and overvalue university customs. This may lead to being critical of family values or even an attempt to ''improve'' the family, which the family naturally resents and resists. Or if the university deliberately or inadvertently influences the student toward a different set of moral values, this may be very upsetting to the family. Although the concept of a school acting *in loco parentis* has waned considerably, even when it existed more strongly the university's version of its role often differed considerably from that of a given set of parents. Sometimes the difficulties may be multigenerational, in that the parents can accept the student's ideas or behavior, but they remain dominated by grandparents who find the student life-style unacceptable, and the grandparental disapproval is transmitted to the student by the parents.

170

Conclusions

The transition from adolescence to adulthood is both an internal and an external process, frequently encompassing mistakes, inefficiencies, and detours as well as successful experimentation, progress, and triumphs. One hopes the process will lead to the establishment of an adult identity which is satisfactory to the individual and which provides a certain stability on which later aspects of adult development can be based. Those who watch the process most closely—notably parents, but also teachers, friends, chaplains, physicians, and counselors—can attempt to help at times by example, advice, or professional skill. Maturity, however, I feel, can only be attained if the individual has selected and consolidated an identity which allows for self-determination and self-fulfillment, making for a sense of direction and personal worth. The university years in our culture seem like a good medium in which to accomplish this process, although the impact on the individual is not always regarded as an unmixed blessing by the family, who may be inclined to blame the university for disruptions in the student's relationship with the family. I feel, however, that in most cases a rapprochement does occur between student and family once the student has achieved some inner stability in the adult role, and the family has more or less accepted the fact that the son or daughter is an independent individual.

REFERENCES

Arnstein, R. L. 1979. The adolescent identity crisis revisited. *Adolescent Psychiatry* 7:71–84.

Blos, P. 1967. The second individuation process of adolescence. *Psychoanalytic Study of the Child* 22:162–186.

Erikson, E. H. 1950. *Childhood and Society*. New York: Norton.

Erikson, E. H. 1968. *Identity: Youth and Crisis*. New York: Norton.

Freud, A. 1958. Adolescence. *Psychoanalytic Study of the Child* 13:255–279.

Freud, S. 1905. Three essays on the theory of sexuality. *Standard Edition* 7:125–243. London: Hogarth, 1953.

Fry, C. C., and Rostow, E. G. 1942. *Mental Health in College*. New York: Commonwealth Fund.

Kernberg, O. F. 1974. Mature love: prerequisites and characteristics. *Journal of the American Psychoanalytic Association* 22:743–769.

Levinson, D. J.; Darrow, C. N.; Klein, E. B.; Levinson, M. H.; and McKee, B. 1978. *The Seasons of a Man's Life*. New York: Knopf.

Lidz, T. 1968. *The Person*. New York: Basic.

Marcia, J. E. 1966. Development and validation of ego-identity status. *Journal of Personality and Social Psychology* 3:551–558.

Offer, D., and Offer, J. 1976. Three developmental routes through normal male adolescence. *Adolescent Psychiatry* 4:121–141.

Prelinger, E. 1974. Crises of identity. In M. D. Keys, ed. *The Identity Crisis*. New York: National Project Center for Film and the Humanities.

Schafer, R. 1973. Concepts of self and identity and the experience of separation-individuation in adolescence. *Psychoanalytic Quarterly* 42:42–60.

Siggins, L. 1973. Women university students and careers. *Australian and New Zealand Journal of Psychiatry* 7:1–4.

Sternschein, I. 1973. The experience of separation-individuation in infancy and its reverberations through the course of life: maturity, senescence and sociological implications. *Journal of the American Psychoanalytic Association* 21:633–646.

Stone, L. J., and Church, J. 1957. *Childhood and Adolescence*. New York: Random House.

Timiras, P. S. 1978. Biological perspectives on aging. *American Scientist* 66:605–614.

Webster's Third New International Dictionary. 1971. Springfield, Mass.: Merriam.

14 ADOLESCENT REBELLION AND THE TASK OF SEPARATION

RICHARD C. MAROHN

"I'm grown-up" may be the excited and enthusiastic exclamation of the girl who eagerly anticipates her future vocation, or the anxious and panicky cry of the frightened boy who feels unable to survive without the consolation and solace of childhood, or the rebellious, defiant challenge of the incorrigible boy or girl who triumphantly asserts his or her independence. It is the latter state of mind I hope to explore in this chapter.

As do Baittle and Offer (1971), I would define "rebellion" as external behavior, directed against the parents or their surrogates, which may include the establishment, society, authority in general, teachers, or therapists. Webster's *New Collegiate Dictionary* (1949) defines "rebellious" as resisting or defying authority, but as a secondary definition includes "resisting treatment or operation," that is, "refractory." I will not describe such behavior in order to elucidate underlying psychodynamics; many authors have done so satisfactorily. To catalog struggles for emancipation, acts of open resistance or defiance, states of negativism, chronic complaints, provocative acts, truculence, nagging, fighting, disobedience, "masculine protest," deidealization, disillusionment, comtemptuous attitudes, assaults, or serious delinquency may aid us in classifying or catagorizing the end result, the phenotype of adolescent rebellion, but not help us to understand the underlying anxieties, impulses, defenses, deficits, and conflicts (Baittle and Offer 1971). I will reconsider, however, the intrapsychic determinants of adolescent rebellion in the context of recent formulations of narcissism and the psychology of the self.

Some apparently rebellious behavior is not, indeed, a rebellion against parental prohibitions and values, but a more honest and open representation of parental wishes and preferences. Johnson and Szurek (1952) showed that delinquent children may often be gratifying the unconscious wishes of their seemingly upright parents. A popular author, Nancy Friday (1977), writes that many girls are taught their mother's attitudes about sexuality; that virginity must be preserved at all costs unless one is to be swept off her feet. Becoming infatuated and losing one's virginity seems to be a rebellion against mother's strict admonitions about premarital intercourse, but in reality is an identification with mother's own wishes to surrender to urges that she finds unacceptable. A similar process of identification is seen in those student activitists who, while attacking the establishment, are not rebelling against parental values and norms, but rather behaving according to their own parental identifications, beliefs that are passively held by the parents but actively lived out by their children.

Other authors have attempted to understand adolescent rebellion as counterdependence, that is, an attempt to separate or individuate and to achieve some autonomy, though spurious. For example, Baittle and Offer (1971) suggest that "the main function of rebellion, in the more or less normal adolescent, is to achieve an initial step in the process of emancipation from the parents. However, not all adolescent rebellion is in the service of emancipation. The concept of emancipation is not inherent in rebellion, though it is often associated with it." Nonetheless, the concept of rebellion is so intimately tied to the idea of the adolescent achieving individuality that Pearson (1958) summarizes his work as a study of "adolescence and the conflict of generations," and many of us believe firmly and teach repeatedly that teenagers need firm limits, boundaries, and parental positions against which they can differentiate themselves. Many times such differentiation appears as the teenager seeks out the firm wall to butt. In the middle adolescence or adolescence proper of Blos (1962), one would expect that such apparent rebellious behavior has diminished, for the adolescent by this time should no longer be beset by preoedipal regressions, and should be comfortably moving away from the intense infantile ties to the parents. Rebellious behavior in a middle or late adolescent would suggest significant psychopathology because in middle adolescence, although it is difficult to ascribe an age to this period, heterosexual experimentation and peer relationships should reach their zenith and the need to separate from parents will be so fulfilled.

Yet Blos (1972) returns to remind us that much of the rebellious behavior seen in later adolescents, especially that of the "angry or activist adolescents who seek the creation of a perfect society," derives from the narcissistic rage provoked by the failure of society to live up to the fantasies of parental perfection. Bettelheim (1971) also notes that such late-adolescent student activist rebellion serves either to provide the youth with a sense of himself or to occupy and define him and save him from a state of psychological emptiness and boredom.

Despite the fact that Anna Freud (1958) advised us that a certain amount of turmoil seems to be the hallmark of adolescent health, it is not clear that such turmoil necessarily expresses itself in overtly tumultuous behavior. In fact, the work of Offer (1969; also Offer and Offer 1975) would suggest that the process of adolescent separation and individuation occurs in some without overt rebellion and in many with rebellion that would hardly be considered a family or social problem. Nonetheless, Wolf, Gedo, and Terman (1972) reemphasized the maturational efficacy of apparent adolescent rebellion when, in their review of the phenomena of adolescent secret academic societies, they not only note how the idealization of literary and cultural heroes facilitates the deidealization of parental imagos and the establishment of internal psychological structure, here specifically one's own ideals, but they state that the further one traverses from an adherence to parental ideals to an adherence to new ideals, the more one has separated and achieved psychological structuralization and psychological maturity. Such is "one measure of a man," and may be a vital determinant of later creativity. They suggest, in fact, that the nature of the peer ties may, in fact, determine the degree to which one makes such a move, just as earlier Anna Freud (1965) suggested that displacement by chance onto a delinquent subculture may result in the internalization of delinquent values. Klumpner (1972) succinctly points out that such displacements do not facilitate changes in internal ideals and psychological structure, but rather are external manifestations that such changes are taking place intrapsychically.

Similarly, I am not so concerned with those familial, social, environmental, cultural, or political factors which sustain, stimulate, or provoke adolescent rebellious behavior. Rather, I am interested in the psychic and psychological configurations which resonate with and precipitate states of mind readily expressed in overt rebellion. Without these, despite any extreme condition or provocation in the external world, such rebellion is not likely to occur.

In fact, Spiegel (1971) suggests that in the United States, large-scale rebellions will "erupt whenever a group in an excluded category (blacks, women, youth, etc) makes its historically appropriate bid for entry into the elitist system." Such rebellion, often spearheaded by youth, does not derive from any attempt to differentiate oneself (or to change the system) but rather from an attempt, at least in this country, to be included in the mainstream. Such phenomena raise the serious question of whether or not rebellion is an attempt to fight or conquer authority, even though its manifest intent seems to be such, or whether it is an attempt to achieve something quite different, something of a highly personal, many times unconscious meaning to the rebel, especially the adolescent rebel.

Anna Freud's classical paper on adolescence (1958) sharply defines the centrality of the adolescent separation process in an understanding of the psychology of this maturational phase. She proposed not only guidelines for the definition of normality versus psychopathology, but constructed a viewpoint of adolescent development that included ego functions and object relations building upon her father's view of the transformations of puberty.

Sigmund Freud (1905) had described the shifts in adolescence from familial attachments to peer attachments as the result of incestuous prohibitions against the now genitalized oedipal wishes. Anna Freud delineates not only the process by which this is accomplished, but also the quantitative and qualitative differences that might determine health or illness. She notes that the primary task of adolescence is to achieve such separation from incestuous, that is, infantile object ties, and defines two general ways in which this is done—that is, by establishing defenses against incestuous ties or by establishing defenses against the instinctual urges themselves. In the former category are the psychological processes of displacement, reversal, withdrawal, and regression, and in the latter category, the ascetic adolescent and the uncompromising adolescent. She notes that these mechanisms are on a continuum from the healthiest—displacement—to the sickest—the uncompromising adolescent. Furthermore, the adolescent who uses any of these mechanisms precipitously or exclusively is more likely to be ill than the adolescent who experiments with a variety of psychological maneuvers or proceeds gradually to separate from the infantile love objects. Her clinical examples, while rich in generalizability and resonating with the clinical experiences of many of us, are tied to a theoretical framework which rests exclusively on libidinal and incestuous object relating. As Hicks (1977) has described, to formulate the negative oedipal attachment of a boy to his father and to make interpretations in his therapy exclusively in terms of homosexual libido may confront the teenage patient not only with an erroneous formulation, but also with the narcissistic injury of being treated by a nonempathic therapist. Homosexual libido it may well be, but it may also be the idealization of a narcissistic object which may yet be experienced with the father, or displaced onto heroes, or repeating itself in a narcissistic idealizing transference.

I have found Anna Freud's formulations to be exquisitely helpful in explaining to students the process of adolescent emancipation, in formulating some ideas about health and sickness, and in raising questions about the treatability of many teenagers. Yet, I believe that these ties to the infantile love objects cannot be described solely in terms of libidinal attachment to incestuous objects, but must also be seen in terms of the narcissistic line of development. After all, a meaningful love relationship includes not only libidinal components, but narcissistic, usually idealizing, and sometimes mirroring components as well.

Kohut (1971) defines and describes the movement from primary or primitive narcissism to a secondary, mature form. He delineates the transformation of the grandiose self and its interactions with the mirroring empathic parent into self-esteem and ambition, as well as the transformation of primitive idealization of the parental self-object into important ideals and values and the respect and admiration of others. In later contributions, Kohut (1977) noted that in addition to understanding narcissistic pathology in terms of personality disorders, one must also think about narcissistic behavior disorders, that is, those people who show their disturbances in terms of behavior. This is particularly germaine to the issue of the rebellious adolescent who may externalize his narcissistic pathology.

Furthermore, Kohut notes that cohesion of the self and organization of the self may occur around one or both aspects of the bipolar self, that is, around either the grandiose self and its transformations, or the idealized parental imago and its transformations. That is to say, one's narcissistic organization may develop either around self-grandiosity or self-esteem, or around idealization or ideals or both, and such interactions may occur with one or both parents. Such theoretical speculation has its limitations and needs to be founded in clinical experience. Suffice it to say, however, that the kinds of ties to the infantile love objects that Anna Freud described cannot be viewed as consisting solely of incestuous libidinal attachments, but include some understanding of the self-object relating that occurs in the child-parent relationship. Consequently, we must also look at how adolescent defensive processes deal with these narcissistic ties, and here, specifically, how such might result in the external manifestations of rebellious behavior.

The adolescent's grandiosity no longer turns to the parents for mirroring or admiration, but instead to peers and groups. Similarly, the adolescent's need to idealize expresses itself no longer with parents, but toward heroes, groups, and new ideals. If gradual displacement from parents to others occurs, psychological structure may be built, as the teenager experiences minimal but tolerable frustrations and disappointments and begins to mirror or idealize his own internal representations.

If displacements, however, are precipitous, the teenager may simply replace the parental self-objects with other self-objects. Such shifts may show themselves in rebellious behavior; the grandiosity may desperately cling to a choice of friends, groups, clothing, or music which is unacceptable to the parents and to society; the need to idealize may focus intently on certain unacceptable heroes, or ideals, or groups, or result in intense infatuations, again, unacceptable to the family. These behaviors may be viewed as defiance, but intrapsychically they may represent a clinging or a repair of the deficit, not a defiance—a healing rather than a vicious attack.

The reversal that Anna Freud describes does not occur solely in libidinal terms, for converting affectionate ties to hostile ties includes more than incestuous wishes. The teenager who has, heretofore, been turning to mother for admiration and reinforcement now becomes hostile to any parental overtures and offers of help, and, in fact, may go so far as to guarantee that his parent will never praise him, but indeed will turn away from him in disgust at his clothing, at his behavior, at his speech, or at his choice of friends. Such disgust is the negation of mirroring; this teenager is not asking to be admired, but rather he is demanding that he not be admired. It seems to me that this is better understood as a negation of the wish for narcissistic supplies from one's parents, rather than a denial of an incestuous libidinal relationship.

Another teenager can no longer idealize his parents, but deidealizes them in the severest degree; he depreciates and disparages them. Such open attacks on parents, such defiance and hostility, can better be understood clinically in terms of disillusionment and depreciation, an inability to idealize one's parents, or rage at one's recognition that parents do have failings, rather than a reversal of libidinal incestuous wishes which are somehow converted from sexual interest to hostile rejection. Although in some instances other people may become idealized by the teenager, there are some adolescents who deidealize all representatives of the parents, and this may include all authority, social institutions, and the establishment. This eventuates in a cynical or a nihilistic adolescent, or one whose rage expresses itself in the destruction of social institutions.

All these reversals of narcissistic bonding may express themselves in rebellion. Such rebellion may result from the teenager denying and reversing his wish to be admired by the parents or his wish to idealize the parents, but it may also be an expression of the narcissistic rage he feels at his parents' failure to admire him or his inability to idealize weak and deficient parents.

A case report may illuminate some of these ideas. Frank is a fifteen-year-old adolescent who came to treatment after several months in a hospital, where the therapist felt that he was a psychopathic individual who adhered to no value system and had no capacity to relate to others except for his own needs. His behavior was opportunistic and manipulative, and he complained bitterly about the restrictions his parents placed on him which kept him from having fun and interfered with his peer experiences.

Frank was involved in multiple delinquencies, including frequent runaways from home, serious school truancy, stealing money from his parents, taking the family car on a number of occasions without permission, sneaking out of the house during the wee hours of the morning, using alcohol and drugs at home and outside of the home against his parents' wishes, selling marijuana and being arrested for it at school, driving a stolen car, driving without a license, and assaulting his older sister with a piece of furniture. All of these behaviors he saw in terms of his parents' refusal to give him freedom and autonomy. It was clear after awhile that his protests of parental control were somewhat shallow, for he consistently provoked more and more parental control by his apparently rebellious behavior. Frank was attempting to ward off a serious depression, presumably related to the loss of nurturing and supportive relationships with both parents, who were heavily invested in his future as their only son.

Any attempt on the part of each parent to try to understand his conflict or empathize with his struggles in achieving meaningful peer relationships was met with denial and rage. Similarly, when later on the therapist interpreted to him how his behavior, though by his claim designed to achieve autonomy, seemed to provoke more and more controlling responses by his parents, he angrily denied any such motivation. Gradually, however, the patient began saying that he had problems and could discuss these only with the therapist. Yet, at other moments, he would state quite openly that though he was pleased with his new school program and the restrictions it entailed, therapy had been of no help to him, despite his parents' insistence that it had been; and, indeed, he insisted that his parents were wasting their money. At the same time he, not defiantly, but quite comfortably, began traveling the substantial distance to the therapist's office by himself, no longer chauffered by his parents. He enjoyed the freedom of exploration he found in taking public transportation, even in the depths of the winter. When spring approached, he talked about bringing his friends to a nearby park to show them the wonders of the city, at the same time indicating that he found that he could have fun, smoke marijuana, go to parties, and engage in what he felt were suitable adolescent activities without provoking parental control or causing parental discomfort. Indeed, although such attitudes had prompted a previous therapist to view him as a manipulator and a psychopath, this young man was beginning to appreciate the failings and unacceptability of his parents' value system, which he no longer needed either to idealize as omniscient or to depreciate as outmoded. He was now developing a belief system of his own. His rebellion indicated that a certain internal readjustment was occurring as he moved away from the sustaining and nurturing self-object support of parental ties, replaced

179

it with that of the therapist, and began to rely on his own values, comfortably and without apology.

In fact, he did bring his friends to a park in the neighborhood of the psychiatrist's office, and, as he described it with enthusiasm in a session a few days later, wondered if I also was there in the park that same day.

At the same time that he expected the therapist to be like him and be in the park at the same time, he denied the value of the sessions, felt that he and his parents were wasting time and money, and confronted the therapist with his explicit belief that "you don't help me." He insisted that all the changes he had made were changes of his own doing and asked for a two- or three-week control period away from treatment where he could demonstrate that he would continue to behave well without the need for therapy. My comments that he had improved were met with statements that he really did not care what I thought; yet his behavior indicated an excitement and an interest in continuing the sessions.

Though it is clear that certain narcissistic ties are expressed clearly in treatment as wishes for mirroring and admiration or wishes to idealize and admire the therapist, the reverse are also transferences; deidealizing the therapist or rejecting his praise are ways of dealing with and expressing intense narcissistic bonds. Many of the delinquent adolescents we treat can engage in meaningful treatment only if they have a capacity to idealize someone. Yet such a capacity may show itself in a depreciation and deidealizing attack on important people in the patient's life. And it seems to me that such ideas about narcissistic bonding are more useful clinically in working with a rebellious or delinquent adolescent than the nature of his heterosexual or homosexual libidinal ties to the therapist. Aichhorn (1925) noted too that with many delinquents, understanding the nature of their narcissistic relationships was more helpful than viewing them as capable of relating in a libidinal manner.

Blos (1977) has delineated the psychological manifestations of the closure of adolescence. Completing the second individuation process must be understood in terms of the mood swings of narcissistic reorganization and the conflicting wishes to "enshrine for good those infantile object attachments" while experiencing "a critical deidealization, or humanization." The continuity of the ego with an individual past, present, and future leading to a "kind of historical reality testing" can be understood in terms of the cohesion of the self. The working through of residual traumata is often seen in the development of compensatory narcissistic structures and shifts between the two poles of the self leading to the formulation of a unique character. And sexual identity, distinguished by Blos from gender identity, involves the

180

establishment of an ego ideal, "abstracted and desexualized," but clearly the result of narcissistic transformation.

Conclusions

Adolescent rebellion is behavior which, though it may provoke a variety of reactions, may betray a myriad of underlying psychological motivations. It may, indeed, represent neither rejection nor defiance, but in fact may be the living out of parental expectations and values. It can be an attempt to protect oneself against dependency longings and tendencies to regress to more infantile attachments. Nonetheless, it is not equal to emancipation. It may be the angry reaction of a disillusioned adolescent confronting the deficiencies and failings of the adult world. It may be the stimulus-seeking response of the bored or empty youth.

Though it may appear to some that adolescent rebellion facilitates the separation process and, indeed, may result in greater autonomy and psychological structuralization, to others it may demonstrate simply that differentiation is taking place. Too often, we may confuse adolescent rebellion with the establishment of a new order through the development of new value systems, when in reality it represents simply an effort to gain one's place in the establishment.

Adolescent rebellion has frequently been understood in terms of Anna Freud's formulations about adolescent separation. Although it is clear that the vicissitudes and varieties of such separation are important to an understanding of adolescent maturation, understanding these movements in terms of libidinal shifts is insufficient. Bonding to infantile incestuous objects occurs and must be understood, particularly as the adolescent achieves first homosexual and then heterosexual displacements. On the other hand, bonding to the parents of infancy involves narcissistic claims—demands for mirroring or admiration and propensities for idealization and respect. To chart the psychological movements of adolescence involves an understanding of the transformations of narcissism and the eventual accretion of internal psychological structure.

To understand adolescent rebellion, one must also look at the displacements or reversals of narcissistic ties as shifts from the parents to parental surrogates, to peers, to values.

Adolescent rebellion may represent a rejection of parental admiration or a disillusionment and depreciation of parental value. Adolescent rebellion may result from narcissistic rage that parents have failed to support and mirror the adolescent, or have failed to live up to his expectations. So may society disappoint the adolescent. But adolescent rebellion as it is an exaggeration and derailment of separation and individuation is more than libidinal shifts. It represents a pathology of the self, expressed externally in a narcissistic behavior disorder.

To treasure and to explore the therapist's turf may enable the adolescent to move away from his parents and their suburb, but at the same time, the adolescent must insist, "I don't care what you think." Such is the paradox of adolescent rebellion; such is the dilemma of narcissistic binding. To be attached is to be submerged; to separate is to die.

REFERENCES

Aichhorn, A. 1925. *Wayward Youth.* New York: Meridian, 1960.

Baittle, B., and Offer, D. 1971. On the nature of male adolescent rebellion. *Adolescent Psychiatry* 1:139–160.

Bettelheim, B. 1971. Obsolete youth: toward a psychograph of adolescent rebellion. *Adolescent Psychiatry* 1:14–39.

Blos, P. 1962. *On Adolescence.* New York: Free Press.

Blos, P. 1972. The function of the ego ideal in adolescence. *Psychoanalytic Study of the Child* 27:93–97.

Blos, P. 1977. When and how does adolescence end: structural criteria for adolescent closure. *Adolescent Psychiatry* 5:5–17.

Freud, A. 1958. Adolescence. *Psychoanalytic Study of the Child* 13:255–278.

Freud, A. 1965. Dissociality, delinquency, criminality as diagnostic categories in childhood. In *Normality and Pathology in Childhood: Assessments of Development.* New York: International Universities Press.

Freud, S. 1905. Three essays on the theory of sexuality. *Standard Edition* 7:132–243. London: Hogarth, 1953.

Friday, N. 1977. *My Mother Myself.* New York: Dell.

Hicks, W. R. 1977. The negative oedipus complex, the idealized parental imago, and the geneology of the ego ideal in adolescence. Paper presented at the Second Annual Central States Conference of the American Society for Adolescent Psychiatry, Dallas, September 10, 1977.

Johnson, A., and Szurek, S. A. 1952. The genesis of antisocial acting out in children and adults. *Psychoanalytic Quarterly* 21:323–343.

Klumpner, G. 1972. Discussion of Wolf, Gedo, and Terman paper. Presented before Chicago Psychoanalytic Society, May 23, 1972.

Kohut, H. 1971. *The Analysis of the Self.* New York: International Universities Press.

Kohut, H. 1977. *The Restoration of the Self.* New York: International Universities Press.

Offer, D. 1969. *The Psychological World of the Teenager.* New York: Basic.

Offer, D., and Offer, J. B. 1975. *From Teenage to Young Manhood: A Psychological Study.* New York: Basic.

Pearson, G. 1958. *Adolescence and the Conflict of Generations.* New York: Norton.

Spiegel, J. P. 1971. Toward a theory of collective violence. In J. Fawcett, ed. *Dynamics of Violence.* Chicago: American Medical Association.

Wolf, E.; Gedo, J. E.; and Terman, D. M. 1972. On the adolescent process as a transformation of the self. *Journal of Youth and Adolescence* 1:257–272.

15 NORMAL FEMALE AND MALE ADOLESCENT PSYCHOLOGICAL DEVELOPMENT: AN OVERVIEW OF THEORY AND RESEARCH

MARK J. BLOTCKY AND JOHN G. LOONEY

Adolescents have always been perplexing to adults who find them frustrating and confounding but likewise enchanting, fascinating, and inspiring. Perceived as impulsive and pleasure seeking, adolescents offer the hope of the future, a sense of immortality, and a vicarious opportunity for those whose youth has been spent. Adolescent idealism becomes the guidelight of the future; their contempt for hypocrisy, the outspoken moral leadership of tomorrow. Through changing times punctuated by despised wars, radical hair styles, miniskirts, and marijuana, certain landmarks of development remain constant.

Adolescent psychological development is a complex, intricate, and tortuous road. Its picture has been painted with only the broadest of strokes with large areas yet to be etched. Normality itself is a difficult concept far overshadowed by interest in pathology, the latter seemingly more easily defined. Nevertheless, a large body of literature touches on many aspects of adolescent development and can be organized into theoretical papers on the one hand and research papers on the other. This discussion of normal adolescent development is, therefore, organized from three major perspectives. The first is theory and encompasses what we think we know—our hypotheses and working formulations supported largely from clinical experience with patients. The second perspective represents what we do know—that is, what research data reveal. The final section integrates theory with research findings and suggests some important areas yet to be explored.

The concept of mental health is both a conceptual and definitional quandary. Normality (Offer and Sabshin 1963) may be defined in at least four ways: health, or the absence of disease; utopia, or optimal functioning; the average, that is a statistical norm; or process, a more complex definition involving change and growth. Normality implies not only adaptive functioning but also the proper integration of psychic agencies. It depends on compromises, an internal balance of forces, and a workable adaptation to external demands. Each developmental stage faces anew the task of harmonizing old fixations, defenses, and drive organization which are now discordant with the new phase's specific task. The result is an increasingly differentiated synthesis. Reviewing normal development, one quickly realizes that authors define normality using various criteria. Psychoanalytic writings usually use the utopia model; researchers, the statistical model. Clinicians pragmatically turn to the model of health.

Theoretical Perspective of Adolescent Development

The traditional psychoanalytic understanding of adolescence has best been articulated by Blos (1962, 1967, 1970), who divides the period into preadolescence, early adolescence, adolescence proper, and late adolescence and who, along with a number of others (Freud 1958; Geleerd 1961; Josselyn 1954; Kestenberg 1967a, 1967b, 1968), offers a rich description of the developmental process. The following discussion draws heavily from these landmark works.

Preadolescence

Defined as roughly that period from nine to eleven years of age, preadolescence is marked by a loosening of the structure of latency just prior to major pubertal changes. While latency has been an age of mastery of social relationships—work, play, and reality—preadolescence is characterized by the resurgence of infantile drives which transiently take precedence over social adaptation and the mastery of current reality. Early on there is a generalized increase in drive activity. The preadolescent becomes hungrier, greedier, nastier, dirtier, more curious, more assertive, and more self-centered than he was the year before. Defensive organization and drive modifications which were previously effective are no longer in harmony with the adolescent's changing physical and social status. The increase in drive intensity clearly occurs before any physical changes are noticeable and revives old

185

wishes, affects, conflicts, and fantasies related to infantile experiences. However, they are clothed in relatively ego-syntonic garb disguising their more primitive origins. Ego organization is, at times, characterized by stringent attempts at warding off impulses, while at other times allowing unrestrained expressions of drive activity.

Preadolescence is marked by changing patterns of identification. Old primary identifications with the family weaken, while new identifications with peers and their values assume greater vitality. Adolescents find themselves conflicted in their loyalty to parents on the one hand and to peers on the other. Peers are often superficially and outspokenly antiadult. Similarly, parents are frequently resentful of the adolescents' new friends. In consequence, adolescents experience shame and guilt in relation to both loyalties. They feel conflicted about their childish dependency and are easily embarrassed when they submit to the rules of adult politeness and good manners. At times they react shamelessly, grossly, and with great bravado extending to counterphobic risk taking such as fast driving, heavy drinking, or gorging. The young adolescent may openly flaunt his abilities to adults in order to enhance his peer relationships but at the cost of being perceived by adults as fresh or a smart aleck. Security is sought in isosexual cliques rather than mixed groups. Within these gangs, bravery and courage are displayed against the enemy usually identified as all adults, parents in particular, but occasionally as the opposite sex. Communication with adults is commonly devalued except during times of serious stress when provocative behavior literally melts away allowing the youngster to turn again to his parents for support.

While both boys and girls show evidence of regression, there are certain fairly typical sex-defined differences. The adolescent boy demonstrates rather massive regression as he fearfully turns away from girls with contempt. This contempt is evidenced in name calling, depreciation of girls as sissies, and repulsion with traditionally feminine traits and activities. Thus dependency, passivity, physical incoordination, concern about dress and manners, and interest in cooking or housework are derogated. While drive diffusion is seen in both sexes, it is far more apparent in boys and, for them, often is the primary preadolescent defense. Drive diffusion may be defined as regression under stress to more primitive areas with more generalized drive discharge. It manifests in increased motor activity particularly in pregenital outlets: toilet jokes and noises, dirty words, messy play, and crude eating fads. The regression defends against pregenital and oedipal threats which are now more alive in reality for the adolescent. He is in a sense an adult, and many of his fantasies could actually be realized.

186

The preadolescent task for the girl is resisting the regressive pull toward her mother and renouncing pregenital gratification. She rarely displays drive diffusion to the depth observed in boys, but instead defends against regression with its attendant homosexual threat using a pseudo-oedipal configuration involving sexual fantasies and wishes. This turn to the opposite sex is not true femininity, but largely defensive. Her interest in boys is heavily colored by a longing for possession and a search for completeness. Her defensive pattern is expressed by increased activity, bossiness, and tomboyish behavior that denies dependence on mother while identifying with father.

Early Adolescence

Roughly the age span of eleven to fourteen, early adolescence is marked by a more specific onslaught of genital impulses. This intensification is a double-edged sword offering the opportunity for increased gratification outside the family while jeopardizing the adolescent's familial ties with incestuous coloring. Disengagement from primary love objects and withdrawal of object libido therefore ensue. Introjects lose some of their former cathexis, weakening the adolescent's control system and allowing a softening of the superego. The adolescent may become inattentive and impulsive at school, continues devaluing his parents, and often appears more overtly rebellious.

The result of loosening parental ties is a growing need to seek out new objects. The adolescent chooses a same-sexed friend whose talents and personality complement his own. The athlete takes up with the bookworm; the introvert, with the extrovert. This idealized friend is perceived as possessing traits the adolescent feels are missing in himself. Internalization of these character traits, values, morals, and achievements result in a new psychic agency, the kindly, noncritical ego ideal. This internalization broadens the youngster's capacity for self-observation and serves as an internal support in contradistinction to the critical superego function. It thus secures esteem from within.

Sexuality during early adolescence makes some rather significant developmental advances. Heterosexual relationships remain tentative, transient if intense, and largely frightening. Nevertheless, there is clearly increased interest if not preoccupation with sexuality. Frank sexual behavior at this age is usually either experimental or defensive, though a few rare early adolescents may be able to form true heterosexual relationships with buds of adult intimacy. The relationship with the special same-sexed chum has both homo-sexual and narcissistic components. The sexual aspects are usually much too frightening for the adolescent boy though it is more common for a thirteen-year-old girl to have a crush on an older adolescent girl.

The early adolescent's bodily concept plays an increasingly important role in his psychic life. Physical attractiveness, disability, or disfigurement come to have new meaning. Internalized dynamic forces influence all those perceptions which are then organized into the body concept or body image. Family attitudes regarding the meaning of the adolescent's body have embossed indelible impressions on him from infancy to his present pubertal state. The way he has been touched, admired, looked at, perceived, all affect his own feelings about his body. Sociocultural ideals, so rigidly conveyed through television and advertising, provide the ideal image the adolescent often uses as a template for comparison.

One final area of early adolescent development is the acquisition of logical, abstract thinking. The youngster now has the ability to reason on pure hypothesis. The latency-age child used more concrete operations related to objects or perceptive events. Thinking processes could not become independent of the concrete. However, the adolescent, now equipped with abstract thinking, is not only able to progress educationally but also able to achieve greater social integration. This new capacity for introspection and self-awareness allows for more intense self-scrutiny. Everything becomes food for thought, for endless discussion and rehashing. Even the youngster's own thought processes are exciting to him. The adolescent critically evaluates the world, ethics, values, science, and religion and out of such questioning slowly discovers an identity. He precipitates a new sense of where and how he belongs within the world of people, organizations, social systems, and generations.

Adolescence Proper

Adolescence proper, or mid adolescence, spanning roughly ages fourteen to seventeen, encompasses most of what is more commonly considered adolescence. By adolescence proper the youngster's emotional life is becoming deeper, richer, wider, and more intense. Four major tasks may be defined in adolescence proper: (1) resolution of the rekindled oedipal complex; (2) separation from parents with new object finding; (3) formation of stable extrafamilial object relationships; and (4) finalization of sexual identification.

Sexual encounters during preadolescence and often early adolescence are best viewed as the psychological equivalent of masturbation, emphasizing their autoerotic and narcissistic components. However, during adolescence proper many youngsters begin to experience true mutuality. Homosexual fears are often as active as castration anxiety or superego anxiety. Incestuous longings are too frightening, and their eruption is often poorly veiled beneath mother-son and father-daughter fights. The excitement can be intense, and the arguments seemingly endless. Triangulation often increases the furor, excitement, and fear.

As the youngster's sexual strivings turn him away from his family, new support is required. Despite all the sputtering, moaning, and cries to the contrary, separation even at this age is threatening. Depreciation and now overt rebellion ease the emancipation process, yet derogation of parents must be carefully titrated. Successful emancipation from the family requires that the adolescent modify his view of his parents as omniscient while maintaining a positive internalized image of them.

Blos (1967), emphasizing the structural changes that accompany this separation process, has termed it "the second individuation process of adolescence." The devaluation of parents during adolescence proper leads to object hunger and an increased investment in self with partial transient identifications. The withdrawal of cathexis from objects results in hyperacuity of the senses with a longing to stimulate them, a reveling in the beauty of nature, and a preoccupation with cosmic concerns. The decathexis of internalized objects also results in an intense longing for cheap thrills and immediate soothing, a turning to drugs, and a surrealistic wonder at the world. Parents' praise if often scorned with such retorts as, "I don't care what you think of me!" This intense resentment belies the youngster's underlying struggle with dependency which is so easily triggered by parental praise. The defensive result then is the stereotyped, cantankerous, and arrogant adolescent.

During adolescence proper, the ego develops a capacity to secure a sense of self-esteem on the basis of realistic achievements. For if the adolescent no longer wishes to depend upon his parents, he must be able to produce in order to maintain self-esteem. Trial action and rich fantasies are typical of this age. Regressive fantasies may delay action, but creative fantasies—practicing in one's head—become a means of actually planning for the future.

Many adolescent relationships are quite intense and have a narcissistic or "as-if" quality reflecting the adolescent's need to relate to others through a longing for completion or possession. Resonance, a major facet of this process, involves the search for a heterosexual partner who possesses all the qualities which the adolescent must relinquish in himself in order to establish firmly his own sexual identity. The boy places his passive, tender qualities onto a girl friend for whom he then has the capacity to care deeply. The girl places her aggressive, sexual qualities onto her boyfriend with whom she can likewise develop a more intense relationship. Through this process adolescents become more definitively identified with their own sexual position, either masculine or feminine, as these identifications are elaborated in their own minds. This crystallization of sexual identity has been facilitated during early adolescence by the internalization of homosexual libido in the ego ideal.

True mutuality is first within reach during adolescence proper. Caring no longer needs to be separated into sexual and tender love. Sex loses much of its anal, messy quality. The adolescent boy no longer needs to villify a girl in order to have sex with her. He now has the capacity to become enthralled with a particular girl friend despite lingering fears of submission and emotional surrender, both of which are equated with the passivity he views as feminine. The adolescent girl struggles with overvaluing and idealizing a boy without acknowledging his sexuality and (like her male counterpart) is only able to enter into a tender, romantic love relationship after finalizing her sexual identity. Promiscuity may reflect both idealization of the male and a defense against regression.

This age also confronts the youngster with many new demands and new situations. Old habits and childhood excuses must be abandoned. There is a disturbing sense of estrangement with soul-searching questions: Who am I? What am I worth? Who cares? The adolescent no longer understands himself or what he is becoming. He is no longer a child, and this causes problems for both himself and his parents. While two years ago his parents were supportive to him, now they are regressive. For support he turns to his peer group, where he is as much a conformist as ever.

Late Adolescence

Encompassing ages seventeen to nineteen, late adolescence is characterized by ego synthesis. The tasks involve real separation from parents, greater autonomy and social responsibility, and a new capacity for intimacy. Lifelong goals and ambitions, as well as education and work options, become important. It is a phase of consolidation similar to that seen in latency with enhancement of the conflict-free sphere of the ego. Affective and volitional processes are better integrated. The adolescent becomes more predictable, more productive, better able to work and to play, and more amenable to negotiation and compromise. Frustration tolerance and the capacity to delay gratification are markedly improved. Self-esteem is more consistent, mood less labile. The adolescent must delineate those things which really matter in life, his philosophy and values, and in accomplishing this solidify his own social identity. This new sense of social integration diminishes the resentment of authority figures. Cathexis of self and objects is now more reliable as narcissism comes under better control. Stabilization of the psychic apparatus results in better drive regulation, harmony of ego defenses, and more modulated and effective superego functions. And the close of adolescence is marked by significant stabilization of character structure which will persist over time.

Review of Research Findings

Over the last fifteen years, a large number of cross-sectional, longitudinal, and epidemiologic studies have focused on defining and understanding normal adolescent development. Most of this work examines the conceptualization of adolescence as a period of inevitable chaos, ego disruption, and maladaptive behavior. This "turmoil view" (Oldham 1978) describes a large number and variety of symptoms which are transient, fluctuating, and essentially benign in most adolescents, but hard to differentiate from true psychiatric illness in others. Precise diagnosis is often held to be difficult and prognosis of symptomatology nearly impossible. It posits, in fact, that adolescents whose development is more level may be at risk for more serious psychopathology than those adolescents who are more symptomatic or chaotic. Biologic factors with the disruptive effects of increased drives, the yet-to-be-consolidated adolescent ego, and the adult-alien behavior of adolescents are all central to this view. Anna Freud (1958) described adolescent development as evidencing symptom formation not only of neurotic configuration but also of borderline and psychotic form and suggested that differential diagnosis between these developmental upheavals and true psychopathology is quite difficult. The research data reviewed here clarify these issues considerably.

Most of the studies involve choosing a sample of adolescents, cross-sectional or longitudinal interviews and questionnaires, and at times psychological testing and/or the collection of data from parents and others. While there are often methodologic liabilities, the findings will merely be presented here as they stand.

Douvan and Adelson (1966) studied a large population of junior high and high school boys and girls using both interviews and questionnaires. These adolescents were generally trusting of their parents, derived much of their self-esteem from parental approval, and shared a core of common values with them. Rebellion was chiefly evident in disagreements about such things as music and dress. They showed little evidence of inner turmoil or ego disruption and, contrariwise, appeared rather conservative and compliant.

Silber, Hamburg, Coelho, Murphey, Rosenberg, and Pearlin (1961) selected fifteen high school seniors on the basis of their academic and social success. These students felt a sense of competence and mastery. They described reaching out for new experiences and saw themselves as gradually evolving in a desired direction.

Grinker (1962), studying an older population of well-adjusted college freshmen, reported similar findings. These late adolescents demonstrated impressive ego strengths, supportive interpersonal relationships, and a healthy sense of self-esteem. There was no indication of severe inner turmoil or identity crisis, and Grinker rather emphasized adaptive coping mechanisms.

Offer and his colleagues (Offer 1967, 1969; Offer, Marcus, and Offer 1970; Offer and Offer 1968, 1969; Offer and Sabshin 1963; Offer, Sabshin, and Marcus 1965) have reported the most comprehensive and convincing studies of normal adolescent development to date. This work focuses on a sample of average or modal adolescent boys over a seven-year period including their four years in high school. Seventy-three boys in two high schools were interviewed six times. They were also administered a self-image questionnaire covering a wide range of variables. The subjects were self-selected and represented normality in the sense of the statistical average; that is, the extremes of psychopathology and superior adjustment were eliminated.

Rebellion during early adolescence (eleven to fourteen years old) was rather undramatic, but noted. Chronic disagreements focused on matters of dress, household chores, and curfew hours. Rebellious behavior did not expand into delinquency or extreme emotional upheaval, but instead was seen as central to the emancipation process. Though there were transient periods of anxiety, depression, guilt, and shame, these adolescents did not suffer serious fluctuation of affect. Mood swings were not overwhelming and were usually related to external stress. Only 7 percent of this normative group evidenced significant emotional problems.

Sexuality was conflicted for these boys who felt uncomfortable about impulses, uneasy and apprehensive with girls, and unable to discuss their concerns with their parents. In early adolescence, sexuality was handled with denial and repression, and there was little dating. However, by their senior year most were dating and enjoying relationships with girls. In this group of boys, sexual intercourse was acknowledged by 10 percent during the third high school year, 30 percent during the first post–high school year, and 50 percent by the third post–high school year. These figures probably underestimate the sexual activity of today's adolescent boys. None of this group described overt homosexual behavior.

Finally, Offer and his associates confirm Douvan and Adelson's (1966) impression that, parental devaluation notwithstanding, adolescents tend to share their parents' core value system. While these boys could be critical of their parents, for the most part they respected them, wanted to be like them, and felt understood by them. Additionally, the vast majority felt their parents disciplined them reasonably and fairly. Complementary to this finding, parents reported a sense of overall satisfaction with their sons.

In summary, Offer reports that normal adolescent boys, while struggling with an upsurgence of drives, were not overwhelmed but instead showed considerable adaptive and coping strength. Heterosexual relations, at first tenuous, became more satisfying in late adolescence. Parental values were generally accepted, and parents perceived as supportive and reasonable. Familial conflict was manageable, and independence was gradually achieved. Self-satisfaction and parental satisfaction were the norms. Identity consolidation and true intimacy were within reach though yet to be achieved. Overall, these findings are consistent with theoretical constructs, but emphasize ego control rather than disintegration. The data do not support speculations proposing severe inner turmoil, significant ego weakness, or terribly conflictual relationships with parents and adults as part of normal adolescence. Offer is at work collecting similar data regarding adolescent girls, for, unfortunately, very little research is available focusing specifically on their developmental process.

Masterson and associates (Masterson 1967a, 1967b, 1968; Masterson and Washburne 1966) matched 101 clinic patients—boys and girls ages twelve to eighteen—with 101 nonpatient controls. Roughly 70 percent of both clinic and control populations experienced symptomatic anxiety, and 40 percent of each group evidenced depressive phenomena expressed as feelings of inadequacy. However, the patient group had about 50 percent more total symptoms than the control group. Also in contrast to the controls, the clinic group demonstrated more acting-out behavior (17 percent vs. 5 percent), more impaired school and social functioning, and more disturbed family relationships. The nonpatient sample displayed minimal symptoms, good social adjustment, and satisfying family relationships. Symptoms in these healthy adolescents were generally single, mild, and episodic. Masterson's five-year follow-up of seventy-two of the clinic patients found that symptom patterns persisted, with two-thirds of the patients remaining moderately or severely impaired. His conclusion is that initial diagnosis in adolescents may be troublesome with regard to the precise illness but not in distinguishing normative adolescent developmental stress from psychiatric disturbance.

Rutter, Graham, Chadwick, and Yule (1976), using interviews and questionnaires, studied a large British sample of rural boys and girls ages fourteen to fifteen. Outer turmoil involving rebellious behavior characterized by verbal disagreements with parents over hair style, clothes, and other relatively trivial matters was common. Feelings of inadequacy occurred in about 20 percent of the sample, but clinical depression occurred much less often. Communication problems with parents were reported by 25 percent of the adolescents. Notably only 4 percent described these as having increased during adolescence. Psychiatric disorder was found in 10 percent of the sample, and altercations with parents were more than twice as frequent in this subgroup. Rutter's findings again suggest that transient symptoms are common in adolescents but are easily distinguishable from psychiatric disturbance.

Weiner and DelGaudio (1976) studied psychopathology and symptomatology with regard to developmental changes and the diagnosis of situational disorder in adolescent patients. Their findings concur with Masterson's that adolescent symptom patterns persist and become more differentiated over time. They disagree with the notion that adolescent developmental turmoil is ubiquitous and question the sometimes glib handling of adolescent symptom formation.

Looney and Gunderson (1978) followed a large sample of young men, most in late adolescence, who had been given the diagnosis of transient situational disturbance. Based on three or more years of follow-up, a substantial proportion of these patients manifested personality disorder and 20 percent required hospitalization. These findings further suggest that adolescent symptomatology should not be too quickly dismissed.

A quite fascinating longitudinal study by Peskin and Livson (1972) examines the relationship of prepubertal, postpubertal, and adult psychological functioning. Their hypothesis was that certain clusters of behavior at specific developmental stages could reliably predict psychological health at adulthood. The results suggest that such a relationship does exist, and that adult psychological health is significantly predictable from multiple behaviors assessed at preadolescence defined as ages eleven through thirteen.

They believe that preadolescent boys were likely to become psychologically healthy adults if they were expressive and outgoing in social situations, had adequate control over aggression, and were free of irritability and temper tantrums. Preadolescent girls who were described as independent, self-confident, and intellectually curious were likely to become healthy adults. Though a less consistent finding, certain early adolescent behaviors tended to be predictive of later mental health but did so in an opposite direction from preadolescent behaviors. For example, four preadolescent to early adolescent patterns which predicted adult psychological health for girls were these reversals: (1) from rare to frequent whining; (2) from high to low self-confidence; (3) from independence to dependence; and (4) from good impulse control to explosive temper. Indeed, the data suggest that psychological health is even more predictable if these sequences take place. For both sexes the pattern is characterized by a move from a more controlled and self-directed preadolescence to a more stressful or crisis-ridden early adolescence. This work is especially reminiscent of theoretical formulations suggesting that a steady equilibrium during adolescence is somewhat abnormal (Freud 1958).

Peskin and Livson (1972) also compared adolescents with early and late pubertal onsets. Early-maturing boys tended to be more inhibited cognitively, socially, and athletically from puberty through adolescence proper. Late-maturing boys evidenced a more intense thrust of activity, more exploratory behavior, greater social initiative, and more intellectual curiosity. From projective testing, the early maturer seemed to struggle with instinctual expression by quite rigid defensiveness accompanied by abrupt, episodic tension-releasing behavior. However, early- and late-maturing males, on reaching adulthood, differ less in degree of psychological health than in character style. The late maturer has prepared himself for greater mastery of and safety in the intrapsychic environment, whereas the early maturer feels safer in his self-definition within the social environment.

The findings regarding girls remain less clear. Peskin and Livson suggest that the early-maturing girl is in an undisguised crisis. She responds to her early maturity neither with her male counterpart's overcontrol nor with his reliance on social supports and rewards. And while the early-maturing girl evidences more whining and explosiveness, diminished sociability and increased introversion, Peskin and Livson emphasize the reversal which takes place by adulthood. In fact, by adulthood, she has surpassed her late-maturing peer in overall psychological health. In summary, early-maturing males control strong pubertal drives by concentrated efforts to master the outside world. Early-maturing females move further into the emotional, introspective sphere and achieve control by directly experiencing affective states.

Conclusions

Adolescence is a period of regression, recapitulation of earlier stages of development, and movement toward autonomy. Contributions to a theory of adolescent development (usually developed by clinicians working with disturbed adolescents) purport serious inner turmoil and powerful forces in conflict. Empirical studies, on the other hand, emphasize adaptive strengths and coping skills.

Theoretical formulations and research findings do not significantly conflict with regard to an understanding of basic adolescent tasks and the stresses of growing up in modern society. However, they differ considerably with respect to their predictions regarding adolescent functioning. Cross-sectional and longitudinal studies find adolescence to be an orderly, modulated process. Reports emphasize ego strength and do not describe psychotic-like regressive phenomena. Serious loss of control and control conflicts with parents are not evident. Data-based reports instead indicate youngsters perceive their parents as supportive and reasonable. Research suggests sexuality is troublesome to the adolescent, but much more manageable than theory predicts. The onslaught of sexual impulses does not result in counterphobic acting out or overt behavioral regression. The reawakening of the oedipal constellation is not normatively associated with behavior reflecting intense excitement, fear, or conflict. And while heterosexual relations are tenuous in early adolescence, there is a steady progression toward intimacy in late adolescence. Likewise, while research finds the emancipation process to be difficult, it is characterized by some order and not torn by excessive rebellion. There may be some minor, early devaluation of parents, and disagreements about day-to-day matters certainly occur, but seriously disruptive conflict is not part of normal adolescent separation. Instead, researchers find parental values accepted. Persistent delinquent acts or extreme emotional upheaval suggest disturbance. Though the stresses of adolescence are substantial, regressive behavior such as drug usage rarely became self-destructive in any of the samples of normal adolescents studied to date.

Important research questions are unanswered. The Committee on Research of the American Society for Adolescent Psychiatry (1977) has outlined three broad areas of needed investigation: (1) further definition of the adolescent developmental process; (2) the assessment of adolescent psychopathology and treatment; and (3) the delineation of special problem areas. With regard to the first area, what would happen to the research data as well as to theoretical formulations if instead of chronologic age, physiologic parameters were used to define developmental stages? Would developmental patterns become clearer and more discrete, and would better staging alter the work which attempts to predict healthy adult outcome based on adolescent variables? Another intriguing problem is the relationship between physiologic change and hormone balance as they relate to psychological integration. Is there some biologically timed triggering in the central nervous system that relates to behavioral changes, or is what is observed primarily related to drive intensification and resultant new defensive patterns? Further, one of the more controversial areas in mental health today is that of sexual orientation. Sexual issues are significantly shaped during adolescence, and one wonders if the work that has been done with children regarding sexual orientation does not need expansion into a more meticulous view of how sexual orientation is influenced by the adolescent process.

With regard to the second area of needed investigation outlined by the Committee on Research, one would like to predict more accurately childhood antecedents of adolescent pathological syndromes, familial and social/cultural factors leading to disturbance, and the course and natural history of psychopathological states. Certainly the effectiveness of our various clinical interventions needs to be documented systematically.

Finally, with regard to special problem areas, a great deal of thought needs to be given to the adolescent's ever-changing place in society. What are his or her needs? What educational and vocational options are available? How is the adolescent affected by the legal system, increased drug abuse, the erosion of the neighborhood school, the availability of birth control and abortion, increased sexual freedom, and the possibly rapidly changing American family structure? How many of today's youths need mental health services? How do physical handicaps and mental retardation affect adolescent development? All these issues and many more remain unclear. It is clear, however, that while we have learned a good deal, there are many large and gaping holes in our knowledge and plenty of work remains for both theoreticians and researchers.

A final observation regarding the theoretical and research literature seems germane. One is struck by the relative paucity of research data available on adolescents when compared to the massive clinical efforts directed toward them, the latter being commonly reported in our literature. As clinicians, we do all kinds of things to help troubled youngsters, but, as noted, we infrequently involve ourselves in research-based efforts to understand the nature of normal adolescent growth and why some teenagers deviate from that progression, or to document the effectiveness of our clinical efforts. Our science is secondary to our art, and it behooves established clinicians to become involved in research to establish more solid scientific underpinnings of knowledge.

REFERENCES

Berman, S. 1970 Alienation: an essential process of the psychology of adolescence. *Journal of the American Academy of Child Psychiatry* 9:233–250.
Blos, P. 1962. *On Adolescence: A Psychoanalytic Interpretation*. New York: Free Press.
Blos, P. 1967. The second individuation process of adolescence. *Psychoanalytic Study of the Child* 22:162–186.
Blos, P. 1970. *The Young Adolescent*. New York: Free Press.
Committee on Research of the American Society for Adolescent Psychiatry 1977. Presented at Annual Meeting, Toronto.
Douvan, E., and Adelson, J. 1966. *The Adolescent Experience*. New York: Wiley.
Freud, A. 1958. Adolescence. *Psychoanalytic Study of the Child* 13:255–278.
Freud, A. 1965. *Normality and Pathology in Childhood*. New York: International Universities Press.
Geleerd, E. R. 1961. Some aspects of ego vicissitudes in adolescence. *Journal of the American Psychoanalytic Association* 9:394–405.
Grinker, R. R., Sr. 1962. Mentally healthy young males (homoclites). *Archives of General Psychiatry* 6:405–453.
Josselyn, I. 1954. The ego in adolescence. *American Journal of Orthopsychiatry* 24:233–237.
Kestenberg, J. 1967a. Phases of adolescence with suggestions for a correlation of psychic and hormonal organizations. I. *Journal of the American Academy of Child Psychiatry* 6:426–463.
Kestenberg, J. 1967b. Phases of adolescence with suggestions for a correlation of psychic and hormonal organizations. II. *Journal of the American Academy of Child Psychiatry* 6:577–614.
Kestenberg, J. 1968. Phases of adolescence with suggestions for a correlation of psychic and hormonal organizations. III. *Journal of the American Academy of Child Psychiatry* 7:108–151.
Looney, J., and Gunderson, E. 1978. Transient situational disturbances: course and outcome. *American Journal of Psychiatry* 135:660–663.
Masterson, J. 1967a. *The Psychiatric Dilemma of Adolescence*. Boston: Little, Brown.

Masterson, J. 1967b. The symptomatic adolescent five years later: he didn't grow out of it. *American Journal of Psychiatry* 123:1338–1345.

Masterson, J. 1968. The psychiatric significance of adolescent turmoil. *American Journal of Psychiatry* 124:1549–1554.

Masterson, J. 1972. *Treatment of the Borderline Adolescent: A Developmental Approach.* New York: Wiley.

Masterson, J., and Washburne, A. 1966. The symptomatic adolescent: psychiatric illness or adolescent turmoil. *American Journal of Psychiatry* 122:1240–1247.

Offer, D. 1967. Normal adolescents: interview, strategy and selected results. *Archives of General Psychiatry* 17:285–290.

Offer, D. 1969. *The Psychological World of the Teenager.* New York: Basic.

Offer, D.; Marcus, D.; and Offer, J. L. 1970. A longitudinal study of normal adolescent boys. *American Journal of Psychiatry* 126(7): 917–924.

Offer, D., and Offer, J. L. 1968. Profiles of normal adolescent girls. *Archives of General Psychiatry* 19:513–522.

Offer, D., and Offer, J. L. 1969. Growing-up: a follow-up study of normal adolescents. *Seminars in Psychiatry* 1:46–56.

Offer, D., and Sabshin, M. 1963. The psychiatrist and the normal adolescent. *Archives of General Psychiatry* 9:427–432.

Offer, D.; Sabshin, M.; and Marcus, D. 1965. Clinical evaluation of normal adolescents. *American Journal of Psychiatry* 121:864–872.

Oldham, D. 1978. Adolescent turmoil: a myth revisited. *Adolescent Psychiatry* 6:267–279.

Peskin, H., and Livson, N. 1972. Pre- and postpubertal personality and adult psychologic functioning. *Seminars in Psychiatry* 4(4): 343–353.

Rutter, M.; Graham, P.; Chadwick, O.; and Yule, W. 1976. Adolescent turmoil: fact or fiction. *Journal of Child Psychology and Psychiatry and Allied Disciplines* 17:35–56.

Silber, E.; Coelho, G. V.; Murphey, E. B.; Hamburg, D. A.; Pearlin, L. I.; and Rosenberg, M. 1961. Competent adolescents coping with college decisions. *Archives of General Psychiatry* 5:517–527.

Silber, E.; Hamburg, D. A.; Coelho, G. V.; Murphey, E. B.; Rosenberg, M.; and Pealin, L. I.. 1961. Adaptive behavior in competent adolescents: coping with the anticipation of college. *Archives of General Psychiatry* 5:354–365.

Weiner, I., and DelGaudio, A. 1976. Psychopathology in adolescence. *Archives of General Psychiatry* 33:187–193.

JEFFREY R. MITCHELL

As part of a growing interest in human development, mental health professionals have focused increasing attention on the adolescent growth period. Early investigators portrayed adolescence as a period of crisis and turbulence. Chaotic behavior was considered normative. Diagnosis and treatment was a hazardous, if not impossible, venture. More recent investigations, however, have challenged the notion of normal turmoil in adolescence. Findings from studies of normal adolescence indicate that the discontinuity between this stage of growth and adjoining stages may not be as extreme and prolonged as implied in earlier writings. Studies also show that many disturbed adolescents do not "grow out of it," as had previously been believed. This chapter will review the conflicting statements made about adolescents and discuss their effects on diagnosis and treatment.

Early Investigations

Although adolescent psychiatry and psychology are relatively new areas of study, the interest and concern of adults about young people is not a recent development. Statements about the vagaries of youth have been attributed to Socrates and Aristotle that could easily be mistaken for modern day complaints. Many of Shakespeare's writings, particularly *Romeo and Juliet* and *Hamlet,* can be viewed as sensitive psychological statements about youthful passions and the passage from adolescence into adulthood. Historical studies (Bakan 1971; Kett 1977) illustrate, however, that the long-standing concern by adults about adolescence became an obsession in the past century—perhaps because social changes such as industrialization, child labor laws, and compulsory school attendance created a large class of unemployed young people who somehow needed to be both restrained and satisfied.

G. Stanley Hall's (1904) two-volume publication is often referred to as the prototypic study of adolescence. In his treatise, Hall described adolescence as a period of *sturm und drang* (storm and stress). He was influenced by phylogenetic theory (ontogeny recapitulates phylogeny), explaining the adolescent growth period as a reincarnation of man's precivilized existence as a primitive, tribal being. Although Hall's attempt to apply embryological theory to human psychological development did not endure, his notion of adolescense as a period of chaos has remained in the minds of scientists and laymen alike. Colorful terms like "turmoil," "turbulence," and "rebellion" have been applied so frequently to adolescents that there seems to be a cultural expectation that anything, and probably everything, will happen with the onset of puberty.

Although Freud did not write at length about puberty, his *Three Essays on Sexuality* (Freud 1905) and his comments on adolescence sprinkled throughout other papers (Klumpner 1978) provided impetus for later, more detailed studies by Jones (1922), Aichorn (1925), and Bernfield (1938). The resulting postoedipal developmental picture was described as one of a long, quiescent latency period, from approximately six to twelve years of age, during which drives and impulses were steadily held in check by repression. With the onset of puberty, however, the psyche undergoes rapid change. Drives increase in strength, with a subsequent reawakening of preoedipal and oedipal conflicts. The ego becomes weakened, owing to a loosening of the repression barrier. Infantile object ties (parents) are no longer adequate or desirable means of support. The developmental goal is separation from the family, but the process of detachment is characterized by ambivalence over dependency, rapid fluctuations in mood, and impulsive behavior.

Anna Freud made important contributions to our understanding of adolescent psychology in her study of ego defense mechanisms (1936) and her later paper on adolescence (1958). She focused on the disruptive influence of the sudden increase of instinctual drives during adolescence and the equally disturbing libidinalization of infantile ties. In her view, a variety of pathological defenses, such as displacement, reversal of affect, withdrawl into the self, regression, asceticism, and inability to compromise may be mobilized to deal with drives and threatening parental attachments.

Although these expositions of defenses were illuminating, her study of adolescence (Freud 1958) has led to confusion and controversy over the issues of normality versus pathology. In that paper, she stated that pathological defenses could combine with other defenses and, if used in moderation, could be part of normal growth, creating a condition that she refers to as "adolescent upset." Commenting upon the prevalence of this condition, she observed that "the upholding of a steady equilibrium during the adolescent process is in itself abnormal." She further comments upon the difficulties clinicians face when attempting to distinquish normal adolescent upset from psychopathology, since "adolescent manifestations come close to the symptom formation of the neurotic, psychotic, or dissocial disorder and merge almost imperceptively into borderline states, initial, frustrated, or fully fledged forms of almost all the mental illnesses."

As for treatment implications, she states that "while an adolescent remains inconsistent and unpredictable in his behavior, he may suffer, but he does not seem to me to be in need of treatment. I think that he should be given time and scope to work out his own solution. Rather, it may be his parents who need help and guidance so as to be able to bear with him."

The themes of normal adolescent turmoil being barely distinguishable from psychopathology and withholding of treatment are common to a number of important psychoanalytic studies. Josselyn (1954) wrote that "typical adolescent behavior seems to be characterized by a lack of integration," and compares this failure of the ego, which she terms "ego exhaustion," with that found in adult neuroses and psychoses. The rejection of dependency upon parental figures was also described by Josselyn as if it were an all-or-nothing phenomenon, making it impossible to use identification as a defense. Sublimation in the form of athletics, work, peer relationships, and experimental sexual play is also an inadequate defense because such activities are "too closely linked to their origin" (i.e., forbidden oedipal and preoedipal drives). Like Anna Freud, Josselyn cautions against vigorous therapeutic efforts because "the [adolescent's] ego is too exhausted to build adequate defenses, and therefore cannot stand the additional strain of further disturbing insight." A wait-and-see attitude is prescribed because adolescence "offers an opportunity for the spontaneous resolution of conflicts."

A number of similar papers—stressing a combination of themes, such as the normal turbulence of adolescence, the rejection of parental figures, the failure of sublimation and identification, the inadvisability of diagnosing and treating adolescents, and the concern about "good" adolescents who are rigidly defending against drives and certain to develop disturbances in later life—have been produced by a number of important analytic writers (Blos 1962, 1967; Erikson 1956; Gardener 1954; Geleerd 1957; Lindemann 1964; Spiegel 1961; and Winnicott 1971). The influence of their thinking can also be seen in the monograph on *Normal Adolescence,* published by the Group for the Advancement of Psychiatry (1968). The analytic writings mentioned contain generalizations about adolescence based upon direct work with adolescent patients and the recollections of adult analysands about their teenage years. Anna Freud (1958) and Josselyn (1954) both preface their papers with comments about the limitations of this kind of study. Adult patients readily produce memories of the events of their adolescence, but the memories are dissociated from the affects which accompanied them at the time. Also, direct analytic work with adolescents can be frustrating because the analyst meets with strong resistances. Despite these reservations, it has been noted (Masterson 1968) that many authors frequently switch, sometimes in midsentence, from descriptions of their young patients to general statements about adolescence without acknowledging that this transformation has occurred. Anthony (1969) criticizes this kind of generalization and views it as a symptom of adult anxiety about adolescents, paralleling the media's tendency to equate adolescence with delinquency:

The clinician does little to correct this misconception since he himself is constantly confronted with extreme reactions and may eventually be led to regard them as typical rather than atypical and infrequent. The "good" adolescent, although representing perhaps three-quarters of the adolescent population, is so effectively camouflaged by his conformity to the standards of a given culture that he is scarcely credited with existence. . . . To compound the mischief further, the stereotypes have also functioned as mirrors held up to the adolescent by society, reflecting an image of himself that the adolescent gradually comes to regard as authentic and according to which he shapes his behavior. In that way, he completes the circle of expectation.

Recent Investigations

The concept of normative adolescent turmoil has not been universally accepted, however, and has undergone critical scrutiny in recent years. Mead's (1928) anthropological studies did not find any evidence of storm and stress among Samoan youth. Grinker, Grinker, and Timberlake (1962) studied a group of male college students and were surprised to note that "with few exceptions [their] passage through puberty and adolescence was smooth and devoid of turbulence." Impulsivity and rebelliousness were not predominant features of their teenage years. Anxiety, depression, and anger were commonly experienced and acknowledged by the subjects, but were transient and related to external stress. Grinker's group observed that sublimatory activities, such as sports, were not "pallid efforts," as stated by Josselyn (1954), but were effective coping mechanisms. They also felt that identification with the father was an extremely significant factor in determining the health of the young male subjects.

Douvan and Adelson (1966) conducted an interview and questionnaire study of over 3,000 boys and girls from secondary schools across the United States. The data obtained did not support a picture of adolescence characterized by rejection of parents and of rebellious behavior. Generally, parents were significant sources of support and approval for these youngsters. Rebelliousness was observed, though it tended to occur in the form of minor disagreements over dress codes, musical taste, and household duties rather than major clashes over relationships and values.

In an attempt to define normal adolescence, Offer (1969) and his colleagues conducted a longitudinal study of 102 boys from suburban middle-class environments. The study began during their subjects' freshman year in high school and continued into their college years. Subjects were statistically selected for normality by virtue of their scores on the Offer Self-Image Questionnaire and their lack of behavioral problems in school. Besides interviews with the subjects and their parents, the boys were evaluated by psychological tests. The findings of this study reconfirmed the studies by Grinker et al. and Douvan and Adelson. Although the boys and their parents reported some difficulties during their earlier adolescent years, ages twelve to fourteen, the problems were usually manifested by struggles over dress and household duties. Parents were not rejected or ignored; their values and opinions strongly influenced their sons. Resistance in the early years could be seen as a transient "negative dependence"; that is, independence was established by taking an equal and opposite position over daily issues.

Eight years after their study began, Offer's group (Offer and Offer 1975) reviewed their data and distinguished three growth patterns in 79 percent of their subjects. Twenty-three percent of their normal males progressed smoothly through adolescence without manifestations of turmoil. This group was labeled the "continuous"-growth group; its members had virtually no contact with mental health workers and were therefore unlikely to be represented in the clinical literature. A second group, 35 percent of the sample, was called the "surgent"-growth group, consisting of boys whose development was characterized by occasional periods of regression and conflict with parents. A third pattern of development was seen in 21 percent of the subjects, and was labeled "tumultuous"-growth. Through a large part of their adolescence, subjects in this group seemed to experience the turmoil that was described by earlier writers: wide mood swings, distrust for adults, conflicts with parents, and inconsistent responses to their environment. A number of subjects in this group had contact with mental health professionals. It is possible, then, that adolescents who use this route for development are overrepresented in the literature.

The picture of adolescence generated by these and other psychosocial studies (Rutter, Graham, Chadwick, and Yule 1976; Silber, Coelho, Murphy, Hamburg, Pearlin, and Rosenberg 1961; Westley and Epstein 1969) is different from one of normative chaos. Psychic equilibrium seems much more stable than implied in earlier descriptions. It seems possible for many individuals to experience their adolescence without turmoil and still be well adjusted.

Diagnosis and Treatment

Formulations of normal adolescence have diagnostic and therapeutic implications. Those who view turmoil as normative for adolescents conclude: (1) diagnostic and prognostic statements about teenage patients are difficult because normal adolescent behavior mimics neurotic and psychotic disorders, and (2) "good" behavior in adolescence foreshadows psychopathology in adulthood. If we examine these two proposals carefully, we see the implications for research. If adolescents showing signs of turbulence are followed into their adulthood, we would speculate that the manifestations of turbulence would disappear with age. Conversely, if a group of adolescents who appear to be adjusted are studied longitudinally, we would expect them to show signs of disturbance in their adulthood.

Vaillant (1978), in a longitudinal study, provides some information about adjustment from adolescence to adulthood. He examined ninety-five male subjects who had been evaluated thirty-five years before as sophomores in college. His findings indicate that good adjustment in adolescence remains quite stable with age. Subjects who showed signs of poor adjustment in adolescence were prone to develop problems with emotional adjustment, occupational success, and family relationships throughout adulthood. More significantly, good object relations in adolescence, as measured in the initial evaluation by psychiatric interview, were strongly predictive of good emotional development, occupational satisfaction, marital harmony, and closeness to offspring.

If good adjustment in adolescence predicts stability throughout the adult years, does psychopathology in adolescence remain stable? This question was addressed by Masterson (1967) and his colleagues in a five-year follow-up study of seventy-two boys and girls, twelve to eighteen years of age, who received outpatient psychiatric treatment and were matched with an equal number of nonpatient controls. The adolescents in the patient group remained more disturbed than controls throughout the follow-up period. Schizophrenia, personality disorders, some neuroses, and acting-out behavior were significantly more prevalent in the patient group after five years. The patients continued to experience difficulties in family relationships, school functioning, and social adjustment. The author concluded that they did not "grow out of it."

Weiner and DelGaudio (1976) conducted a ten-year follow-up study of 1,334 adolescents who received psychiatric care. Ten years later, 723 subjects (54 percent) had reappeared on the case registers. The investigators found that schizophrenia showed a diagnostic stability (62.2 percent) that approximated the stability of that diagnosis in adults (70.4 percent). Furthermore, 14.1 percent of those diagnosed as neurotics and 11.2 percent of those diagnosed as situational disorders were later diagnosed as schizophrenic. These data belie the notion that emotional upset in adolescents will disappear with time.

Other studies (Henderson, Krupinski, and Stoller 1971; Rosen, Bahn, Shellow, and Bower 1965) have examined the frequency of the use of transient situational disturbance—adolescent adjustment reaction—as a diagnosis for adolescents. These studies report that it accounts for approximately one-third of the diagnoses made in that age group, compared with a five percent utilization with adult patients (Weiner 1970). A three-year follow-up study by Looney and Gunderson (1978) revealed that 41 percent of 1,874 young naval personnel receiving this diagnosis were later found to have protracted difficulties. Twenty-seven percent were hosptialized for psychiatric reasons, another 10 percent were prematurely discharged from military service for administrative reasons, and an additional 4 percent were not recommended for reenlistment because of substandard performance. Of the rehospitalized patients, almost half were diagnosed as having personality disorders.

By definition (*Diagnostic and Statistical Manual—II* 1968), diagnoses of transient situational disturbances should only be applied to temporary disturbances in behavior, responding to environmental stress and occurring in individuals without any apparent underlying disorders. Feinstein (1975a) points out that chronic regressive behavior with severe or multiple symptoms should lead the clinician to consider a more serious mental illness. Kernberg (1978) suggests that the adjustment reaction label in adolescence ''is not so much a diagnosis as an alarm signal in dictating the need to evaluate in depth the personality structure of an adolescent in social conflicts.'' Selzer (1960), using strict criteria for diagnosis, noted that, although his subjects often presented with symptoms that appeared acute, careful histories often revealed chronic symptoms that warranted more serious diagnoses. He diagnosed adjustment reactions in only 3.8 percent of one group of 288 students and in 14.2 percent of another group of 218. These figures are much closer to the 5 percent figure for adults noted above and considerably less than the usual one-third in other studies of adolescent groups.

Discussion

Is psychiatry enhanced or hurt by the disparate views of adolescent psychological development? We might look at the divergent opinions generated by the earlier analytic writings on one hand and empirical studies on the other and attribute them simply to differences in methodology. However, while it is true that two different approaches are liable to produce two sets of data that do not agree, they should at least parallel, if not complement each other. Shapiro and Perry (1976), in their comprehensive study of the midlatency growth period, have shown that information obtained from psychoanalysis, developmental psychology, and neurobiological science can be complementary. A similar synthesis of data obtained from various scientific disciplines was accomplished by Kestenberg (1967, 1968) in her description of the phases of adolescence.

A complete description of the developmental data may not be possible until various subgroups within the adolescent population are examined as thoroughly as white, middle-class, male high school students have been studied. There are in fact no well-known longitudinal studies of youth from the lower classes or minority groups, and females have been the subjects of only a few important investigations. Hamburg (1974) and Miller (1978) suggest that early adolescence may be characterized by the turmoil previously ascribed to all adolescents, but before we make generalizations about early adolescents we must realize that studies of this age group are as rare as studies of female and disadvantaged youngsters.

Even if future investigations show that early adolescents are experiencing turbulence it may well be that the manifestations of turbulence are not as disruptive as reflected in the literature. Perhaps young people enter their adolescence more psychologically equipped than we had originally believed. For instance, Salzman (1974) and Spiegel (1951) suggest that the latency stage of development, far from being a dormant phase, is characterized by conflicts and behaviors that serve to prepare young people for the stresses they may experience in adolescence. Douvan and Adelson (1966) believe that "the specific disengagement techniques that the adolescent discovers, tests, and employs contain sources from the past and provide bridges to the future." It seems plausible, therefore, that the ego functions obtained from earlier developmental stages normally serve to dampen drives and keep impulsivity from becoming too disruptive while young adolescents develop new and more sophisticated functions. Although there may be some disturbance of equilibrium in early adolescence, continuity with earlier and later phases may outweigh discontinuity.

Giovacchini (1973), using object-relations theory in combination with ego psychology, seems to have a sense of continuity in mind in his essay on adolescence and character formation. He states:

Though there seems to be a discontinuity in the developmental process during adolescence, from the viewpoint of ego processes, structural changes occur in a relatively smooth, continuous fashion. The old introjects do not conflict with the new introjects required to deal with the tasks of the adult world. . . . The new introjects are not discontinuous and are not essentially different from the old ones; they become structural extensions of the latter, which, during childhood, help the ego develop executive techniques appropriate to that period of life. Now executive techniques become refined in order to deal with adult complexities.

Clinicians who view normal adolescence as a long period of discontinuity and disorganization are not likely to look beyond the symptoms of a disturbed adolescent. The patient's past, early developmental history, and previous level of functioning are meaningless if normal and abnormal are going to converge during adolescence. On the other hand, if clinicians believe that normal adolescence is continuous with earlier stages, that behavioral disturbances are usually kept within limits, and that ego functioning remains essentially intact, they are likely to be careful to evaluate the chronicity and severity of disturbing behavior in adolescent patients and will try to understand the patient's symptoms in the context of the developmental history. Meeks (1973) and Oldham (1978) see this approach as essential to good diagnosis with adolescents, reducing the possibility that serious pathology will be confused with transient disturbances.

Although nosology in adolescence is still imprecise, there has been some progress in the understanding of disturbing behavior in this age group. Besides the recognition of criteria for the diagnosis of organic and functional psychoses (Meeks 1973), clinicians are beginning to take a closer look at the so-called acting-out disorders of adolescence. Masterson (1973), for instance, describes wide fluctuations in emotions and behavior plus chronic impulsivity as possible signs of borderline personality organization. Anthony (1970) and Feinstein (1975b) have noted that affective disorders in young patients may be masked by impulsivity, irritability, and other forms of disruptive behavior. Studies of children with histories of hyperactivity and attention deficits (Gross and Wilson 1974; Mann and Greenspan 1976) have found that many young people with this syndrome do not "get better" with the onset of puberty, as had previously been believed. Rather, there may be continued problems in adolescence and adulthood with impulsivity, temper control, and concentration.

Nosology, then, may be progressing, but there still exists the problem that a significant number of adolescent patients will present with symptoms that confuse the most astute diagnostician. In such cases, it does not seem helpful to apply a diagnosis that creates a veneer of certainty over an uncertain situation, such as the imprecise use of adjustment reaction. It seems better in such cases to use categories that reflect an appropriate amount of concern about the patient's condition but do not close out the diagnosis. Looney and Gunderson (1978), for instance, suggest the use of *Diagnostic and Statistical Manual—III* categories of "atypical psychosis" or "unspecified mental disorder (not psychotic)" when the diagnosis with young people is unclear. The use of such categories would allow clinicians to admit their confusion while emphasizing the need for continued contact and evaluation.

Conclusions

Trying to determine what constitutes normality and pathology in mental function is a difficult task, but for the adolescent age group this seems to have been especially enigmatic. Studies of adolescents using empirical methods produced findings that did not agree with earlier conclusions by prominent psychoanalysts and others; in fact, there seemed to be a deviation in directions. What was abnormal for one group was considered normal by the other. These differences have practical implications in that the belief that adolescence is normally chaotic may cause a clinician to (1) neglect the patient's developmental history and the chronicity of symptoms, (2) use an imprecise diagnosis for a precise problem, and (3) prescribe a wait-and-see therapeutic approach to a problem requiring more vigorous intervention.

Besides the consistent findings by empirical studies that social and emotional adjustment is the norm in adolescence, psychoanalytic theory has progressed in such a way that growth can be viewed as an essentially continuous process. Future studies, it is hoped, will aim toward integrating developmental theory with empirical findings. In the meantime, there is a need for clinicians to reexamine their views of adolescence, to take adolescent disturbance more seriously, and to be more circumspect in their use of vague diagnostic categories with their adolescent patients.

REFERENCES

Aichhorn, A. 1925. *Wayward Youth*. New York: Viking, 1974.
Anthony, E. J. 1969. The reactions of adults to adolescents and their behavior. In A. H. Esman, ed. *The Psychology of Adolescence*. New York: International Universities Press, 1975.
Anthony, E. J. 1970. Two contrasting types of adolescent depression and their treatment. *Journal of the American Psychoanalytic Association* 18:841–859.
Bakan, D. 1971. Adolescence in America: from idea to social fact. *Daedalus* 100:979–995.
Bernfield, S. 1938. Types of adolescence. *Psychoanalytic Quarterly* 7:243–253.
Blos, P. 1962. *On Adolescence*. New York: Free Press.
Blos, P. 1967. The second individuation process of adolescence. *Psychoanalytic Study of the Child* 22:162–186.
Diagnostic and Statistical Manual—II. 1968. Washington, D.C.: American Psychiatric Association.
Diagnostic and Statistical Manual—III (Draft). 1978. Washington, D.C.: American Psychiatric Association.
Douvan, E., and Adelson, J. 1966. *The Adolescent Experience*. New York: Wiley.
Erikson, E. 1956. The problem of ego identity. *Journal of the American Psychoanalytic Association* 4:56–121.
Feinstein, S. 1975a. Adjustment reaction of adolescence. In A. Freedman,

H. Kaplan, and B. Sadock, eds. *Comprehensive Textbook of Psychiatry*. Vol. 2. Baltimore: Williams & Wilkens.

Feinstein, S. 1975b. Adolescent depression. In E. J. Anthony and T. Benedek, eds. *Depression and Human Existence*. Boston: Little, Brown.

Freud, A. 1936. *The Ego and the Mechanisms of Defense*. New York: International Universities Press, 1966.

Freud, A. 1958. Adolescence. *Psychoanalytic Study of the Child* 13:255–278.

Freud, S. 1905. Three essays on the theory of sexuality. *Standard Edition* 7:130–243. London: Hogarth, 1955.

Gardener, G. E. 1954. The mental health of normal adolescents. *Mental Hygiene* 31:529–540.

Geleerd, E. 1957. Some aspects of psychoanalytic technique in adolescence. *Psychoanalytic Study of the Child* 12:263–283.

Giovacchini, P. 1973. The adolescent process and character formation: clinical aspects. *Adolescent Psychiatry* 2:404–414.

Grinker, R. R., Sr.; Grinker, R. R., Jr.; and Timberlake, J. 1962. Mentally healthy young males (homoclites). *Archives of General Psychiatry* 6:405–453.

Gross, M., and Wilson, W. 1974. *Minimal Brain Dysfunction*. New York: Brunner/Mazel.

Group for the Advancement of Psychiatry. 1968. *Normal Adolescence*. New York: Scribner's.

Hall, G. S. 1904. *Adolescence: Its Psychology and Its Relations to Physiology, Sociobiology, Sex, Crime, Religion and Education*. 2 vols. New York: Appelton.

Hamburg, B. 1974. Early adolescence: a specific and stressful stage of the life cycle. In G. Coelho, D. Hamburg, and J. Adams, eds. *Coping and Adaptation*. New York: Basic.

Henderson, A.; Krupinski, J.; and Stoller, A. 1971. The epidemiological aspects of adolescent psychiatry. In J. G. Howells, ed. *Modern Perspectives in Adolescent Psychiatry*. New York: Brunner/Mazel.

Jones, E. 1922. Some problems of adolescence. *Papers on Adolescence*. London: Baillere, Tindall, & Cox, 1948.

Josselyn, I. 1954. The ego in adolescence. *American Journal of Orthopsychiatry* 24:233–237.

Kernberg, O. 1978. Diagnosis of borderline conditions in adolescence. *Adolescent Psychiatry* 6:298–319.

Kestenberg, J. 1967. Phases of adolescence: with suggestions for a correlation of psychic and hormonal organizations, part II. *Journal of the American Academy of Child Psychiatry* 6:577–614.

Kestenberg, J. 1968. Phases of adolescence: with suggestions for a correlation of psychic and hormonal organizations, part III. *Journal of the American Academy of Child Psychiatry* 7:108–151.

Kett, J. F. 1977. *Rites of Passage*. New York: Basic.

Klumpner, G. H. 1978. A review of Freud's writings on adolescence. *Adolescent Psychiatry* 6:59–74.

Lindemann, E. 1964. Adolescent behavior as a community concern. *American Journal of Psychotherapy* 18:405–417.

Looney, J., and Gunderson, E. 1978. Transient situational disturbances: course and outcome. *American Journal of Psychiatry* 135:660–663.

Mann, H., and Greenspan, S. 1976. The identification and treatment of adult brain dysfunction. *American Journal of Psychiatry* 133:1013–1017.

Masterson, J. F. 1967. The symptomatic adolescent five years later: he didn't grow out of it. *American Journal of Psychiatry* 123:1338–1345.

Masterson, J. F. 1968. The psychiatric significance of adolescent turmoil. *American Journal of Psychiatry* 124:1549–1554.

Masterson, J. F. 1973. The borderline adolescent. *Adolescent Psychiatry* 2:240–268.

Mead, M. 1928. *Coming of Age in Samoa*. New York: Morrow.

Meeks, J. 1973. Nosology in adolescent psychiatry: an enigma wrapped in a whirlwind. In J. Schoolar, ed. *Current Issues in Adolescent Psychiatry*. New York: Bunner/Mazel.

Miller, D. 1978. Early adolescence: its psychology, psychopathology, and implications for therapy. *Adolescent Psychiatry* 6:434–448.

Offer, D. 1969. *The Psychological World of the Teenager*. New York: Basic.

Offer, D., and Offer, J. 1975. Three developmental routes through normal male adolescence. *Adolescent Psychiatry* 4:121–141.

Oldham, D. 1978. Adolescent turmoil: a myth revisited. *Adolescent Psychiatry* 6:267–279.

Rosen, B. M.; Bahn, A. K.; Shellow, R.; and Bower, E. 1965. Adolescent patients served in outpatient psychiatric clinics. *American Journal of Public Health* 55:1563–1577.

Rutter, M.; Graham, P.; Chadwick, O.; and Yule, W. 1976. Adolescent turmoil: fact or fiction. *Journal of Child Psychology and Psychiatry and Allied Disciplines* 17:35–56.

Salzman, L. 1974. Adolescence: epoch or disease. *Adolescent Psychiatry* 3:128–139.

Selzer, M. 1960. The happy college student myth. *Archives of General Psychiatry* 2:131–136.

Shapiro, T., and Perry, R. 1976. Latency revisited: the age 7 plus or minus 1. *Psychoanalytic Study of the Child* 31:79–106.

Silber, E.; Coelho, G.; Murphy, E.; Hamburg, D.; Pearlin, L.; and Rosenberg, M. 1961. Competent adolescents coping with college decisions. *Archives of General Psychiatry* 5:517–527.

Spiegel, L. 1951. A review of contributions to a psychoanalytic theory of adolescence. *Psychoanalytic Study of the Child* 6:375–393.

Spiegel, L. 1961. Identity and adolescence. In S. Lorand and H. I. Schneer, eds. *Adolescents: Psychoanalytic Approach to Problems and Therapy.* New York: Hoeber.

Vaillant, G. 1978. The natural history of male psychological health. *American Journal of Psychiatry* 135:653–659.

Weiner, I. 1970. *Psychological Disturbance in Adolescence.* New York: Wiley.

Weiner, I., and DelGaudio, A. 1976. Psychopathology in adolescence. *Archives of General Psychiatry* 33:187–193.

Westley, W., and Epstein, N. 1969. *The Silent Majority.* San Francisco: Jossey-Bass.

Winnicott, D. W. 1971. Adolescence: struggling through the doldrums. *Adolescent Psychiatry* 1:40–49.

17 RECENT CONTRIBUTIONS TO THE THEORY OF FEMALE ADOLESCENT PSYCHOLOGICAL DEVELOPMENT

SIDNEY WEISSMAN AND PETER BARGLOW

Adolescence since the time of Freud has been conceptualized as a recapitulation of earlier psychological phases of development. The resulting progressive and regressive shifts in personality, with restructuring leading to new personality configurations, are marked by a wealth of clinical phenomena that have been extensively detailed in the psychoanalytic literature and organized theoretically by the landmark work on adolescence by Blos (1962).

Classical psychoanalytic theory, when it addresses the complex biopsychosocial developmental processes of adolescence, confronts the same problems that it has had in describing accurately the schizophrenic process. In discussing schizophrenia, analysts have frequently resorted to considering energy forces and counterforces. This language allegedly explains psychoanalytic theory but does not explain specific clinical phenomena (Holzman 1976).

The same problem in comprehending schizophrenia would appear relevant to the understanding of adolescence. Clinical phenomena derived from outside psychoanalysis are too often excluded as being nonanalytic and therefore not studied as relevant to understanding the adolescent's development. In contrast, we emphasize the necessity to examine all relevant behavioral sciences to determine the possible impact of current research findings on psychoanalytic theory. Cognitive development, neuroendocrine feedback mechanisms, and brain lateralization afford insights relevant to groups of adolescent girls. Advances in the fields of endocrinology, neurosciences, and developmental psychology (Piaget) are presented because they enable us to develop a psychoanalytic model which does not conflict with our sister science of behavior.

In the same vein we propose that the psychology of the self is a valuable addition to earlier psychoanalytic models in integrating and organizing the complex behavior of adolescence.

Traditional Psychoanalytic Theory of Adolescence

The well-known regression-progression sequence accords three major viewpoints of classical analytic theory: the libidinal stages, the view of object relations, and the structural (id, ego, superego) schema. According to the writings of Freud (1905a), Deutsch (1945), and Blos (1951), the profound physical changes in bodily size and shape and the onset of menstruation recreate oedipal conflicts, revive female castration anxiety, and reinforce penis envy. As a result, there is also a reproduction of phallic-, anal-, and oral-phase phenomena that typified the adolescent girl's psychology during the early infantile years of life. Classical theory claims that the girl's envy of the male genital is a crucial constant pressure and fosters adolescent personality change and growth. In adolescence her lack of a penis motivates her to turn away from her mother to pursue the adolescent boy who possesses the prized penis. This narcissistic disappointment in the mother (Blos 1962) is considered also to reinitiate a deep, internal struggle for the girl's emancipation and independence. The resulting move away from mother contributes to a transitory, defensive, masculine identification and is considered the major contributor to the tomboy period of adolescence. The girl experiences and expresses her heightened libidinal drives through a variety of sexual fantasies and activities or defends against sexual urgency through innumerable inappropriate methods. Later in adolescence, she is said to give up her pursuit of the penis by attaching herself to a male and by planning to have a baby (Deutsch 1945; Freud 1914; Nagera 1976).

A libidinal (and aggressive) decathexis of both parental imagoes occurs with a reversal of the introjective processes through which identifications took place. The entire object-relinquishment process is accompanied by a search for new external (to become internal) objects. The chief clinical phenomenon marking efforts to establish freedom from parental intrapsychic objects is said to be adolescent rebellion. One frequent clinical manifestation of object finding (recathexis) is intense attachment to admired folk heroes, new friends, famous athletes, or popular movie heroines. New object relations are demonstrated also during middle adolescence by deep group loyalties and

215

in late adolescence and early adulthood by long-lasting, more realistic sexual, social, or even marital relationships.

Id regression, discussed previously, and heightened pregenital and oedipal drive urgency may be accompanied by relative ego weakness. In addition, some adolescent theoreticians (Freud 1958; Kestenberg 1976) find evidence of extensive loss in previously established object constancy and ego boundaries. Geleerd (1957), for instance, believes that the normative regression is to the undifferentiated phase of object relations. There may be apparent diminution in the strength of previously secure countercathectic defensive forces or a reinstinctualization of autonomous ego functions such as judgment, reality testing, and perception. The besieged ego may lose some capacity to maintain drive and affect thresholds. Instinctual breakthroughs are expressed through adolescent masturbation, sexual or violent fantasies and fears, and often premature sexual activity that in turn may lead to venereal disease or pregnancy (Barglow, Wright, Bornstein, and Visotsky 1968). Drive intensity may also be managed by phobic defenses and massive ad hoc or characterological inhibitions of many psychological functions.

But most attention in psychoanalytic adolescent theory has been devoted to the changes in the superego structure. Gradolph (1979) has described a phase-appropriate breakdown of the superego-ego ideal system into its primitive prohibitive and idealized components. He also noted a partial externalization of these superego precursors onto popular contemporary figures treated with awe-inspiring reverence. For girls, stage, screen, and musical heroines are said to absorb idealizing libido. Temporary weakening of inner moral behests and a disbelief in the validity of parents' values often facilitate drive expression and may account for sexual acting out. Ego efforts to cope with the force of projected superego precursors may be reflected in allegiance to cults, adherence to ascetic religious movements, or even in masochistic submission to fanatical leaders of either sex. Such culturally sanctioned movements may provide considerable protection against adolescent anxiety and fear caused by the threat of newly unleashed instinctual forces.

Later in adolescence there occurs a reinternalization of the superego, sometimes with considerable imprint and modification of the qualities of idealized objects that were so crucial. There is also a restoration of consistent, persistent goals, values, and ideals. Not infrequently, the latter may not differ so much from the standards that have identified and colored the particular life-style of the late-adolescent girl's parents and older siblings. The generations some have called "warring" have again made relative peace, to the welcome relief of both parent and child.

216

The Libido Concept in Light of Contemporary
Neurophysiological Research

Although Freud depicted several adolescent patients in his famous case studies, he devoted little theoretical attention to this developmental period. In his essays on sexuality Freud (1905a) introduced an unmistakable somatic emphasis that is well represented in most classical writings and is present also in contemporary adolescent literature. He emphasized particularly the important psychic changes initiated by the physiology of puberty. Pubescent hormonal factors, he felt, strengthened libidinal instincts, initiating both regressive and defensive responses. Contemporary theory still relies on the conceptualization that the motivating force behind sexuality is the sexual instinct or libido. Freud (1905b) had tentatively defined instinct as "an endosomatic, continually flowing source of stimulation . . . on the frontier between the mental and physical." It is not clear from his description if he considered the sexual instinct to be derived from the excitability of the erotogenic zones or if the sexual instinct took on the character of the various erotogenic zones in a phasic fashion. Recent authors (Klein 1976; Schafer 1974) have criticized the concept that libido is a motive force or energy source for the psychic apparatus.

Klein (1976) criticizes a number of crucial assumptions that Freud made in his development of drive-libido theory: "The model of drive discharge is not specific to sexuality, but refers to a more general regulative process concerning what Freud considered to be the basic aim of the nervous system, the discharge of excessive energic accumulation" (p. 47). However, if libido is conceptualized as a motive force, it would theoretically be increased by the sexual maturation of the individual and profoundly depleted by damaging the genitals. For example, consistent with Freud's theory, castrating a male would lead to a profound decrease in his sexual urges, which, in fact does happen when we find a boy castrated before puberty. However, this is not necessarily true of individuals castrated after puberty since such males continue to maintain sexual interests even in the absence of gonadal sexual hormones. It seems likely that the psychologic experience, identifications, mental representations, and conflicts experienced in childhood related to sexuality are not fixed in the mental life of the child unless it has experienced puberty with its accompanying upsurge in sexual hormones. The sexual hormones necessary to establish the "drivenness" of adolescent sexuality probably are not essential for their maintenance after the desires are firmly established. This view is further supported by the finding that women, after a bilateral oopherectomy, may not sustain any loss in sexual drive. Likewise, the work of Masters and Johnson (1970) does not indicate any necessary decline in sexual interest in postmenopausal women.

The interaction of the sexual hormones with the psychic content of the adolescent's self-system leads to numerous qualitative changes in the individual's psychologic structures. We cannot now describe the mechanism of how sex hormones affect these changes, which can be described from a classical, an ego psychological, or a self-psychology perspective, but we want to emphasize the importance of organic variables and the implications of this factor for the theory of libido. Clinical observations suggest that although the unconscious psychological content of an individual's sexual urges may be constant from childhood to adulthood, the hypothetical quantity called "libido" or the "sexual drive" or "instinct" may have a different quality during the two periods. This conclusion is quite different from traditional psychoanalytic theories of sexuality which consider the libido, as Freud did, simply to be quantitatively accentuated after puberty. In contrast, we propose the possibilities that the quality of the libido, as related to sexual drivenness, is in fact quite different in children and adults. The theoretical problem in conceptually relating quantity and quality in psychoanalysis has been recently clarified by Galatzer-Levy (1978).

A review of our present understanding of the neuroendocrine changes which propel the developing girl into puberty also raises doubts about the validity of the classical view of libido. From 1932 to 1970, the age of onset of menarche in the United States declined from 13.5 in 1932 to 12.6 years in 1970 (Zacharias and Wortman 1969). Regardless of what factors trigger menarche, scientists agree that prior to menarche the level of gonadotrophic hormones released by the pituitary gland increases and there already exists some cyclicity of this release. The pituitary gland is under the control of the hypothalamus, and this control is mediated through a portal system which transports gonadotrophin-releasing factors from the hypothalamus to the pituitary. At the start of each menstrual cycle, the hypothalamus produces follicle-stimulating hormone release factors (FSHRF) which stimulates the pituitary to release follicle stimulating hormone (FSH). These factors, in turn, stimulate the ovary to develop a follicle which, in turn, produces estrogen. The estrogen inhibits, through a negative feedback, the production of FSH in the pituitary, but the estrogen levels that rise through a positive feedback mechanism trigger the release of luteinizing hormone (LH). The LH causes the follicle to rupture and initiates luteinization of the ruptured follicle with the result that the follicle (known now as the corpus luteum) produces estrogen and progesterone. The progesterone inhibits the production of further LH through a negative feedback mechanism. The cyclic changes in estrogen and progesterone have well-known specific effects on the uterus.

Benedek and Rubenstein (1952) demonstrated that the hormonal phases of the menstrual cycle affect the quantitative and qualitative aspects of sexual interests as manifested in thought content reported in analysis. A potential fruitful area of analytic inquiry would be to explore further the interface between hormonal shifts and changes in an individual's thought processes. Particularly important in understanding the essence of adolescence is comprehending the means through which the adolescent girl integrates changes in the experiencing of her body. The adolescent boy without a hormonal cycle clearly has an easier task than the girl. Perhaps by focusing on the unique developmental tasks which face the girl in this psychosomatic area, the student of intrapsychic experience can make his most valuable contribution.

Central Nervous System Factors

In traditional psychoanalytic theory it has been assumed implicitly that the cortical areas of males and females are equivalent and that early development leads to the internalization of external behavior patterns of influential objects which are both unique for a given individual and clearly identified with one or the other gender. In this theory males are seen as active and aggressive as an outgrowth of a major central identification with the father resulting from the resolution of the Oedipus complex. Females are considered passive and submissive as a result of identification with their mothers and as a result of the psychic structures laid down as the products of the resolution of the Oedipus complex. However, recent findings indicate that cerebral cortical functioning may not be equipotential in males and females.

Significant behavioral differences observed between boys and girls may reflect a biologic basis, not solely a psychologic one. The careful systematic observations of girls and boys identifying developmental differences indicate that girls are developmentally advanced compared with boys in onset of speech articulation, verbal fluency, expressive use of language, and lateralization of speech perception (Petersen and Wittig 1979). Restated briefly, girls are superior to boys in mental functions associated with the left cerebral hemisphere. These female advantages occur early in childhood and are sus-

219

tained after puberty (Wolff and Hurwitz 1976). However, boys older than eleven years generally are superior to girls in spatial visualization and the perception of part/whole relationships, functions associated with the right cerebral cortical hemisphere.

These findings have a great potential impact on psychoanalytic theories of sexuality. Erikson (1968) describes how latency-aged children, eleven years old, given blocks for observed play, organize them in a predictable fashion linked to gender. Girls use the blocks to define closed, controlled spaces; boys use them to build towers. Classically, this finding has been taken to represent a projective expression of the girl who symbolically represents her inner genital space and maternal concerns. The boys' upright constructions are said to represent symbolic representation of phallic concerns. While cultural contributions must also be considered, in light of new findings regarding brain functions, we could argue that the girl focuses on closed, controlled spaces because of subtle differences in her biologically determined capacity which leaves her less capable than the boy in integrating larger, uncontrolled spatial configurations. This possibility does not tell us much about the specific child's association to individual construction but does permit an important generalization. It is quite possible that the distinctions between the play of boys and girls observed in the laboratory are less the result of some inner sense of genital space and more related to basic cerebral functions.

The same reasoning may apply to the classical attribution of passivity to girls, a trait which might be related to their heightened verbal skills compared with males at a particular age. Language ability offers the girl greater opportunity to express verbally diverse affective states and to modulate her response to the environment and the urgency of adolescent needs. This enables her to react less than boys with physical activity and motoric protest to stressful environment inputs. Girls are assumed to have weaker superegos and to be less aggressive than boys. Again, such observations could well derive from the girl's biologically determined, better verbal ability. The oedipal girl with her superior verbal skills could react to complex situations in a more subtle fashion. This special capability could easily have been mistaken as a sign of a weaker superego by past observers. We might emphasize that these preliminary hypotheses obviously do not account for the specific motivations of a given individual, but they do describe clearly the potential influences of biologic systems when the girl enters puberty. Behaviors which previously have been considered psychological are probably more physiologically determined and less psychologically shaped than previously thought.

Developmental Contributions

Nearly parallel with the development of psychoanalysis has been the work of Jean Piaget (Piaget and Inhelder 1969), who, through repeated careful observations, placed at age eleven and thirteen years the onset of the child's capacity to perform certain tasks signaling the intrapsychic achievement of "formal operations" or "abstract thought" (Basch 1977). This refers to thought in which relationships can be examined independent of concrete observations. Piaget's observation that the individual develops the cognitive capacity for formal thought in early adolescence initially appears to be contradicted by the appearance of so-called ego-centered thought in the early adolescent, which is unaffected by the rules of formal thought. The young adolescent is convinced that his or her idiosyncratic view of the world is the correct one and that he or she alone comprehends the appropriate response to the crises that occur around them. The adults' repeated presentation of the laws of logic (formal thought) will not prevent the adolescent from believing intensely the rightness (or righteousness) of his or her view of the world.

The early-adolescent girl develops the appropriate cognitive skills to assess the subtlety of the world around her but would appear to lack the capacity for empathy. We define "empathy" in Kohut's (1971) sense as a means of observation using vicarious introspection which includes "the capacity to detect the other person's state of mind through identificatory processes" (Gedo 1979). In contrast, the late adolescent appears to have this capacity. This distinction can be seen in the contrast between the early adolescent's loud complaints upon being told by parents what time to be home, and the later adolescent's appreciation or at least acknowledged awareness of the parents' concern for his or her well being. Recent attention has been drawn to the cognitive skills that are needed for the empathic process. We propose that these skills are those of formal thought. An appropriate research domain for the psychoanalyst is to discover what developmental achievements occur in the adolescent which enable his empathic capacity to flower in late adolescence although the cognitive capacity for it exists much earlier.

When this cognitive milestone has been attained, the adolescent can interpret and grasp concrete and symbolic meanings of events or experiences in the lives of other individuals and can identify a similar event in her own life. Yet to be truly empathic, the process of self-examination requires not only recall of cognitive experiences but also recall of affective experiences, and the latter capacity signals another separate developmental step. In an analytic setting, for instance, the analyst must be cognizant of and utilize both these capacities that originate during adolescence. An adolescent girl can examine her own feelings cognitively only if she first acquires control of her impulses and inner tension states. The bodily changes and hormonal shifts of early adolescence may leave the girl in such an unstable situation that she may not feel adequately in control of her body and the experience of new impulses may become frightening and dangerous.

The early adolescent often responds to intense affects and inner pressures by utilizing her newly developed cognitive capacity in a defensive fashion to avoid acknowledging her lack of an integrated, cohesive self. As she proceeds through adolescence, the girl develops gradually the capacity to modulate her sexual urges, to integrate a new bodily self-image, and to utilize her new cognitive capacities. Only after these cognitive, affective, and physiologic changes have attained stability can she begin to examine more realistically and effectively her own motives and to compare them more accurately with the outside world. Only after she accomplishes this can she introspect and develop the capacity for empathy.

While it is possible to describe the role of formal thought in the adolescent's development of empathy, how does the development of this capacity affect other psychological processes seen in adolescence? Psychoanalytic theory assumes that the heightened sexual drive attributed to adolescence contributes to the configuration of the total personality through the integrative capacities of the ego. The progressive changes in the ego allow also a new resolution of the oedipal conflicts of childhood, a process demonstrated clearly through observations of adolescents in analysis. Clearly, the successful outcome of adolescence does require the integration of sexuality with the total personality. But that function traditionally described as the ego's increased capacity to deal with sexual concerns may be understood profitably also in Piaget's (Piaget and Inhelder 1969) terms as the individual's new capacity for formal thought. The individual is partially freed from the demands of concrete connections to intrapsychic objects and is better able to assess the implications of desires in reference not to one object but to a universe of objects sharing abstract similarities.

When she begins dating, the girl interacts with a variety of different boys and can begin to compare them with each other and with her own idealized fantasies of males. While the content of her fantasies is, of course, unique for each girl, the capacity for formal thought facilitates the girl's establishment of new, more complex relationships based on values, ideals, and goals of her own. She no longer needs to continue utilizing concrete internalized aspects of her parents and progressively has the cognitive capacity to distinguish clearly herself from her parents and to assess the total inner world and outer environment in her own right. Why some adolescent girls do not do this, or may be incapable of taking such steps, is an appropriate and important domain for psychoanalysis. By exploring this area, psychoanalysis can supply some explanations of the idiosyncratic thinking of our patients. But Piagetian psychology is a useful conceptual tool to account for generalizations that explain the adolescents girl's progressive capacity to assess these new crucial interpersonal relationships and to make increasingly fine distinctions.

The previous discussion has assumed that the adolescent develops the capacity for formal thought as initially described by Piaget between the ages of eleven and thirteen. More recent work raises some doubt about the timing of onset of the development of formal thought and indicates that some individuals may never develop this capacity (Dulit 1972). These findings do not contradict our stated assumptions but might explain why the capacity for empathy sometimes is not attained at all by some and appears at different ages for others.

The preceding developmental considerations differ in perspective from the genetic viewpoint of Freud that views adolescence as principally a recapitulation or revival of infantile developmental phenomena. The vantage point of Piaget emphasized new psychological additions, transformations, and organizations. "A good deal of the behavior of teenagers can be explained on the basis of the impact of these new emergences rather than earlier determinants" (Abrams 1978, p. 394).

Psychology of the Self

After the preceding behavioral science focus on areas somewhat distant from psychoanalysis, we return to the realm of introspective psychology and inspect recent changes in the field of psychoanalysis. The classical analytic views of female adolescence utilize principally the drive-conflict theory of Freud in conjunction with the structural model of the mind as applied to object relations. Freud's theoretical model relied heavily on energy concepts. The validity of several alternative psychoanalytic models has been presented recently in the psychoanalytic literature (Basch 1977; Schafer 1974).

One of the most influential and widely utilized of such efforts has been the self-psychology framework pioneered by Kohut. This is a model which we consider especially suitable for comprehending further the various clinical phenomena universally associated with female adolescence. Kohut (1972) wrote: "Extensive changes of the self must . . . be achieved in the transition from early childhood to latency, from latency to puberty, and from adolescence to young adulthood . . ." (p. 367). Utilizing understanding of development derived from self-psychology, a narcissistic line of development can be outlined specifically for the adolescent girl as follows:

1. Preadolescence: Self-esteem regulation, which has been dependent on both parents, becomes unstable as disillusionment and deidealization with both parents begins. Substitutes for the mother are intensely sought after and are often provided by slightly older girls—career counselors, friends, a sister with a more secure social or career identity, or a young protective teacher. The preadolescent girl appears to need such idealized female figures somewhat less than do normal, adolescent boys and moves into adolescence earlier and easier. We speculate that this slight difference might repeat a timetable distinction between boys and girls in the first year of life. Tolpin (1971) has written, "It is simply impossible for the mother to hold and calm the larger, more active, and alert infant of the second half of the first year in exactly the way that she held and cradled the physically more immature infant with whom an almost complete sense of physical merger is possible. This condition would be exacerbated for the boy because he is larger, more active, more aggressive, and probably less soothable than the girl during the earliest six or eight months of life." If this is so, the girl infant could linger longer within the confines of the mother-infant symbiosis. This potential, gender-linked, developmental difference could support the girl's progress earlier than the boy's, in areas of conation, cognition, autonomy, and verbal fluency (Barglow and Schaefer 1976). The mother similarly can be more helpful for a longer period to her adolescent girl than to her male child, who often turns fiercely against her with revived aggressiveness and rage.

The use of the function and appearance of the physical self to maintain self-esteem becomes crucial with development and menstruation, symbolizing both a new possibility and a major challenge. Many new responses and sublimations are now needed to maintain narcissistic balances. For example, athletics, traditionally the province of males, has become for adolescent girls a means of reaffirming the integrity and stability of the threatened, latency bodily self. Athletic performance can channel narcissistic tensions while providing gratification of heightened exhibitionistic needs.

2. Early adolescence: As in boys, the ego ideal and superego which modulate self-esteem may undergo some phase-appropriate dissolution with the appearance of a regressive diffusion into precursors (Blos 1962). The loss of stabilization of the ego ideal leads to increased feminine vulnerability and

to narcissistic injury. Here the girl seems initially to suffer more than the boy. The reexperiencing of the critical preoedipal change of object (from mother to father) produces separation anxiety with the risk of experiencing traumatic disillusionment (Gedo and Goldberg 1973).

The lifelong, intense, dependent attachment of the girl to her mother no longer has the protective, comfortable merger quality (just we two females) of early childhood or, to a lesser extent, of normal latency. Now regressive and anaclitic longings for maternal closeness and soothing come into conflict with the adolescent heterosexual self-image. Wishes for maternal intimacy may be interpreted by the girl not only as infantile (childish) but also as homosexual and dangerous to the establishment of a heterosexual adolescent identity crucial as a stepping-stone to adult femininity. One common defensive maneuver against regressive homosexual strivings is seen in the activities of the superfeminine or promiscuous teenager whose frantic need for boys may end in adolescent pregnancy (Barglow et al. 1968; Blos 1951).

Difficulties in transformation of the homosexual or nonsexual self-object relationship to the mother into the self-representation and perception compatible with the heterosexually oriented self of early adolescence contributes to self-esteem vulnerability or even transitory states of fragmentation during this normative time period. For instance, breast development may paradoxically be viewed by the adolescent girl as a humiliation rather than as an advantage. Breasts may be perceived as smaller and less attractive than those of friends or older girls who have become unconscious representatives of the oedipal mother. This may lead to brooding feelings of inferiority and obsessional preoccupation with these body elements. Or the visible evidence of puberty may be misinterpreted as revealing to everyone concealed, embarrassing sexual fantasies, daydreams, and forbidden activities. Likewise, menarche, rather than viewed as signaling potential emergence of future motherhood, may be psychologically equated to dirty anal products or may be considered to reveal loss of control over bodily fluids and functions, triggering latent fears of bodily disease or deterioration. These meanings of physical development may then motivate efforts to conceal and disguise developmental physical changes associated with negative self-images or to retain characteristics of the relative stability of the younger girl's latency mind-body-self.

On the other hand, considerable protection against the threat of narcissistic disequilibrium, and also against the dangers of regressive homosexual defenses against heterosexual impulses, is provided by the sublimations characterizing early adolescent homosexual peer-group culture with culturally determined rituals, clubs, clothing, music, and so forth. These group activities were well described for male adolescents in the description of Wolf, Gedo, and Terman (1972).

Other defensive or compensatory mental activities include polymorphously perverse fantasies or behavior that may be expressed in solitary masturbation or masochistic submission to inappropriate males. Religious fervor, as mentioned, may conceal or substitute for erupting sexual impulses, blunting and controlling sexual impulses while simultaneously expressing a culturally sanctioned grandiosity. Religion may also shore up the cohesive self by establishing a continuity with cultural and familial traditions associated with the history of one or both of the parents.

3. Middle adolescence: The inevitable, seemingly heterosexual crushes of this period, are, of course, revivals of intense oedipal longings. These familiar romantic attachments also serve as idealizing transferences to nonincestuous objects that compensate the adolescent personality for the "sharp decrease in the continuity, stability and cohesiveness of the self" (Gradolph 1979). Such characteristic addiction-like attachments also buttress defensive efforts to buffer painful failures in achieving adequate mirroring of the grandiose self. Without such idealized passionate involvements with nonsexual objects there may occur partial "mini" fragmentations of self-structures with an ominous threat to self-cohesion (Wolf 1979). This precarious state is manifested clinically by transitory episodes of profound loneliness, pessimism, and strange fleeting sensations of inner emptiness that could progress to the perception of deadness characteristic of schizophrenic experience in pathologically vulnerable adolescents. Perhaps this could be conceptualized metapsychologically as a temporary undoing of structures created by transmuting internalization. This would be comparable to the traditionally utilized concept of superego and ego ideal externalization or projection traditionally applied to mid-adolescence.

The use of intense musical, sexual, or drug stimulation can undo the danger of this disintegrating self-experience through repeating the early soothing, comforting infantile environment once provided by the maternal self-object. Obviously, the emotional availability of an empathic idealized maternal substitute provides needed protection against the possibility of psychotic regressions or preoedipal fixations that could lead to serious adult psychopathology. We doubt that marked id or ego regression described in the summary of classical theory characterizes normal mid adolescence at all (Barglow and Schaefer 1979), a view consistent with Offer and Offer's (1975) research with male normal adolescents.

4. Late adolescence: The adolescent girl begins to make peace with her parents, and the gulf between old and new generations diminishes. Disillu-

sionment with childhood ego ideals is soon replaced by other new, lifelong identifications, based on shared intellectual and emotional goals and values that continue to function as permanent, externalized, self-objects. This provides optimal assistance to the adolescent maintenance of narcissistic balance (Wolf, Gedo, and Terman 1972). The rehabilitation of the self-structures weakened in early adolescence is accelerated through the reactivation of the process of transmuting internalization, utilizing the beneficial input of new objects, and prior mastery of adolescent emotional challenges. "The self-structure becomes more stable and cohesive allowing a continuity and predictability of the late adolescent's experience" (Gradolph 1979). Freud's eloquent prediction for the termination of mourning describes this adolescent achievement: "We shall build up again all that war has destroyed, and perhaps on a firmer ground and more lastingly than before" (Freud 1916).

Cultural factors as noted by Benedek and Rubenstein (1952) are considered more important than was true of the classical view of adolescence. For example, diminished prestige accorded motherhood, an increase of worry about population control, and admiration for the career woman—fostered by feminism or economic and political factors—may have had some reactive impact diminishing the centrality of the goal of parenthood in the ambitions and ideals of late female adolescence (Ritvo 1976; Schafer 1974). The biological contributions considered in this chapter certainly also contribute to alter adult feminine gender identity. But the idealized parental imagoes must be the most important source of the adolescent's ideals and the idealization. Since "both parents foster and orient the feminine individuation of their daughter" (Blum 1976), the core personality structures of both mother and father, as well as major adolescent "new objects," will determine the adult outcome of late adolescent career versus motherhood conflicts.

We have not yet commented on the importance attributed to the alleged female adolescent resolution of the stigma of penis envy through the solid establishment of a substitute wish for pregnancy and motherhood (Deutsch 1945; Freud 1914; Kestenberg 1976; Nagera 1976). Kohut (1969) has written: "I believe that the healthy woman's wish for a child is, in psychological terms, grasped much more adequately as a manifestation of her nuclear self, as a manifestation of her most central ambitions and ideals—in short, as the high point of a development that has its beginning in the archaic self's urge toward self-expression . . . when the convergence of *biological* and *cultural* factors may give this concretely defined content to women's self-expressive needs" (p. 786; our emphasis). We feel this comment summarizes our view that the pregnancy wish is a primary feminine attribute. This does not preclude the possibility that in certain individuals the pregnancy wish can serve the defensive task of neutralizing pathological penis envy.

227

Conclusions

In this chapter we reviewed briefly the classical psychoanalytic conceptualization of female adolescent psychological growth and development and inspected the concept of libido in light of new contributions to psychoanalytic literature and recent advances in the biologic and behavioral sciences. We examined contemporary research into aspects of adolescents' cerebral and cortical functioning, which seems to be gender linked and developmentally distinguishable from birth onward through adolescence; and we explored the application of Piaget's concepts to adolescent development. All the contributions clarify crucial aspects of female adolescent behavior and provide potential bridges between contemporary advances in the biological and behavioral sciences and recent psychoanalytic work emphasizing concepts of narcissism.

REFERENCES

Abrams, S. 1978. The teaching and learning of psychoanalytic developmental psychology. *Journal of the American Psychoanalytic Association* 26:387–406.

Barglow, P., and Schaefer, M. 1976. A new female psychology? *Journal of the American Psychoanalytic Association* 24(5): 305–350.

Barglow, P., and Schaefer, M. 1979. The fate of the feminine self in normative adolescent regression. In M. Sugar, ed. *Female Adolescent Development*. New York: Bruner/Mazel.

Barglow, P.; Wright, M.; Bornstein, M.; and Visotsky, H. 1968. Some psychiatric aspects of illegitimate pregnancy in early adolescence. *American Journal of Orthopsychiatry* 38:672–687.

Basch, M. F. 1977. Developmental psychology and analytic theory. *Annual of Psychoanalysis* 5:229–263. New York: International Universities Press.

Benedek, T., and Rubenstein, B. B. 1952. *Psychosexual Functions in Women*. New York: Ronald.

Blos, P. 1951. Preoedipal factors in the etiology of female delinquency. *Psychoanalytic Study of the Child* 12:229–249.

Blos, P. 1962. *On Adolescence*. New York: Free Press.

Blum, H. 1976. Masochism, the ego ideal, and the psychology of women. *Journal of the American Psychoanalytic Association* 24(5): 157–192.

Deutsch, J. 1945. The psychology of women in relation to the functions of reproduction. *International Journal of Psychoanalysis* 6:405–418.

Dulit, E. 1972. Adolescent thinking à la Piaget: the formal state. *Journal of Youth and Adolescence* 4:281–301.

Erikson, E. 1968. *Identity, Youth and Crisis.* New York: Norton.

Freud, A. 1958. Adolescence. *Psychoanalytic Study of the Child* 13:255–278.

Freud, S. 1905a. Three essays on the theory of sexuality. *Standard Edition* 7:135–245. London: Hogarth, 1953.

Freud, S. 1905b. Fragment of an analysis of a case of hysteria. *Standard Edition* 7:7–122. London: Hogarth, 1953.

Freud, S. 1914. On narcissism: an introduction. *Standard Edition* 14:73–102. London: Hogarth, 1957.

Freud, S. 1916. On transcience. *Standard Edition* 14:305–307. London: Hogarth, 1955.

Galatzer-Levy, R. M. 1978. Qualitative change from quantitative change: mathematical catastrophe theory in relation to psychoanalysis. *Journal of the American Psychoanalytic Association* 26:921–935.

Gedo, J. 1979. Less is more. Paper presented at the American Psychoanalytic Society, September 25, 1972.

Gedo, J., and Goldberg, A. 1973. *Models of the Mind.* Chicago: University of Chicago Press.

Geleerd, R. R. 1957. Some aspects of psychoanalytic technique in adolescence. *Psychoanalytic Study of the Child* 12:263–283.

Gradolph, P. 1979. Developmental vicissitudes of the self and the ego ideal during adolescence. Paper presented at the winter meetings of the American Psychoanalytic Association, New York, December 1979.

Holzman, P. S. 1976. Theoretical models and the treatment of schizophrenia. *Psychological Issues* 9(4): 134–157. New York: International Universities Press.

Kestenberg, J. S. 1976. Regression and integration in pregnancy. *Journal of the American Psychoanalytic Association* 24(5): 213–250.

Klein, G. S. 1976. Freud's two theories of sexuality. In M. M. Gill and P. S. Holzman, eds. *Psychology vs. Metapsychology: Psychoanalytic Essays in Memory of George S. Klein.* New York: International Universities Press.

Kohut, H. 1969. A note on female sexuality. In P. H. Ornstein, ed. *The Search for the Self.* Vol. 2. New York: International Universities Press, 1978.

Kohut, H. 1971. *The Analysis of the Self.* New York: International Universities Press.

Kohut, H. 1972. Thoughts on narcissism and narcissistic rage. *Psychoanalytic Study of the Child* 27:360–400.

Masters, W. H., and Johnson, V. E. 1970. *Human Sexual Inadequacy*. Boston: Little, Brown.

Nagera, H. 1976. *Female Sexuality and the Oedipus Complex*. New York: Aronson.

Offer, D., and Offer, J. 1975. *From Teenage to Young Manhood: A Psychological Study*. New York: Basic.

Petersen, A. C., and Wittig, M. C. 1979. *Sex-related Differences in Cognitive Functioning: Developmental Issues*. New York: Academic Press.

Piaget, J., and Inhelder, B. 1969. *The Psychology of the Child*. New York: Basic.

Ritvo, S. 1976. Adolescent to woman. *Journal of the American Psychoanalytic Association* 24(5): 127–138.

Schafer, R. 1974. Problems in Freud's psychology of women. *Journal of the American Psychoanalytic Association* 22:459–485.

Tolpin, M. 1971. On the beginnings of a cohesive self. *Psychoanalytic Study of the Child* 26:316–352.

Wolf, E. 1979. Paper presented to the Psychology of the Self workshop at the Chicago Institute for Psychoanalysis, Chicago, February 1979.

Wolf, E.; Gedo, J.; and Terman, D. 1972. On the adolescent process as a transformation of the self. *Journal of Youth and Adolescence* 1:257–272.

Wolff, P. H., and Hurwitz, I. 1976. Sex differences in finger tapping: a developmental study. *Neuropsychologia* 14:35–41.

Zacharias, L., and Wortman, R. J. 1969. Age at menarche: genetic and environmental influences. *New England Journal of Medicine* 280:860–868.

18 OPPORTUNITIES IN ADOLESCENCE TO RECTIFY DEVELOPMENTAL FAILURES

IRVING N. BERLIN

The developmental tasks of adolescence have been described by many authors as the working through of individuation and independence from family, the capacity for expressing and accepting feelings of closeness and intimacy, and the mastery of sexual urges brought on by hormonal changes at puberty so that sexual experiences also express loving, close, and tender feelings. The adolescent must develop a capacity to utilize formal operational thinking to open new vistas and desires for learning, use scientific methods to solve problems, and acquire skills for productive work in order to become an independent, effective adult (Blos 1967; Erikson 1963, 1968; White 1960).

The stresses, both physiological and psychological which occur in adolescence, may also foster a plasticity and capacity for new solutions to some previous failures in adaptation. For example, the hunger of many female adolescents for intimacy and closeness often leads to nonfulfilling sexual relations and pregnancy. These events can lead to catastrophic mother-child relations because of the burdens placed on a not yet mature and developmentally delayed young woman who has been deprived of maternal nurturance. However, with proper help over time, personal growth, and maturation a capacity for mothering can be stimulated and sustained. Methods of encouraging the capacity for close relationships with persons of both sexes will be described in this chapter in the context of adolescent development and growth (Giovacchini 1977; Kohler 1971).

Ravenscroft (1974) and others have described the adolescent period as one of normal regression in which young persons, like children, strive for autonomy, make demands, and try to impose their will. At the same time, these adolescents are implicitly asking adults to be clear and firm about the areas in which their development does not give them sufficient judgment to make decisions. Thus, like the young child searching for autonomy who needs a

231

firm "No!" to prevent impulsive and destructive behavior, the adolescent requires adult acknowledgment and evidence of respect for developing capacities, areas of maturity, and clear supportive limits where judgment has not yet fully matured. Such recognition of the adolescent's dual needs promotes growth. Those adolescents who previously have had few limits placed upon them may experience major developmental growth when parents are helped to understand their tasks (Derdeyn and Waters 1977; Gutmann 1973; Masterson 1967; Offer 1969).

Developmental Continuity

In the last decade as developmental processes in infancy and childhood have been studied from a variety of biological, psychosocial, cognitive, and sensorimotor aspects, adolescence emerges as a continuity in development to be understood in the context of previous developmental experiences. Inquiry into early phases of development of troubled adolescents reveals difficulties in resolution of earlier developmental conflicts. It must be emphasized, however, that most adolescents have few problems and resolve adolescence in a reasonable manner.

In retrospective analysis of problems in adolescent development data emerge concerning preschool problems, problems in separation, failures in socializing, handicaps in cognitive learning, and failure to resolve oedipal conflicts. A developmental framework views the present troubles of the adolescent in term of both current developmental stress and the need to reduce the deficits which have occurred in earlier development. The essential goals of adolescent development must include a viable work or productive role. Some adolescents' troubles appear to stem from the fact that society has no real use for them. The adolescent is not wanted as a potential contributor of either his labor or his mental energies. Massive unemployment, lack of effort in schools to help adolescents learn to think in problem-solving terms, or failure to learn viable work skills contributes to adolescents' sense of not being needed in the adult world and often results in escape to the more hospitable world of alcohol and drugs (Adams 1973; Blos 1962; Nagera 1966; Offer and Offer 1973; White 1960).

Conflicts around Sexual Maturation

The physiological surge owing to sexual maturation has a great impact on the adolescent. The rapid body changes and total body growth in the direction of adult body habitus are viewed with pleasure by most adolescents. In some, however, such bodily alterations seem to indicate loss of any chance to make up for the closeness and tenderness missed as a child and pose the threat of becoming an adult deficient in these areas of interpersonal development (Benedek, Poznanski, and Mason 1979; Gutmann 1973).

Adolescence most often produces an exacerbation of previous oedipal conflicts. This is especially noted in the authority conflicts between parent and adolescent of the same sex. Sexuality is often a major area of conflict for parents as well. Many parents have not achieved mutual sexual enjoyment, a sense of intimacy and closeness, and, therefore, they are envious that their adolescent may experience feelings unknown to them.

The capacity for expressing and feeling tenderness and reducing conflict with the parent of the same sex in part depends upon an understanding of how these previous conflicts evolved and were handled. The conflicts which result from overt seductive behavior by the parent of the opposite sex reinforce and exaggerate conflicts. The opposite-sex parent's seductive behaviors are usually indicative of various alliances between parent and child which exclude the other parent. Alliances may occur in cognitive and intellectual areas, affective relationships, and even in the sharing of particular sensorimotor experiences (i.e., sports and hobbies).

In family therapy, when such oedipal triangles exist it becomes possible to trace the history of these alliances, their effect on the adolescent and the family, and to examine their consequences on current development. It also becomes possible to focus on the role changes required of each parent to facilitate the adolescent's development. Such a focus also requires behavioral changes in the adolescent in order to reduce the previous conflictful interactions. In many such efforts notable changes in the parents' relationships with each other as well as the adolescent occur (Anthony 1969; Derdeyn and Waters 1977).

Case Vignette 1

Julie, age fourteen, was failing in school. She started out each semester well and then rapidly went downhill. She had also made some suicidal threats when her mother would not allow her to stay home and avoid school.

In family therapy it was clear that mother had had a very poor relationship with Julie since preschool when she had been Dad's girl. Mother and Julie fought about clothes, friends, school work, and chores. Somehow, whenever Dad was turned to, he resolved matters Julie's way. Mother and father's sexual and social relationships deteriorated, and often Dad took Julie out alone to a concert or movie.

As each described memories of past and recent events, it became clear that Julie's troubles in school were in part related to father's expectations that she do well and go to college. Previously father had excused her nonlearning as "too much to expect"; now she really did not have the background to succeed. We began to examine Julie's early developmental experiences with each parent. We noted especially the failure of both parents to support each other around learning in school and undertaking age-appropriate tasks at home. Each parent, but especially father, vied for Julie's favor and did not deal with her playing one against the other to avoid work, learning, and the social discomforts which occur in each phase of development. Julie had few friends, few social, academic, or interpersonal skills, and a poor self-image.

We began to outline a program in each area of retarded development which required parental cooperation and Julie's agreement. Special tutoring, working after school in mother's day-care center with other girls, and permitting mother to help her with some of her school work began to shift relationships. Father gave Julie driving lessons so she could get her license and, despite several fights because he demanded a very high level of performance, they were pleased with her skills and she acquired her license. After several months both parents went away for a week to learn to be together and to get to know each other. During that week they resumed sexual relations.

Another crisis occurred when Julie began dating. Father was irate because she stayed out late after a rock concert. Mother felt the parents had not been clear about a curfew and sided with Julie. Again oedipal problems were reduced as mother helped father and Julie find a reasonable resolution of the problem.

In one year Julie made up many academic deficits so that she could begin a realistic high school curriculum. She developed friends of both sexes and began getting along better with mother. Her relationship with father was less close but easier. It seemed to the family that problems were greatly reduced and developmental gains were made by Julie. Both parents slowly became aware of how their mutual relationship had duplicated previous relationships with their parents and siblings. They began to examine ways of avoiding these old behaviors by recognizing and labeling destructive interactions in terms of their origins. Thus when mother was depressed and rageful when father had to miss dinner in order to complete some work, she recognized her own mother's silent rages when her father frequently failed to notify that he would not be home for dinner. Father also recognized that his belated notifying mother of his absence acted out his own father's grandiose role where no one dared question his actions.

They could also help Julie identify hostile or potentially destructive actions in behaviors they had let her get away with in the past, recognizing similar feelings and behavior in their adolescence when acting out against their parents. Such insights and discoveries became tinged with less hostility and more humorous glimpses from present to past and back again. The increased capacity of each family member for expressing warm and tender feelings was greatly increased. The parents' obvious new-found pleasure in each other seemed to free Julie to try out new relationships with peers of both sexes.

Case Vignette 2

A black pregnant fifteen-year-old was hospitalized with a serious depression. It became clear that Frances had been a seriously abused and neglected child. She ran away from home at eleven and lived with friends and relatives. In each setting, while she yearned for the love and closeness she had not experienced with her own mother and father, her angry behavior always resulted in rejection and being ousted from the home. She was, at an early age, involved sexually with the older men in each household in which she lived. She described the seduction by the adult male in each instance as the "greatest" feeling of being wanted and loved that she had experienced. In each instance she discovered that there was not much love and that she was being used. Her anger would then lead to being rejected by the foster father. She got pregnant when she felt she and an eighteen-year-old boyfriend really loved each other. Wistfully, Frances recounted that in their continued sexual relationships she enjoyed the cuddling and not the intercourse. When Joe left her for another girl after she became pregnant, Frances slashed her wrists in a serious suicide attempt.

The victim of a nonnurturing parental relationship, it was clear that when her baby was born she needed to learn to relate to it in a much more maternal fashion than her mother had interacted with her. She was enrolled in a group of pregnant adolescents from similar circumstances. Group therapy with exceptionally open and honest young male and female group leaders permitted a great deal of catharsis and repeated discussions of past relationships with parents and men. A growing recognition occurred of how much she needed and wanted to be loved. She also recognized through discussions of her expectations that she expected responsiveness and love and was likely to be angry at her baby for its constant demanding attention.

These young women, as they studied infant and child development, learned how helpless and in need of care an infant was. The normal development of the infant and how to facilitate it were common concerns.

Once the babies were born, an infant-stimulation group was formed. The bonds from the prenatal group held this group together. Each mother was helped to recognize how much her talking, singing, and handling of the baby resulted in the infant's happy reaction and was important to its develoment. This was reinforced in the group discussions. Each mother was asked to spend an hour each week with someone else's baby. Thus they recognized the individual differences in temperament and capacity for interaction and how each mother had to work individually with her child.

These young women not only became proud of their mothering abilities as measured by predictable developmental steps and their enjoyment of their infant, but in the group they experienced closeness and intimacy as they faced mutual problems and could openly talk about their feelings and be supported by women of similar age.

The group therapists were able to model honest male and female relationships. They could express open disagreement. When a therapist was attacked by group members for failures in understanding or giving enough, he could allow the other therapist to bear the brunt of any feelings expressed until it escalated so that no one could be heard, then the other therapist would be interpretively supportive. Thus they demonstrated that they were neither fragile, overprotective of each other, or repressive in shutting off discussion and yet could come to each other's aid as needed.

Most of these young women became affectionate and effective mothers and thus were able to experience tangible evidence of their child's love for them.

The Peer Group and Adolescent Development

For most adolescents their friends or gang become very important in sustaining them. The peer group serves as a support system in sharing problems and troubles with their family and attempts to find ways of solving these issues. Close relationships with one or two adolescents of the same sex provide allies in exploratory sexual relationships with adolescents of the opposite sex. Peer concern around clothes, make-up, cars, dating, music, athletics, hobbies, and other interests permits closeness.

For some adolescents such peer closeness is difficult to attain. They remain alone and lonely despite their competence in many areas that could be shared. These young people have never learned to socialize during preschool and primary school ages. They never learned the skills of forming relationships and sharing and enjoying play with someone else because of shy withdrawn behavior. Frequently they manifested overly active aggressive behavior which turned age mates away.

Learning social skills is a major developmental task in adolescence and requires organized opportunities for activities under the guidance and help of adults. The anxieties of forming new relationships must be reduced over time until friendships can be experienced positively. Social activities for remediation must be of sufficient duration so that one is certain the adolescent has acquired the new skills. Such development is particularly critical to resolution of schizoid and depressive disturbances in some adolescents. These symptoms may reflect developmental delays not only in social relations but also in problems about feeling closeness with others resulting from difficulties in early parent-child relationships (Berlin 1978; Malmquist 1979; Offer 1969; Peterson and Offer 1979).

Cognitive Development

Most adolescents are increasingly effective and competent cognitively. They move from concrete operational thinking into formal operations and can thus reason scientifically utilizing deductive, inductive reasoning and conceptual thinking. Some adolescents, however, never attain the state of formal thinking and remain at the concrete operational stage for the rest of their lives. Here there has been no encouragement in the home or school to develop abstract thinking and to learn to problem solve. It is clear from many studies that such development can be fostered in the school setting through use of practical experience in certain interest areas coupled with courses which promote problem solving.

One such example has been demonstrated around adolescents working in caring for children in day-care settings and learning child development. These adolescents wanted to understand the causes for certain behaviors, attitudes, and severe problems noted in day-care children. They related their developmental knowledge to themselves and their own families. They eventually demanded better care for the children, and especially parental participation in the day-care activities to help parents better understand and relate to children with behavioral problems.

237

Through practice in actual life situations, young people begin to problem solve and think in logical, deductive, and inductive ways, thus altering previous cognitive developmental sets. In one project, it became clear that ghetto youth could conceptualize urban-renewal ideas which were much more meaningful and effective than those of some city planners (Block 1971; Piaget and Inhelder 1969).

Learning potential in school and college can be maximized if the curriculum is stimulating and promotes problem-solving thinking. Learning, in adolescence, becomes an essential aspect of beginning to regard oneself as an effective and competent person who can become independent and self-reliant. Adolescence and young adulthood are potentially creative periods as formal operational thinking becomes primary. Many of our youth are not helped to find ways to learn and feel competent and thus do not develop into effective, independent adults. Adolescence permits an opportunity, because of the fluidity of the period, to master a variety of new information and to develop a new cognitive style of thinking. A society that has no place for adolescents in its work force and does not use their problem-solving capacities condemns adolescents to passive helpless roles in an indifferent society. Their alternatives are often drugs, alcohol, and dropping out of society (Elkind 1975; Erikson 1968; Kohlberg and Gilliam 1971; Silber, Coelho, Murphey, Hamburg, Pearlin, and Rosenberg 1961).

Intimacy and Closeness as an Adolescent Goal

For sexual relationships to be meaningful they must provide opportunities to feel close to another person without fear of ridicule, exploitation, or incorporation. Adolescents who have had good early object relations, which makes feeling close possible, may subsequently have experienced parental violence, parental psychosis with consequent irrational relationships, or may have been deprived of continued close relationships with parents and siblings by divorce, separation, or death, resulting in adolescent upset. Adolescence permits experimentation with closeness which, if well handled by therapeutic figures, provides models for nondestructive close relationships. In our experience this has been especially true for schizoid, depressed, or violently aggressive youth where the violence masks depression. These young people do well in a supportive, firm milieu with therapists who in group and individual therapy can support and sustain the struggles to feel close and to

238

overcome the fears of being devoured or destroyed (Anthony 1969; Blos 1962; Caplan and Lebovici 1969; Giovacchini 1977).

Case Vignette 3

Sandy, a schizoid seventeen-year-old, was hospitalized because of psychotic anxieties that school friends were accusing him of sexually promiscuous behavior. Thus he had withdrawn to his room and refused to go to school. On the ward at first he regarded any friendly approaches as seductive. He was fearful that anyone who knew him would hate him and be derisive. Eventually his artistic talents were used as an entry into the group. In the group, his fears were opened for exploration and reality testing. In family therapy his very paranoid father, an effective professional, was helped to talk of his childhood and youth during which he had similar feelings. Father was also helped to test reality by his wife and Sandy's sister who understood father's sensitivity to criticism and fear that people would not like him. Father was slowly able to examine incidents in the family and in his practice where his suspicions were not borne out by subsequent behavior of people around him.

Sandy's tenuous relationship with Leah, a depressed girl, was carefully scrutinized, and this girl's dependence on Sandy for understanding and reassurance slowly reduced his fears that someone would exploit him as he believed his mother must have exploited his father.

In family therapy he learned about his mother's supportive role with father. He was finally able to express anger that when mother was depressed during a phase of father's illness and incapacitation she had neglected him. He slowly began to see himself as not so vulnerable. On the ward as he tried to master new skills and make new relationships, he found that he regarded himself as a more confident young person. On discharge he was able to continue his relationship with Leah and make other friends in the day treatment program.

Chronic Illness and Development

Many adolescents with chronic illnesses (asthma, arthritis, ulcerative colitis, diabetes) have used them as part of an environmental conspiracy to ignore the serious conflicts between parents, and parents and child, which seriously interfered with development and permitted the child to avoid responsibilities at home and learning in school. Any difficult task or relationship was reacted to with exacerbation of illness. In adolescence, family therapy makes it possible to delineate the role of the child and family members in maintaining these maladaptive behaviors. It also permits assigning new roles to family members, with opportunities for role playing and modeling in the session and analysis of what facilitated or prevented enactment of new roles that would reduce the chronic illness role of the adolescent and facilitate new development.

The need for independence, new peer relationships, and an adequate sexual role becomes the dynamic force behind the efforts to alter the previous sick role. Our own work with diabetes and anorexia nervosa, as well as Minuchin's (1974), indicates the importance of assigning new roles and constantly assessing the obstacles to their attainment until these new roles result in effective new living and relating in and outside of the family (Malmquist 1979; Offer 1969; Offer and Offer 1973; Peterson and Offer 1979).

Authoritative versus Authoritarian Roles as an Adolescent Developmental Goal

Most troubled adolescents are either very passive and wait to be told what to do or are very authoritarian and dictatorial in imitation of adult figures in their lives. The goal of adolescence is to become authoritative and productive. As a result of feeling competent and effective in work or learning it becomes easier to feel close to others and thus to be less fearful of sexuality as exploitative. There is therefore less need to dictate like a small fearful child and more need to be aware that being a benign authority is more effective in promoting relationships and feeling good about oneself. Such a shift from authoritarian, antagonistic positions to becoming authoritative is in part a function of how adults in the environment acknowledge the knowledge and competence of the adolescent and behave with respect and regard for his competencies. Such respect encourages self-respect and enhances the self-image of the adolescent as a potentially effective person with an important place in the world. That shift is one of the key developmental changes that can be facilitated by teachers, parents, adult friends, and therapists who can demonstrate their regard for the adolescent's capacities. Also inherent in these attitudes is the expressed hope of the adults to see the adolescent take a place as an adult who can have an impact on the world. It is that belief in the potential of the adolescent coupled with willingness to help him learn to become effective without fear that he will surpass the adult that completes this developmental stage (Szurek 1969; White 1960).

Conclusions

The plasticity of adolescence, the energies mobilized and available due to sexual maturation, the transition from concrete to formal operational thinking all provide opportunities for new growth. Many adolescents have few problems in this phase of development; however, many troubled adolescents, in addition to the stress of this developmental period, must deal with deficits arising in previous developmental periods.

Adolescence is an opportunity to find new solutions to past developmental delays or arrests and to emerge a more effective and less conflictful person. Illustrations given indicate that with the help of adults new and effective role models can be found. Opportunities for successful learning and work experiences can produce dramatic developmental shifts in every area of adolescent development. Family, group, and individual therapy help work through previous developmental obstacles to effective socialization, sexual intimacy, close relationships, as well as independent strivings.

REFERENCES

Adams, P. L. 1973. *Obsessive Children: A Sociopsychiatric Study*. New York: Brunner/Mazel.

Anthony, E. J. 1969. The reactions of adults to adolescents and their behavior. In G. Caplan and S. Lebovici, eds. *Adolescence*. New York: Basic.

Benedek, E. P.; Poznanski, E.; and Mason, S. 1979. A note on the female adolescents' psychological reaction to breast development. *American Journal of Child Psychiatry* 18:537–545.

Berlin, I. N. 1978. Some implications of the developmental process for treatment of depression in adolescence. *Journal of Adolescence* 1:134–145.

Block, J. 1971. *Mastery Learning: Theory and Practice*. New York: Holt, Rinehart & Winston.

Blos, P. 1962. *On Adolescence: A Psychoanalytic Interpretation*. New York: Free Press.

Blos, P. 1967. Second individuation process of adolescence. *Psychoanalytic Study of the Child* 22:162–186.

Caplan, G., and Lebovici, S. 1969. *Adolescence: Psychosocial Perspectives.* New York: Basic.

Derdeyn, A., and Waters, D. B. 1977. Parents and adolescents: empathy and vicissitudes of development. *Adolescent Psychiatry* 5:175–185.

Elkind, D. 1975. Recent research in cognitive development in adolescence. In S. E. Drogastin and G. H. Elder, Jr., eds. *Adolescence in the Life Cycle.* New York: Halsted.

Erikson, E. 1963. *Childhood and Society.* New York: Norton.

Erikson, E. 1968. *Identity, Youth, and Crisis.* New York: Norton.

Giovacchini, P. L. 1977. Psychoanalytic perspectives on adolescence: psychic development and narcissism. *Adolescent Psychiatry* 5:113–142.

Gutmann, D. 1973. The vicissitudes of ego identity: some consequences of the new morality. In J. C. Schoolar, ed., *Current Issues in Adolescent Psychiatry.* New York: Brunner/Mazel.

Kohlberg, L., and Gillian, C. 1971. The adolescent as philosopher: the discovery of self in a post-conventional world. *Daedalus* 100:1031–1086.

Kohler, M. 1971. The rights of children: an unexplored constituency. *Social Policy* 1:36–43.

Malmquist, C. P. 1979. Development: thirteen to sixteen years. In J. D. Call, ed. *Basic Handbook of Child Psychiatry.* New York: Basic.

Masterson, J. F., Jr. 1967. *The Psychiatric Dilemma of Adolescence.* Boston: Little, Brown.

Minuchin, S. 1974. *Families and Family Therapy.* Cambridge, Mass.: Harvard University Press.

Nagera, H. 1966. *Early Childhood Disturbances, the Infantile Neurosis and the Adulthood Disturbances.* New York: International Universities Press.

Offer, D. 1969. *The Psychological World of the Teenager: A Study of Normal Adolescent Boys.* New York: Basic.

Offer, D., and Offer, J. 1973. Normal adolescence in perspective. In J. C. Schoolar, ed. *Current Issues in Adolescent Psychiatry.* New York: Brunner/Mazel.

Peterson, A. C., and Offer, D. 1979. Adolescent development: sixteen to nineteen years. In J. D. Call, ed., *Basic Handbook of Child Psychiatry.* Vol. 1. New York: Basic.

Piaget, J., and Inhelder, B. 1969. *The Psychology of the Child.* New York: Basic.

Ravenscroft, R., Jr. 1974. Normal family regression at adolescence. *American Journal of Psychiatry* 131:31–35.

Silber, E.; Coelho, G. V.; Murphey, E. G.; Hamburg, D. A.; Pearlin, L. I.; and Rosenberg, M. 1961. Competent adolescents coping with college decisions. *Archives of General Psychiatry* 5:517–527.

Szurek, S. A. 1969. Emotional factors in the use of authority. In S. A. Szurek and I. N. Berlin, eds. *The Antisocial Child, His Family and His Community*. Palo Alto, Calif.: Science & Behavior.

White, R. W. 1960. Competence and the psychosexual stages of development. *Nebraska Symposium on Motivation* 8:97–141.

19 ADOLESCENT DEVELOPMENTAL ISSUES IN MARITAL THERAPY

JOHN TOEWS

The first years of marriage present their own special stresses, which may produce severe problems for some couples. One of these stresses is the need to resolve an apparent paradox, the poles of which are the need to share intimately with the marital partner while at the same time maintaining and enhancing individual autonomy. A requirement for successful resolution of this paradox is that both of the marital partners have successfully completed their adolescent tasks of separation from the parental home and the formation of secure identities as autonomous people. A significant number of young adults have not completed these tasks successfully; as a result, when this paradoxical set of demands is encountered, a severe crisis follows. This crisis, often poorly identified, is the issue that frequently sends young couples for therapeutic help. Signs of this crisis may be interminable arguments, loss of all ability to negotiate constructively, and major battles over issues of dominance. Attempts to preserve or restructure a premarital life-style, infidelity, and fully developed extramarital affairs may also result.

Too often, therapists seem only dimly aware of the developmental tasks that underlie the apparent conflict in such a couple. Instead, they react to the anger and hurt expressed or respond to the overt behavior of the pair and attempt to deal with the problems by merely manipulating the behavior or communication of the couple. This effort may result in a therapeutic impasse which leads a frustrated therapist to make premature comments concerning the viability of the marriage and the need for separation. This therapeutic pessimism may cause irreparable damage to the marriage of a young couple struggling to remain together.

It is my experience that, if the disturbing behavior and emotional turmoil of the couple are seen as evidence of a developmental crisis owing to incomplete resolution of the developmental conflicts of adolescence, a whole new range of therapeutic interventions is suggested. Treating couples by utilizing a developmental perspective in therapy allows the couples to view themselves at their own particular stage of the life cycle. Each may then see that establishing an identity as an autonomous adult, combined with the ability to relate intimately to one's marital partner, is a desirable goal, attainable through the successful resolution of this crisis.

Marriage as a Transitional Stage

The developmental crisis underlying the first years of marriage can best be understood if one views the period immediately preceding and following the act of marriage as a transitional stage between families of origin and the family of marriage. Normally, during adolescence, individuals acquire a sense of identity which includes the realization that the course of one's life is uniquely one's own, separate and distinct from the family of origin. This growing autonomy from the parental home leaves young people free to separate from home, choose mates, and establish independent homes of their making.

Separation from the families of origin has not been fully achieved by many couples who run into severe problems early in marriage. There is little evidence that, during adolescence, a period of slowly increasing independence accompanied by gradual working through of the loss of the childhood home has occurred. Instead, some of these young people appear to have denied their dependence on home and suddenly wrenched away to adopt a pseudoautonomous life-style. Others appear to have denied their need for separation from home and have left home only to form a rapid union with a partner in order to re-create a home like the one just left.

Despite a successful separation process, the young adult, as noted by Erikson (1963), still struggles with the conflict between intimacy and isolation. This struggle appears most intense during the period of youth prior to marriage and in the first years of marriage. It is related to the life stage just completed, in that one fears that the experience of intimacy will mean the loss of the independence and autonomy so recently acquired during adolescence. If one has not successfully attained independence of home, or if marriage is entered too rapidly, the struggle between intimacy and isolation is intensified. This is the basis for the conflict acted out by the couples being described. Its seriousness lies in the fact that, when this conflict is dramatically expressed, it may result in separation or divorce.

245

Autonomy and Intimacy

Prior to a discussion of the particular aspects of marriage that heighten the intimacy-versus-isolation conflict of these youths, it is necessary to consider the concepts of autonomy and intimacy.

Autonomy refers to a state of being independent of the control or direction of others. From this perspective, to achieve autonomy during adolescence means to gain independence of parental controls and of undue dependence on the supports of home.

Autonomy in adults has been defined as "the ability to make separate, responsible choices. The ability is demonstrated by the feeling of being a separate person rather than an extension of the other, an awareness of freedom to make choices in selecting or rejecting outside influences and assuming responsibility for one's decisions" (Murphy, Sibler, Coelho, Hamburg, and Greenberg 1963). It is apparent that mature autonomy does not demand isolation. Rather, the autonomous person has the ability to choose freely whether to relate intimately to another.

Intimacy is a similar concept. Erikson (1963) describes it as "the capacity to commit oneself to concrete affiliations or partnerships and to develop the ethical strength to abide by such commitments even though they may call for significant sacrifices and conflicts." Intimacy stems from a mature, certain sense of self. An examination of the definitions of autonomy and intimacy suggests that the realization of adult autonomy by an individual is a prerequisite for establishing a marital relationship in which full intimacy is expressed.

The early intense marital relationship contains certain characteristic stresses, which may severely threaten the young adult still unsure of the autonomy so recently acquired in late adolescence. Among these stresses unique to marriage are the intensity of the relationship, the marked interdependence of the mates, the duration of the relationship, and the legal fact of marriage with its connotations of loss of personal freedom.

The youth experiences threats to his or her autonomy even as early as the periods of serious dating and mate selection. It is well recognized that a major determinant in mate selection is the degree of similarity or dissimilarity to one's parents that is seen in the prospective mate. The selection of the mate may be influenced by recognizing the qualities of the parent in the potential partner. Alternatively, a partner may be selected in a negative reaction to parental characteristics, that is, a partner may be chosen who specifically does not resemble the parents in certain key respects. In each of these instances, the parental home so recently left may, in a figurative sense, be transferred into the marital relationship. The youth then displaces the struggle for independence from parents to marital partner.

This commonly accepted observation has been given a more intense cast by Sager (1976) in his observation that each partner projects simultaneously the transference reactions related to early experiences with both parents onto the other partner. The implications of this double parental transference for a young person unsure of his adult autonomy are clear. The tendency to regress pathologically within the marital relationship is enhanced. In these situations, the family just left has been indelibly transposed into the marital relationship. This may serve as a powerful stimulus for one to withdraw from intimacy to demonstrate independence of the marital partner and thereby demonstrate independence of one's parents.

Isolation and Marital Symbiosis

Individuals who have inadequately separated may respond to the threat marriage poses to their autonomy in unfortunate ways. One response may be to assume a pseudoindependent stance that may ultimately result in a flight from the marriage. Another response is to yield to the pressures toward regression that are present in marriage and fuse with the partner in an overly dependent relationship.

It is important to examine the clinical manifestations of both these responses. Autonomy and intimacy have their pathological counterparts in the isolation and marital symbiosis that appear almost as caricatures or parodies of the healthier, more adult traits. Isolation may be perceived as autonomy by someone who fears the demands on individual freedom that marrige imposes. Symbiosis may replace intimacy in a relationship where the marital partners feel that autonomy is incompatible with marriage.

Thus, isolation may give the illusion of autonomy and symbiosis the illusion of intimacy. The difference between the real and illusory states may be noted in the attainment during adolescence of a good measure of autonomy as a precondition for experiencing intimacy as a young adult in a marital relationship. No such relationship or precondition exists between isolation and symbiosis.

The presenting problems of many young couples who request marital therapy are related to the expression of isolation. Many of these couples are in a crisis precipitated by one partner's expressing in words or actions that he is a separate individual not bound to the demands or considerations of the other. Such expression ranges from marked discord to marital separation. In such relationships, compromise is seen as capitulation and loss of autonomy.

In these relationships, the premarital life-style of the partner is carried into the marriage, with each partner not willing to make concessions to the fact of marriage. The tendency of one toward isolation is often accentuated by the demands of the other for intimacy.

Extramarital affairs are another common route by which isolation rather than autonomy is expressed. In these instances, intimacy is impeded because the commitment to the relationship that is a necessary part of intimacy is denied. Sexual involvement with others is used to state one's autonomy from one's mate rather than to realize the inability to achieve genuine intimacy.

Marital symbiosis may also be evident in couples who present for therapy. Courtship and the early period of marriage for these couples are characterized by an intensely dependent involvement with each other. These couples reveal a strong identity as a couple accompanied by minimal identities as individuals. They share most activities and interests and reveal a curious lack of conflict, despite stresses that would ordinarily produce conflict in other couples. There is often no clear precipitant in these couples that causes them to seek therapy. There may be a gradually increasing feeling of uneasiness in one partner. This feeling is often produced by the realization that the marital relationship is not as fulfilling as originally hoped. Couples may present for therapy at this stage or, as discussed earlier, in a crisis following one partner's suddenly wrenching free of the symbiotic relationship. Then behavior ranging through repeated fights to extramarital affairs and threatened separation may be a precipitant of therapy.

Techniques of Therapy

The therapist is often tempted to focus on overt behavior rather than on the more subtle underlying developmental crisis when facing young couples who are ambivalent about remaining together and whose behavior seriously threatens their marital relationship. When therapists make this error, both they and the couple may experience an increasing frustration with treatment that can easily result in a failed therapeutic contract or, what is worse, a failed marriage that could have continued had the issues been recognized. The therapist often responds to his own frustration by overtly or covertly working toward dissolution of the marriage. In this way, independence for each partner (including the therapist) is achieved at the expense of intimacy and marriage. If, instead, the focus in therapy is on the marital relationship as an implement of emotional growth in which the uncompleted task of adolescence can be addressed in the exploration of autonomy, commitment, and intimacy, the marital relationship will be strengthened rather than weakened by each individual's maturational growth.

Therapy with these and similar young couples can be conveniently divided into three stages. The first stage, problem identification and contract formation, provides the necessary structure for the stages that follow. The second stage focuses extensively on the individuals' need for autonomy from their families of origin as well as from each other. The third stage uses the realization of this autonomy as a base from which to explore the experience of intimacy within the marital relationship.

STAGE 1

Marital therapy begins with the identification of the problems that bring the young couple to seek help. These problems are often presented as though centered in one person. However, the fact that each contributes to the problems and that the problems are shared is strongly underscored. This is necessary since it leads to the first stating of a theme that will recur throughout therapy. Simply stated, the theme is that marriage, once entered, must retain both individual and shared dimensions for each partner. Now the contract can be set. It must be strong enough to provide a structure for therapy and support for the couple during the stage of therapy where individual autonomy and separateness are stressed. It differs from other therapy contracts in certain key respects. The members of the couple are asked to make their wish to remain in the marriage explicit. They are further asked to commit themselves to continue in their marriage at least as long as therapy continues. These stated commitments serve to give the therapy a direction and a goal. Other clauses are specific for each couple and arise out of a consideration of the behaviors that are considered by the couple to be the most destructive to the relationship.

The formation of the contract for therapy may precipitate a crisis that may be understood as a reaction to the fact that the shared aspects of marriage have been reinforced by the commitment implied by the contract. The specific stipulations of the contract may then be rapidly transgressed. When this happens, it is viewed and interpreted as a reaction to the feared loss of identity within the intimacy of marriage. While the fact that these actions arise from the individual's wish to show his maturity by being autonomous is acknowledged, the isolation that results from these actions is also strongly interpreted and the contract reestablished.

STAGE 2

The strategy of the second stage of therapy is to focus on each individual's autonomy. The autonomy of the person as an adult, free from the infantalizing ties with the parental home, is stressed. The fact that a new home has been established that is separate and distinct from the parental home is emphasized. The wish of the individual to be free from the infantalizing and symbiotic ties present within his own marriage is also addressed. Then, within the conjoint sessions, each individual is helped to see himself as a separate person with the freedom to determine his own future.

It is helpful to select the developmental issues of youth and young adulthood as the major focus for interpretation. Restricting the interpretations or explanations to this single area allows comprehensive maturational work while the explanations are kept simple and readily understandable by the couple. Another advantage of using life tasks as a focus for interpretation is that it allows the therapist to comment on individual reactions that are destructive to the relationship within a supportive and positive context.

This method of intervention has the effect of allowing each to see the reactions that have been problems in the marriage in a new light. While these reactions are still perceived as painful and destructive, the maturational intent of the behavior can be understood. The partners are then in a better position to discuss and explore actions that will lead them closer to their life-stage goals.

A major goal of this therapy is to enable the individual to complete the tasks not completed during adolescence. During this stage, each partner is helped to work through residual attachments to the parental home that interfere with independent adult functioning. Each is encouraged, as well, to consider himself as separate from the mate. Individual autonomous choices are supported. Each is actively encouraged to state his own feelings, reactions, and wishes in areas where disagreement is likely. Views of marriage that do not allow this degree of separation are challenged. In couples with symbiotic relationships, it is during this period that their myth of the ideal marriage fades away. As this stage progresses, arguments may become more frequent. Intense struggles between the partners are apparent as each partner attempts to experience and express autonomy. This stage of therapy may end in a therapeutic crisis in which both members of the pair realize that they can separate and survive independently. They may even wonder if this may not be a necessary step in order for each to be an autonomous adult.

During this stage, it is often the contract and the active intervention of the therapist that keep the couple together. During this crisis, one partner may state emphatically the need to be separate. If this statement goes unchallenged, the couple may separate. Instead, the therapist must challenge this statement and explore actively why adult autonomy cannot be experienced within the marriage. This intervention often allows the individual to realize that autonomy and marriage are not incompatible and that the marriage could continue. Alternately, this stage may fade imperceptibly into the third phase—the stage of exploration of intimacy.

STAGE 3

While the second stage of therapy dealt with reworking and completing many of the maturational issues of adolescence, the third stage focuses on young adulthood by exploring the recommitment to the marriage. Overtly or covertly, each member of the pair has chosen to remain married. If these decisions are made covertly, the therapist aids the overt expression of the wish. Couples in this stage usually move rapidly to termination of therapy. The therapist's main tasks are to continue to emphasize each individual's contribution to the marriage and to support the growing comfort both feel with the concept of themselves as autonomous individuals actively deciding to spend their futures together in marriage.

During termination with these couples, individual freedom and responsibility are again emphasized. Leaving therapy is often discussed as analogous to each partner's earlier decision, as a youth, to leave the parental home where others unduly interfere with, influence, and control him. Each is helped to realize that he no longer requires either parent or therapist to direct him.

Conclusions

This chapter emphasizes the clinical manifestations of a common developmental crisis encountered by young married couples. It suggests techniques of intervention whereby isolation and symbiosis can be replaced by autonomy

251

and intimacy. The chapter also emphasizes that, in order to relate intimately, one must have a firm idea of one's own identity. A component of one's identity is a view of oneself as an autonomous person. The definition of autonomy used suggests that the autonomous person is one who views himself as separate rather than as an extension of others, be it parents or spouse. He sees freedom in choices and assumes responsibility for his decisions. Such a person, as an adult, can commit himself to partnerships and have the ethical strength to abide by such commitments. This, Erikson (1963) says, is intimacy.. In reworking and completing the adolescent life tasks of separation from home and the formation of an identity as an autonomous person, the couples described are helped to discover that autonomy is not isolation and that intimacy is not symbiosis. They realize that, for intimacy to flourish, a high degree of responsible autonomy must find expression.

REFERENCES

Erikson, E. H. 1963. *Childhood and Society*. 2d ed. New York: Norton.
Murphy, E. B.; Sibler, E.; Coelho, G. V.; Hamburg, D. A.; and Greenberg, I. 1963. Development of autonomy and parent-child interaction in late adolescence. *American Journal of Orthopsychiatry* 33:643–652.
Sager, C. J. 1976. *Marriage Contracts and Couple Therapy: Hidden Forces in Intimate Relationships*. New York: Brunner/Mazel.

20 NARCISSISTIC GUARDIANS: DEVELOPMENTAL ASPECTS OF TRANSITIONAL OBJECTS, IMAGINARY COMPANIONS, AND CAREER FANTASIES

RONALD M. BENSON

At a panel on the vicissitudes of infantile omnipotence, Ritvo (1974) presented a developmental formulation of omnipotence based on a lifelong tendency to attempt to regain the lost primary narcissism of infancy. He considered normal and deviant adolescence rich fields for the study of this subject. He contrasted those adolescents who persisted in exaggerated fantasies of omnipotence with those able to restructure the psychic apparatus with a shift of power to the ego.

Blos (1974) has commented upon the relative lack of analytic attention to the vicissitudes of narcissism in adolescence. He states that while fantasies about fame, greatness, and perfect love are common features of adolescence, the pervasive obsession with such fantasies and their affinity to primitive narcissistic states characterize them as pathological.

Kernberg (1975) has also called attention to the practical problems of differentiating normal from pathological narcissistic developments in adolescence. Recognizing the quantitative increases in narcissism at this stage of life, he suggests there is also a qualitative distinction to be made. He says that self-absorption, increased concern over the self, and grandiose exhibitionistic and power-oriented fantasies are a normal manifestation of the adolescent increase in narcissism. This reflects a regressive shift to more infantile relations between self and object with a greater libidinal investment of self-representations.

In this chapter, I will describe a particular type of idealized vocational fantasy that—though exaggerated, fanciful, grandiose, and formally regressive—is used for a progressive developmental purpose. I will attempt to compare these fantasies with the imaginary companions and transitional objects of younger children, particularly to demonstrate the essential similarities in their psychic functions from the point of view of the developmental line of narcissism and the establishment of the cohesive self (Kohut 1971).

Illustrative Examples

CASE 1. ADOLESCENT DEPRESSION AND PARENT LOSS

Boyd was sixteen years old, in the eleventh grade, and not doing well academically. His father had engaged a tutor, who felt the boy was depressed. This eventually led to his entering psychotherapy. Boyd was the youngest of three siblings; the older two were out of the home. The household consisted of just himself and his father, his mother having died of cancer when Boyd was eleven.

The boy's conflicts centered around his struggle for autonomy and independence opposed by dependent needs. The father's inability to relate to his son in terms of the youth's own personality, capacities, and stage of development functioned as a severe developmental interference (Nagera 1966). For example, as graduation from high school drew nearer, father felt strongly that Boyd should attend a major university and prepare for an intellectual profession. Boyd had accepted this goal partially and superficially, despite knowledge that he had only average intelligence, was not interested in intellectual pursuits, and would probably be better suited for a job (similar to his brother's) as a clerk in a governmental agency. In fact, Boyd had investigated the requirements for such work and was constructively pursuing those courses in high school that would prepare him for this kind of employment.

Despite realistic awareness of his limitations, Boyd liked to think of himself as a great sports star. He idolized sports figures, and believed that he could be a professional football quarterback. In gym class, he played basketball and would tell with a half-apologetic smile of his activities ''around the league.'' All this was said in a tone of self-mocking irony, yet it was clear that it was as important for him to believe himself a sports star someday as it was for him to avoid any action to implement his dream. He did not try out for varsity athletics despite quite good athletic skills. With his friends,

254

he would express this fantasy only by saying in a joking way, "Here comes the great Boyd, champion quarterback," as they prepared for a ball game.

The importance of this fantasy is illustrated by this vignette from one therapy hour. Boyd was musing about what it would be like to be a college or professional quarterback. He felt that his ability was good enough to make it, but that he had made a mistake by not going out for high school varsity football, and now it was too late. I agreed that since he had not chosen this route earlier, it was not likely he would be able to realize this dream. I inquired regarding any awareness he had of his motives for not choosing to try out for either football or basketball. Boyd's face immediately fell and he looked depressed. He grew silent for the remainder of that hour and the start of the next. When verbal associations were resumed, they centered around some dumb guy who was ignorant about sports and everything else. Only when I pointed out his feelings of self-depreciation in reaction to my earlier comments could he acknowledge that he felt as if I were saying that "he'd never make it at anything."

Although this great sports-star fantasy appeared during many therapy hours, filled part of his thinking on many days, and probably increased in times of stress, it never seemed to interfere with his everyday life. He continued to prepare for college and, in general, functioned at an age-appropriate level.

As Boyd progressed through high school, his academic work improved and his relationship with his father changed. He began consciously to be aware of his father's limitations as a parent and to accept his own responsibility for his future. Along with these changes, his use of the sports-star fantasy minimized and gradually disappeared. It was not forgotten but simply no longer used.

CASE 2. A LEARNING-DISABLED CHILD

Brenda was thirteen years old when her mother called for an evaluation of her "intelligence and stubbornness." Psychological testing revealed borderline normal intelligence, concrete thinking, and function limited by a characteristic stance of withdrawal or stubborn opposition when confronted with any anxiety-evoking situations. Brenda had experienced academic difficulties since kindergarten, and her mother had resisted efforts to have her placed in special education classes. With the onset of puberty, Brenda's attendance at junior high school, and the increasingly obvious differences in

Brenda's development from her very bright siblings, mother felt that psychiatric help was required.

The vicissitudes of Brenda's evaluation and the beginning of psychotherapy are not relevant here. However, during the first year of the work, her self-image—that of an awkward, damaged, lumplike creature who was unacceptable to her family—emerged. Despite often vociferous denials, it was clear that she realized that she was not sufficiently bright to keep up with her peers at her grade level in her upper-middle-class school. Furthermore, she knew that she could learn in a slower classroom more geared to her needs and that, had this kind of program started sooner, she would be better off now.

This conflict came to a crisis when the school demanded a change of program. Brenda acknowledged to her counselor and to her therapist that she knew that this was best for her. Yet to her mother she was evasive.

Eventually, in subtle ways, Brenda forced her mother to decide upon a special program. She was much happier after the change and openly acknowledged her full awareness of her intellectual handicap. She was also well aware that, for her, college and academic intellectual pursuits were unrealistic. Strikingly, along with all the aforementioned awareness, Brenda, at very frequent intervals, would talk of her future life in terms of attending a particular college and becoming a teacher. She idealized the teacher's role, but not any particular teacher. She would playfully make up lesson plans to show me. There was never any acknowledgment directly that this fantasy was in any way in contradiction to her other knowledge of herself or of her actions taken to insure placement in classes for the educationally handicapped. This fantasy remained with her throughout her two-and-a-half years of psychotherapy. Toward the end of treatment, I gently confronted the contradiction, but she told me quite explicitly not to discuss this with her yet, as she still needed it.

Two years after termination, I saw Brenda at her request. She was near graduation and one reason for returning was to have me confirm her view of herself as greatly improved. At the time of that interview, she presented herself as a quite self-possessed seventeen-year-old. School had gone well, and she was working with a special education teacher on a program of vocational training which was satisfying to her and within her capabilities. She felt that she could graduate and find work which she could accomplish. Her social life remained somewhat limited, but some friendships had been established and now she sought out social situations instead of retreating from them. Near the end of that interview, Brenda told me that she still remembered her idea of going to college and being a teacher and that she realized that her handicap did not permit it. "Funny," she said, "I just don't think of that anymore."

CASE 3. NORMAL ADOLESCENT

I knew Quentin from the time he was twelve. He was bright, did well in school, had many friends, and from all outward appearances seemed to be a typical, normally developing youngster. I knew him in a personal context, so I depended for knowledge of him on what he cared to reveal about himself to me of his inner life. His parents felt that his development was unremarkable when we discussed it in retrospect. When I spoke to Quentin about his early adolescence from the perspective of his adulthood, he felt that it was an uncertain time for him, but he did not believe that it was especially troubled when compared with those of his peers, or, for that matter, with his later-gained knowledge of normal development.

However, he remembered that from at least the age of twelve until that of fourteen or fifteen he had a favorite conscious fantasy that he would become the playing manager and second baseman for the local major-league baseball team. He knew that he had few extraordinary skills in athletics but, even though this gave him slight pause, he consciously preferred to overlook that reality. Sometimes he would use a game board with a baseball diamond printed upon it to play out, in the manner of a schematic diagram, his fantasy of the "big game" in which he would be the manager planning the strategy.

He never revealed his fantasy directly to anyone. For example, he never told anyone that he wanted to be a ball player when he grew up. On the other hand, he would make occasional jokes about the great life he thought professional ball players had and how he would "sure like to do that when he was old enough." He always said this in an ironic, joking way so that no one would ever know he really meant it.

Quentin does not recall exactly how the fantasy diminished in importance, but he does know that by the time he graduated with honors from high school, more realistic goals formed the basis of his daydreams. He says that he never entirely forgot the boyhood fantasy. He maintains an interest in sports and baseball as a spectator, but it is quite casual. As an adult, Quentin says that he does not even harbor a single feeling of nostalgia for the old dream. He graduated from college and joined the profession he had planned in late adolescence. Now a husband and father, he is successful in his occupation, which is totally unconnected with sports.

257

Discussion

Blos (1967) conceptualized the adolescent period as a second individuation process akin to that of the first three years of life. He pointed out that extensive structural reorganization is required and that definite limits to self- and object-representations emerge only upon the termination of adolescence. At that point the narcissistic institution of the ego ideal becomes more lasting and important and influences the internalization of responsibility for narcissistic balance.

Kohut (1971) has revised Freud's classic conception of libidinal development from autoerotism via narcissism to object love. He suggests another set of developmental phases which lead from autoerotism via narcissism to higher forms and transformations of narcissism. Crucial to Kohut's thinking is his concept of the development of the cohesive self and of "self-objection," something or someone subjectively experienced as part of the self. Over the course of development and various developmental crises, an overall sense of self evolves, gradually achieving a cohesiveness. The concept of the cohesive self, a product of various enduring and crucial self-objects, endows traditional notions of psychoanalytic development with a new perspective, that of identifying a separate narcissistic line of development.

My studies suggest that there are a series of aids affecting the establishment of a cohesive self. These aids, normative in development with some individual variations, can be described in a sequential, developmental series. These narcissistic guardians are used for the purpose of protecting the development of the self-representation, particularly when it is vulnerable to age- or stage-appropriate psychological stresses. Essentially milestones in the developmental line of narcissism, narcissistic guardians become more abstract and serve multiple developmental adaptive purposes. They would appear, from the observer's point of view, to be increasingly syntonic with reality (Benson and Pryor 1973).

One striking example of a narcissistic guardian is the imaginary companion of childhood already preceded developmentally by the transitional object (Busch 1974; Tolpin 1971; Winnicott 1953). The imaginary companion, like the transitional object, represents a self-object in the transitional zone of experience and from the viewpoints of narcissistic development is instrumental in self-esteem regulation.

Winnicott (1953), in describing his concept of transitional object and the transitional zone of experience, notes that the transitional zone is "an area which is not to be challenged, because no claim is made on its behalf except that it exists as a resting place for the individual engaged in the perpetual human task of keeping inner and outer reality separate yet inter-related.''

Tolpin (1971) relates the transitional zone experience in the transitional object to Kohut's concept of the self-object. She writes, ''The transitional object is thus heir to a part of the infant's original narcissism that was preserved when it is assigned to the idealized parent image . . . the metaphysical basis for its unique role in mental development and for its distinction from the 'pacifer.' '' The transitional object represents those soothing aspects of mother which are cathected with narcissistic libido and experienced as part of the psychic structure of the subject.

This self-mirroring with approval conveys what the child requires (Benson and Pryor 1973). Both the imaginary companion and the transitional object seem to function to permit the self to develop to the point where object love, in contrast with relations with the self-object, are tolerable, safe, and not a threat to the integrity of the self (Kohut 1971). The transitional object and imaginary companion, through their soothing or approving function, provide a transitional form of mental structure until those functions become part of the child's own psychic structure through transmuting internalization (Tolpin 1971).

The transitional object and imaginary companion serve to protect the self-representation during periods of developmental conflict (Nagera 1966). Being under the child's control and not involved in typical conflicts, as are real objects, these constructs serve to protect the child from narcissistic injury when parents can not (Benson and Pryor 1973). That purpose accomplished and the functions they fulfilled internalized, the defenses lose their importance.

It is from the point of view of these concepts that I would like now to consider these illustrative examples, especially to try to understand why each of these youngsters had such a need for their conscious, treasured, and grandiose vocational fantasies. In choosing to focus attention on the narcissistic aspects of their functioning, I do not mean to imply that the youth's developing cognitive abilities or object relations were unimportant in determining the specific content of their fantasies; quite the contrary was probably true in each instance. However, to view these constructs essentially in terms of their object-related meaning would obscure their unique role in the development of the self.

Douvan and Adelson (1966) and Offer (1969) have noted that for normative adolescents, especially adolescent boys, the future is frequently conceived and organized around an occupational identity and occupational choice. That choice, however, is consistent with the realistic assessment of the adolescent's capabilities and is pursued realistically. In each of the illustrations, such occupational choices and planning were occurring, yet despite this, the youngster still required the fantasy as well. The realistic goal, planned for and pursued, existed side by side with the idealized vocational role fantasy, which was used by the adolescent but not pursued. This idealized role, however, did not simply represent high and noble ambitions in a youngster who was so conflicted that he was paralyzed in his efforts to accomplish and achieve those goals (Blos 1974). These adolescents were as successful in actual advancement toward a career and consolidation of identity as their abilities, intellect, and cognitive capacities permitted.

What each of these youngsters had in common was that they each created and used for a period of several months to a few years a fantasy of an idealized and grandiose (from the viewpoint of their actual personal characteristics and abilities) vocational role. It is notable that it was a role and not a particular person or even a real class of persons that was idealized. The characteristics in each role were, in their essentials, created by the adolescent and only in the most superficial details drawn from the real or the object world.

When Winnicott (1953) described transitional object, he said, "It is a matter of agreement between us and the baby that we will never ask the question, 'Did you conceive of this or was it presented to you from without?'" Tolpin (1971) also called attention to this aspect of the transitional object by saying that "when the infant begins to use his blanket . . . he has created something—that is, he has endowed an inconsequential bit of the external world with a capacity to restore or improve his inner equilibrium." Busch (1974), describing the same phenomena, says that all transitional objects are chosen for reasons relating to their availability and familiarity as well as certain qualities of their own and also related to the link with mother's soothing functions.

Nagera (1969), speaking of the imaginary companion, says that the importance is not the content of the fantasy associated with the imaginary companion but the developmental purpose it is designed to fulfill. Thus, for example, Brenda did not pattern her idealization after any of her teachers or even after the way she really felt about teaching as a profession. She felt ambivalent about both the individuals and the profession. Yet, the idealized role was assigned the value of perfection.

Furthermore, the adolescent experienced the role as identical with himself or herself and not truly as a goal to be worked for and reached. Boyd demonstrated this clearly in his ironic references to himself as a champion, demonstrating his inner belief in the oneness of himself and the idealized sports-star role. It was as if in each instance the youth reasoned, ''Perfection and admiration are ceded to my ideal vocation, but I am part of it and therefore admired and perfect.'' In this context, the role represents a self-object, cathected with narcissistic libido and used by the adolescent to achieve a sense of perfection, approval, and worth.

During early and middle adolescence, the youth cannot gain a sense of perfection and narcissistic well-being from his parents because he is actively engaged in diminishing their importance to himself and, besides, due to regressive forces at work, they are once again drawn into the sphere of his conflictual life (Blos 1962, 1967). His own superego is in a similar process of devaluation. No longer will following the rules be sufficient to establish a sense of narcissistic goodness. Peers and others in the object world, like the parents, are conflictual. The youth has not yet matured and developed to the point where either love or friendship is possible without a threat to the integrity of the self (Kohut 1971). The real occupational choice is also part of the object world and involved in conflicts, especially those involving success and competition.

These idealized vocational fantasies, in contrast, were not conflicted. The youths did not truly treat them as public, to be shared indiscriminantly with one and all. However, they did not keep them a closely guarded secret as is usual with adolescent fantasies related to impulses involved in internalized conflict (Freud 1965).

Relations with the self-object were safe for the adolescent involved since the construct was under the complete and total control of its creator. It existed in the ''transitional zone'' (Winnicott 1953) and was relatively immune from acquiring any meaning which would challenge the adolecent's need for a reflection of his worth and goodness.

In this regard it is important to note how directly Brenda insisted that her ''teacher fantasy'' was not to be analyzed because she ''needed it.'' Boyd reacted dramatically to my treating his fantasy as if it reflected reality and was, therefore, part of the objective world instead of the world of his own making. When I inquired about the contradiction between his fantasy and his actions, he experienced a narcissistic rebuff and could say he experienced my remarks ''as if he would never succeed at anything.'' In other terms, it was as if so much narcissistic cathexis was attached to this (self-object) fantasy that to interefere with it was to inflict a narcissistic injury and leave its creator devasted, depressed, and feeling hopeless and worthless.

These idealized vocational fantasies are not to be confused with the ego ideal. They do not represent a goal for the attainment of narcissistic perfection and gratification. Rather, they are in the nature of self-idealizations representing the maintenance of an illusion of perfection as already achieved and existing parallel with other progressive development.

Conclusions

Idealized vocational fantasies are, like the transitional object and imaginary companion, another in the developmental series of narcissistic guardians. They are created by their user, are under his complete control, and are self-objects in the transitional zone of experience. They are used to protect the self-representation at a time of vulnerability due to developmental conflicts. These fantasies permit the adolescent a degree of independence from the object world at a time when all aspects of that world are a threat to self-esteem. Yet, because of their illusory qualities, they provide a means of maintaining a cohesive and satisfying self and help to prevent more regressed and disruptive solutions to the threats of this stage of development.

The fantasies appear very similar in form to constructs that might be highly pathologic in another phase of the life cycle. However, this is no less true of the transitional object and imaginary companion, about which there is increasing agreement that they do not serve as pathologic regulators of self-esteem (Reich 1969), but as transient detours on the way to maturity (Benson and Pryor 1973; Busch 1974; Busch, Nagera, McKnight, and Pezzarossi 1973; Nagera 1969; Tolpin 1971).

Finally, the purpose of these mental creations of adolescents seems to permit progressive development and not to maintain a fixated regressed position. The young person's use of these fantasies, which are self-idealizing and provide an infantile illusion of perfection, seems to be a detour through fantasy, promoting growth (Hartman 1939).

Interference with such fantasies by a parent, teacher, or therapist might serve as an interference to normal development, since these fantasies fulfill their purpose and disappear (Nagera 1966). They are, at times, very close to symptomatic and pathologic constructs. This differentiation, however, is not made on their formal qualities, but requires an assessment of purpose and especially of the progressive versus regressive trends in the totality of personality functioning.

Narcissistic guardians are created by children and by adolescents in response to developmental needs. They permit the growing young persons some immunity from the too soon and too stark realization of his limitations. Yet, all people, throughout the life cycle, are similarly faced with threats to their very sense of existence. It seems likely that the creation of narcissistic guardians may be found in all stages of the life cycle. Their form may become more subtle and they may be more mature. I believe that a further search for such constructs in other developmental stages will prove useful in further understanding the developmental aspects of the self and its maintenance.

REFERENCES

Benson, R. M., and Pryor, D. B. 1973. "When friends fall out": developmental interference with the function of some imaginary companions. *Journal of the American Psychoanalytic Association* 21:457–473.

Blos, P. 1967. The second individuation process of adolescence. *Psychoanalytic Study of the Child* 22:162–186.

Blos, P. 1962. *On Adolescence.* New York: Free Press.

Blos, P. 1974. The genealogy of the ego ideal. *Psychoanalytic Study of the Child* 29:83–88.

Busch, F. 1974. Dimensions of the first transitional object. *Psychoanalytic Study of the Child* 12:193–214.

Busch, F.; Nagera, H.; McKnight, J.; and Pezzarossi, G. 1973. Primary transitional objects. *Journal of the American Academy of Child Psychiatry* 12:193–214.

Douvan, E., and Adelson, J. 1966. *The Adolescent Experience.* New York: Wiley.

Freud, A. 1965. *Normality and Pathology in Children.* New York: International Universities Press.

Hartman, J. 1939. *Ego Psychology and the Problem of Adaption.* New York: International Universities Press.

Kernberg, O. 1975. *Borderline Conditions and Pathological Narcissism.* New York: Aronson.

Kohut, H. 1971. *The Analysis of the Self.* New York: International Universities Press.

Nagera, H. 1966. *Early Childhood Disturbances, the Infantile Neuroses and the Adult Disturbances.* New York: International Universities Press.

Nagera, H. 1969. The imaginary companion. *Psychoanalytic Study of the Child* 24:165–196.

Offer, D. 1969. *The Psychological World of the Teen-Ager.* New York: Basic.

Reich, A. 1969. Pathologic forms of self-esteem regulation. In *Psychoanalytic Contribution*. New York: International Universities Press, 1973.

Ritvo, S. 1974. Vicissitudes of infantile omnipotence. *Journal of the American Psychoanalytic Association* 22:558–602.

Tolpin, M. 1971. On the beginnings of the cohesive self. *Psychoanalytic Study of the Child* 26:316–352.

Winnicott, D. W. 1953. Transitional objects and transitional phenomena. *International Journal of Psycho-Analysis* 34:89–97.

VULNERABLE YOUTH: HOPE, DESPAIR, AND RENEWAL

INTRODUCTION—VULNERABLE YOUTH: HOPE, DESPAIR, AND RENEWAL

MIRIAM ELSON AND JOHN F. KRAMER

We view youth as a time of energy, strength, and vibrancy, yet the problems of our time have precipitated mounting sadness and depressive episodes among young people. A period of disorganization and reorganization in society has an especially severe impact since they are still in the process of defining life-style and vocational goals. New freedoms in personal relationships have emerged which, when abused, seem to emphasize superficiality and transience, not only among their peers but among older adults to whom they look for support. Vastly changing needs for traditional vocations and worsening economic conditions have seriously eroded options for study and training. Possessing genuine talent and skill, young people confront a society which seems to block the very goals toward which their education propelled them. Lacking sufficient depth of experience, they grow despairing.

For almost a quarter of a century, through the University of Chicago Student Mental Health Clinic, we have been privileged to work with over 9,000 students in the undergraduate years, the graduate divisions, and the professional schools. Through their eyes we have witnessed the spiraling intensity of change marked by violence abroad and in our own country. Their vigorous protests to an unjust war and to the massive denial of civil rights for a large segment of citizens had a profound impact on events in our own country.

During the 1960s, when news and TV media were reporting box scores of campuses involved in uprisings and violence, we observed that the exposure itself created an epidemic effect. But it masked the destructive impact on those young people whose lack of attachment and goals could be dispelled briefly by feeling a part of something alive and real and expressive of strong feeling. When the excitement subsided, they were left with apathy and depression and continued to drift in a purposeless way. Little observed, and almost never reported with the same extensive coverage, were thousands of young

267

students who were able to continue striving to complete their education and to succeed in professionalizing their talents and skills.

We have only begun to understand the profound need for attachment which young people particularly require in order to accomplish their transition to adult commitments.

A mental health clinic is only one of many services available to young people on a university campus. Academic deans and advisers, faculty, house-heads, pastoral counselors, and physicians offer a broad range of relationships which can be effective in freeing energy to meet the challenges of our difficult times.

In working with students who sought our help when they were at an impasse in their personal lives or their academic pursuits, we were able to absorb their confusion, rage, and despair. Without intruding upon their initiative, we could provide them the opportunity to clear away crippling doubts and to reengage themselves in making difficult choices and pursuing the goals that were open to them. What seemed to be crucial was the opportunity for a relationship with concerned adults.

Although depression, anxiety, and immobilization are common among university students, this population does not contribute with any significance to the appalling death rate found in the general population of male youth fifteen to twenty-four years of age. In that cohort, three out of four deaths are due to violence—accidents, homicide, and suicide. The death rate among young women is far lower, but depressive symptoms occur much more frequently. There is some evidence that, when the depressive equivalent of drug and alcohol abuse and delinquency—more common among young men—is better understood, we may find a lower differential between the sexes in the rate of depression.

Accordingly, in April 1978 we assembled a distinguished panel to consider the impact of broad social change on youth and the impact of youth on society.

Philip M. Hauser, sociologist and demographer, compared the experiences of Depression-born youth and the baby-boom cohort and defined the difficult burdens the latter bear.

From the viewpoint of contemporary religious trends, Irving I. Zaretsky, anthropologist, placed in historical context youth's search for faith and community.

John Cawelti identified three broad trends in contemporary literature to which youth turns.

Gerald L. Klerman, director of the Alcohol, Drug Abuse, and Mental Health Administration, documented the increasing prevalence of depression

268

in youth and noted the adaptive function of depression as a signal for alerting the environment to the need for nurturance.

Philip S. Holzman, psychologist and psychoanalyst, identified the underlying theme in these chapters: attachments are required for growth, for maturation, and for well-being, and we are seeing an increase in psychopathology because of the loosening of societal supports for youth.

This special section will be of value to all who work with young people. The challenges posed by society require solutions which must be vigorously pursued. We have learned through our own work that it is in the warm acceptance of others that hope can be defined, despair can be overcome, and a renewal of purpose and discovery can ensue.

21 OUR ANGUISHED YOUTH: BABY BOOM UNDER STRESS

PHILIP M. HAUSER

With the demobilization of the armed forces following World War II, the United States was among those nations which experienced a postwar "baby boom." Substantial increases in marriage rates and birthrates after the war produced an unprecedentedly large postwar cohort. The boom began in the year 1946–1947 (July 1–June 30) when the absolute number of annual births increased by more than 1 million, rising from about 2.9 million in 1945–1946 to 3.9 million. Beginning with 1953–1954, the number of births per annum did not drop below the 4 million level until 1964, although the crude birthrate, which had peaked at 27.5 in 1946–1947, dropped to 21.6 by 1953–1954, a little above the average for the years 1941–1945. In the eighteen years between 1946 and 1964 some 72.9 million infants joined the American population. As of July 1, 1978, the Bureau of the Census estimated that 41.5 million persons would be fifteen to twenty-four years of age, virtually all of them members of the postwar baby crop, 49.5 percent of them female, and 13.3 percent of them black. This is the cohort of youth that has probably experienced greater stress and anguish than any previous cohort in American history (U.S. Bureau of the Census 1977).

The youngest of this group were born in 1963; the eldest were born in 1953. Those born before 1953 but after the end of World War II as of this year will be the younger adult population. They too experienced stressful times when they were adolescents and may combine with the late-adolescent group of today to form a significant political bloc in the years ahead—a bloc

Presented at the Conference on Vulnerable Youth, University of Chicago Student Mental Health Clinic, April 3, 1978; written while the author was Senior Fellow, East-West Population Institute, Honolulu, March 1978.

not only more receptive to basic social, economic, and political change but perhaps even insistent upon it.

The Exposure Milieu: Social, Economic, and Political Aspects

Young persons in the United States, those born since the end of World War II, are in many respects a unique generation of Americans. They were born into a society, largely an urban mass society, in which a high premium was placed on education. In consequence, measured by years of schooling they are the most educated cohort of Americans in our history. Moreover, they are the first generation of humankind who from the moment of birth have been exposed to electronic communication, both radio and television. Experiencing socialization as members of a mass society, acquiring relatively high education, and being exposed to worldwide, as well as national and local, events in vivid audiovisual form, they represent a combination of backgrounds in which social heritage may have played a lesser role in influencing values, norms, attitudes, and forms of behavior than has been the case in any previous generation. Permit me to elaborate on the impact of these three elements of the background of contemporary youth.

To begin with, it is important to recognize that persons born between 1946 and 1963 were born into an America that had become 61–71 percent urban. Since the U.S. population did not become more than half urban (51.2 percent) until 1920, populations born prior to that date may be described as having been born into a rural society, and persons born since that date were more likely to be born into an urban society.[1] The postwar baby crop thus contained a larger proportion of youngsters born into an urban society than any previous comparable group. This is a significant fact when it is interpreted to mean that the postwar babies were less likely than previous infants to be subject to socialization in a rural milieu—one in which values, attitudes, and behaviors were likely to conform with tradition as embodied in the social heritage. The youngsters we are considering, then, were more subject than previous cohorts to the acquisition of values, attitudes, and forms of behavior dependent on the contemporary, rather than on the traditional, order.

Next, the relatively high level of formal schooling attained by the baby-boom youngsters, averaging more than a high school education (persons twenty-five to twenty-nine in 1975, born between 1946 and 1950, had a median of 12.8 years of schooling) also made them less susceptible to traditional constraints in behavior (U.S. Bureau of the Census 1976). This follows to the extent that formal schooling produces an open mind—that is, a mind that is not closed by blind acceptance of values, attitudes, and norms of behavior of the past. Presumably the educated person is more likely to be subject to rational, that is, decision-making, behavior than to mechanical acceptance of traditional forms of behavior.

Third, the postwar youngsters were the first generation in the experience of humankind to be reared in a social environment which from the moment of their birth, or at least their attainment of social consciousness, included exposure to audiovisual electronic communication—radio and television. Despite a large content of "wasteland," this exposure also involved an unprecedented amount of information on international, national, and local happenings. There was a disproportionate focus on the most severe problems of the times—international tensions, confrontations, and bloody riots and wars; racial and ethnic tensions and internecine brutal hostilities; international and national economic problems, including recessions, high-level unemployment, and currency depreciation; the North-South confrontation, the tensions between "have" and "have-not" nations; domestic problems, including racial and ethnic tensions and overt conflicts, political corruption, labor-management struggles, ravages of organized crime in its continued control of gambling, prostitution, the drug traffic, and its successful invasion of respectable business enterprises. More specifically, this generation of youth was exposed in a more direct and intense audiovisual way to the atrocities of the undeclared Vietnam War; to the brutalities of the fratricidal conflicts in Northern Ireland, West and East Pakistan, and the Nigerian-Biafran holocaust; the Arab-Israeli wars and PLO atrocities and Israeli responses; the accelerating worldwide terrorist activities, including hijacking; the white-black confrontations, not only in the Union of South Africa and Rhodesia but also in the United Kingdom and the United States; the "cold-war" tensions between the capitalist and Communist states; the bloody invasion by the USSR of Hungary and Czechoslovakia; the gory events in the People's Republic of China connected with the "great leap forward" and the "Great Proletarian Cultural Revolution." Also, during this period problems of environmental degradation and explosive population growth were brought into world, national, and local consciousness in graphic and frightening ways.

On the domestic front there was exposure to the succession of assassinations of major national personalities—John and Robert Kennedy and Martin Luther King; the political corruption in Chicago, New York, Philadelphia, New Orleans, and elsewhere; the inglorious Watergate episode, forcing the first resignation of a president who, apart from personal derelictions as a law-breaker, threatened the constitutional integrity of the nation; the illegalities and immoralities of dozens of high-ranking federal officials, most of whom were members of the bar; the involvement of top leaders of the business community and dozens of corporate giants in shady, illegal political practices at home and immoral practices of bribery and other forms of corruption abroad. A relatively minor episode was the forced resignation of the vice-president of the same administration for political corruption. Also not to be overlooked was the tragic sequence of events involved in the civil rights movement—the revolt of blacks, followed by the revolt of persons of Hispanic origin, Chicanos and Puerto Ricans; the mass burnings and riots in major cities, highlighting the plight of disadvantaged minority groups. Finally, it would be remiss not to mention the student unrest and revolt in the late sixties in which members of the postwar cohorts were active participants. The on-slaughts against universities and even secondary schools and, at the extremes, the activities of the Students for a Democratic Society and the Weathermen such as the Chicago "days of rage" may well be interpreted as forms of violent expression of an anguished youth unable to cope with the stresses to which they were subjected.

This list of events is by no means complete, but perhaps it reflects enough of the stressful milieu in which the present generation of youth was reared to be representative. Moreover, in addition to the real violence and tragedy reported in the mass media, they—and especially television—also presented an unprecedented brand of synthetic violence, entertainment designed to obtain maximum audiences and ratings for commercial purposes, without concern for its possible impact on the attitudes, values, and behavior of young viewers.

Cohort Experience

Let us turn next to some of the actual difficult experiences of the members of this postwar cohort, which in some way are more crucial in explaining their anguish than the milieu to which they were exposed. A good way to do this is to contrast their experiences with those of the group which preceded them—the cohort of youngsters born mainly during the Depression decade of the thirties. Comparisons will be made between the cohort fifteen to twenty-four years of age in 1955 (those born between 1930 and 1940) and the cohort fifteen to twenty-four years of age in 1960 (those born between 1945 and 1955).

To begin with, consider the different experience of these respective groups in school. When the Depression-born cohort reached elementary school age (taken for convenience to be five to fourteen as presented in the census tables), they attended schools in which the number of persons in their age group actually declined. That is, the number of five- to fourteen-year-olds in 1945 (born between 1930 and 1940) decreased by 11 percent from that in 1935 (born between 1920 and 1930) (U.S. Bureau of the Census 1975a, 1975b). In contrast, the postwar cohort of children of elementary school age, those aged five to fourteen in 1960 (born 1945–1955), increased by 45.1 percent between 1950 and 1960 (U.S. Bureau of the Census 1960). Elementary schools were hard-pressed to adjust to the tidal wave of postwar enrollees— a swamping which, it is generally agreed, resulted in a depreciation in the quality of education as well as in a more stressful atmosphere than that experienced by the earlier cohort.

The more stressful climate included more intense competition in the classroom, on the playing field, in organized athletics, and in other extracurricular activities. Much more intensive competition induced by cohort size was undoubtedly accompanied by greater stress and anguish for the postwar-born than for the Depression-born students.

Similarly, a depreciated quality of education and greater stress were experienced by the postwar cohort as compared with Depression-born youngsters throughout their school experience—in high school and in college as well as in the primary grades. Each level of school was, in turn, inundated as the postwar cohort advanced in age.

Next let us consider the labor-force experience of these respective groups. In 1955, at sixteen to nineteen years of age, the Depression-born cohort (born 1935–1941) had an 11 percent unemployment rate (U.S. Bureau of the Census 1970a). In 1972, the postwar cohort (born 1953–1956) had an unemployment rate of 26.9 percent, more than double that of the comparable Depression-born group. And peak unemployment, in the worst recession since the 1930s, was not reached until 1974–1975 (U.S. Bureau of the Census 1970a).

Unemployment rates alone, however, do not tell the whole story of the relatively disadvantaged position of the postwar cohort. Although the data are hard to come by, postwar youth undoubtedly had greater difficulty entering the work force or were more often discounted from the labor force because they had given up as hopeless their search for jobs. Although it cannot be quantified, we can infer that competition at work must have been much more intense for the larger postwar than for the smaller Depression cohort. Opportunities for promotion must have been slower for the postwar youth, even while their prospects for unemployment and underemployment were greater.

With unemployment and underemployment greater, it should not be too surprising that median age at marriage was higher for the postwar than for the Depression cohort, rising from 20.3 for females in the 1950s (when babies born during the 1930s began their first marriages) to 20.8 in the 1970s (when the postwar babies born in the 1950s began their first marriages). This difference may appear small, but its significance is better appreciated when it is realized that age of women at marriage decreased between 1890 and 1950 by 1.7 years and then turned upward from 1960 (U.S. Bureau of the Census 1970a). Women aged twenty to twenty-four in 1960, born between 1935 and 1940, experienced their first marriage at the rate of 264 per 1,000 single women (National Center for Health Statistics 1960). In contrast, women of that age born in 1950–54 experienced a rate of first marriage of 143.8—down 39 percent (U.S. Bureau of the Census 1975a). Similarly, it should not be surprising that age at birth of first child was higher for the postwar than for the Depression cohort, rising from 21.4 in the 1950s to 22.7 in the 1970s (Glick 1976).

If one examines the number of children ever born to women twenty-five to twenty-nine years of age in the respective cohorts, the decline in births is clearly evident. Women aged twenty-five to twenty-nine in 1960 (born between 1930 and 1935) had borne 2,007 children per 1,000. In contrast, women twenty-five to twenty-nine in 1975 (born between 1947 and 1951) had given birth to only 1,360 children per 1,000. At age twenty-five to twenty-nine, then, the postwar cohort of women had only about two-thirds of the children ever born (67.7 percent) to comparable Depression-born women (U.S. Bureau of the Census 1975a, p. 7). Although these census data exclude births to single women and illegitimate births, the decline in fertility is nevertheless substantial.

Another measurement of the difference in childbearing between the two cohorts is given by the percentage of ever-married, twenty-five to twenty-nine-year-old women who are childless. In 1960 only 12.6 percent of the Depression-born cohort of such women were childless (U.S. Bureau of the Census 1970a, p. 54), as contrasted with 21.1 percent in 1975 for the postwar cohort (U.S. Bureau of the Census 1975b, p. 56).

The cohorts differ also in stability of marriages as measured by divorce. Marriages of women born between 1930 and 1934, the Depression cohort, were less likely to end in divorce than those of women born between 1945 and 1949, the postwar cohort. Twenty-one percent of the marriages of the Depression-born women had ended in divorce by 1975, and a total of 26 percent would ultimately end in divorce if their future divorce experience matched the 1969–1974 experience of older persons. For the postwar cohort of women (born 1945–1949), 17 percent of marriages had ended in divorce by 1975 (after a much shorter period of marriage than was experienced by the Depression-born women), but the same projection assumptions suggested that their final divorce rate would be as high as 38 percent (U.S. Bureau of the Census 1978).

Such data certainly help to explain the "sexual revolution" experienced by the postwar cohort. Various aspects of that revolution can be quantified. First of all, illegitimacy is much greater for the postwar cohort of white women than for their Depression-born predecessors. Among white adolescent (age fifteen to nineteen) women in 1955 (born 1935–1939), the out-of-wedlock birthrate was 6.0 per 100. In 1970 the same age group (born 1950–1954) had an out-of-wedlock birthrate of 10.9, 82 percent higher. Similarly, white women aged twenty to twenty-four (born 1930–1934) had an illegitimacy birthrate of 15.0, whereas the same group in 1970 (born 1945–1949) had an illegitimacy birthrate of 22.5, 50 percent higher. Nonwhites had much higher out-of-wedlock birthrates by reason of their history in the United States. Nonwhite women aged fifteen to nineteen in 1970 had an illegitimacy rate of 90.8, compared with 77.6 for the Depression-born. However, for nonwhite women aged twenty to twenty-four, the postwar-born had a lower illegitimacy birthrate, 121.0 compared with 133.0 for the Depression-born cohort, which undoubtedly reflect the influence of increased social work, family planning education, and some advances in integration (U.S. Bureau of the Census 1970a, p. 52).

Premarital sex practices have been measured also by the timing of first births. Six percent of the women first married in 1950–1954, largely Depression-born women, had their first child before marriage. In contrast, 9 percent of the women first married in 1970–1974, postwar-born, had their first child before marriage, a proportion 50 percent greater than was the case for the earlier group. Moreover, 24 percent of the postwar cohort of women, as compared with 17 percent of the Depression-born women, had their first child eight months or less after marriage (U.S. Bureau of the Census 1977, p. 15).

Another index of the sexual revolution is given by the number of unmarried couples living together. Although the available data do not permit a direct comparison of the two cohorts in this respect, they do permit the conclusion that such living arrangements have increased and are more frequently to be found among the postwar cohort than the Depression-born cohort. In 1960, the U.S. Census Bureau reported that there were 439,000 unmarried couples living together; by 1970, 523,000; and by 1977, 957,000. Unmarried adults living together in 1977 made up 0.9 percent of the total population and 3.6 percent of the unmarried adults. That this living arrangement is to be found among younger rather than older people is suggested by the fact that 5.4 percent of divorced men but 8.3 percent of divorced men under thirty-five, were living in such arrangements.[2] These data do not necessarily prove that living as unmarried couples is more apt to be the practice of the postwar than of the Depression-born cohort, but they strongly point to this possibility. Further support for this inference is given by the fact that one-fourth of the unmarried couples under twenty-five included one or both who were enrolled in college.

Readily available data on differential delinquency and suicide rates of the respective cohorts also point up the more disadvantaged position of the postwar cohort. Delinquency rates as measured by cases handled by juvenile courts were more than twice as high for the postwar than for the Depression-born cohort. In 1970 persons ten to seventeen years of age (born 1953–1960) had a delinquency rate of 32.3 (cases per 100 persons in the age group) as contrasted with a delinquency rate of 15.1 in 1947 (persons born 1930–1937) (U.S. Bureau of the Census 1970a, p. 419).

Similarly, the suicide rate of persons aged fifteen to twenty-four in 1970 (born 1945–1955), at 8.8 per 100,000 persons, was double that for the Depression-born group at the same age (born 1930–1940), which was 4.3 per 100,000.[3]

Conclusions

From the available data it is my opinion that the postwar generation experienced more stress and anguish than did Depression-born youth, owing to a doleful world and domestic happenings and intense audiovisual exposure to such happenings. Given the predominantly urban milieu in which the postwar cohort was socialized and the relatively high level of education it achieved, it is not surprising that this cohort was much less subject to the influence of tradition, the values, attitudes, behavior norms, and ideology of the past, than any previous generation of American youth. They are, therefore, much more sensitive and responsive to the worldwide and domestic chaotic setting in which they were raised. Furthermore, their own life experiences as teenagers and young adults were much more arduous, certainly than those of Depression-born youth and probably of any previous generation of American youth.

The experience of college and university mental health services seems to confirm these conclusions, as does the evidence of increased pathology as manifest in increased delinquency and crime, and a suicide rate for the postwar cohort more than double that of the earlier group.

It may be said that the generation of youth born during the Depression decade of the 1930s was always in short supply and experienced a seller's market up to this point in their life cycles—that is, they enjoyed all the advantages of being in short supply relative to the demand for their services. Furthermore, they faced a more tranquil world and national social, economic, and political climate in which to be reared as they reached the teen ages—a world and nation from whose troubles they were relatively insulated before the advent of television. To be sure, World War II occurred while they were growing up, but the Depression cohort was below military age throughout that conflict, and in the absence of hostilities on this continent the war had relatively little conscious impact on the largely preadolescent population. As young adults they were able to obtain employment with little experience of unemployment, enjoy relatively early promotion, and live through a relatively prosperous post–World War II economy characterized by an almost thirty-year period of strong economic growth. To be sure some economic recessions occurred, but they were relatively minor, so much so that economists talked about "fine-tuning" the economy. For the Depression-born cohort the American free enterprise economy and democratic political system really worked.

In contrast, the postwar cohort was in large supply relative to the demand for their services. They inundated the schools at all levels, to the detriment of educational quality. They had trouble finding employment, as evidenced by soaring unemployment rates, while the highly educated among them had increasing difficulty in finding employment that was suitable. Age at marriage and age at birth of first child rose. Those who did marry increasingly failed to remain married, as manifest in the increased divorce rate. A sexual revolution occurred, evident in increasing out-of-wedlock births, increasing numbers of couples living together without benefit of marriage, greater premarital sexual activity, and greatly decreased marital fertility. Undoubtedly, increasing concern about environmental degradation and the consequences of excessively rapid population growth also contributed to decreased fertility. Finally, as incontrovertible evidence of greater stress and anguish, the delinquency and suicide rates of postwar-born youth were more than double those of the Depression-born cohort. For the postwar youth, the American free enterprise economy and democratic system of government did not work well, as is evident in the emergence of such activities as the New Left, the Students for a Democratic Society, and the Weathermen. The failure of the American system was also to be observed in the frictions of the civil rights movement and in the racial and ethnic violence of the late sixties.

What does the future hold? One can only speculate. One possible consequence may be drastic social, economic, and political change, aspects of which are already visible on the horizon. The over 70 million Americans who can be considered part of the postwar baby bulge may conceivably be less resistant to major changes in the American system than was any previous

278

cohort. Moreover, they may not only be less resistant to change, they may be increasingly insistent upon it. Certainly, the growing evidence of the misconduct of corporate enterprise and business and labor leaders, the growing rapaciousness of both business and labor, and the increasing exposure of the misdeeds of politicians and government officials do not lead to greater admiration of the American system as it has evolved to date.

It is possible, of course, that the future may yet improve the lot of our postwar cohort—perhaps enough to enable them to forget their difficult experiences to date. But it is hard to find any evidence of great improvement in the prospect. In the meantime the personnel in agencies with responsibilities to help stressed and anguished people to cope can look forward to secure futures based on a continued large growth of target clientele.

NOTES

1. Percent urban for 1946 and 1963 were interpolated using data from U.S. Bureau of the Census (1970b, pt. 1, U.S. summary, table 3).

2. The 1960 figure was obtained from U.S. Bureau of the Census (1960, vol. 2-B, table 15). The 1970 figure was obtained from U.S. Bureau of the Census (1970a, table 2). The 1977 figure was obtained from unpublished Bureau of the Census survey data.

3. Suicide rates were calculated using data from National Center for Health Statistics (1955, p. 98; 1970, p. 1–246/247). Also see U.S. Bureau of the Census (1970b, table 49; 1975b, table 3).

REFERENCES

Glick, P. C. 1976. Updating life cycle of the family. Paper presented before the Meeting of the Population Association of America, Toronto, April 1976.

National Center for Health Statistics. 1955. *Vital Statistics of the United States*. Vol. 2, *Mortality*. Washington, D.C.: Government Printing Office.

National Center for Health Statistics. 1960. *Vital Statistics of the United States*. Vol. 3, *Marriage and Divorce*. Washington, D.C.: Government Printing Office.

National Center for Health Statistics. 1970. *Vital Statistics of the United States*. Vol. 2, *Mortality*. Washington, D.C.: Government Printing Office.

U.S. Bureau of the Census. 1960. *1960 Census of the Population.* Vol. 1, *Characteristics of the Population.* Vol. 2, *Persons by Family Character- istics.* Washington, D.C.: Government Printing Office.

U.S. Bureau of the Census. 1970a. *Historical Statistics of the United States: Colonial Times to 1970.* Washington, D.C.: Government Printing Office.

U.S. Bureau of the Census. 1970b. *1970 Census of the Population.* Vol. 1, *Characteristics of the Population.* Washington, D.C.: Government Printing Office.

U.S. Bureau of the Census. 1975a. *Current Population Reports: Population Profile of the United States.* Washington, D.C.: Government Printing Of- fice.

U.S. Bureau of the Census. 1975b. *Monthly Vital Statistics Report.* Advance report, final marriage statistics 26 (suppl.): 2, table 4. Washington, D.C.: Government Printing Office.

U.S. Bureau of the Census. 1976. *Statistical Abstract of the United States.* Washington, D.C.: Government Printing Office.

U.S. Bureau of the Census. 1977. *Current Population Reports.* Washington, D.C.: Government Printing Office.

U.S. Bureau of the Census. 1978. *Current Population Reports: Perspectives on American Fertility.* Washington, D.C.: Government Printing Office.

IRVING I. ZARETSKY

As an anthropologist, I have studied religious movements in contemporary America for the past ten years. Young people involved in such movements have a special language, a special way of relating to others. One must learn to listen creatively, to learn to decipher a new linguistic code and its grammar, and to understand how it is acquired and used. It is also important to understand how an individual uses his personal idiosyncrasies in dealing with the real world through the medium of a contemporary religious movement.

In this country, from about 1860 on, approximately every twenty years we have had a religious renaissance, a religious awakening. It is usually correlated with political conditions such as war; with economic conditions such as recessions, depressions, and unemployment; with urban migrations; or with any kind of event that is dislocating to the nuclear family. Today we have been experiencing the most recent form of religious awakening, with our youth joining a wide variety of religious cults. Since the early 1960s and, in greater intensity, since 1969, we have been reaching a period of stabilization, and it is toward that stabilization that we have to direct our attention.

Today's religious renaissance is composed of religious, secular, and quasi-religious groups. There are groups self-described as religious. There are groups (like those within the Human Potential Movement) that describe themselves as completely secular, although they do follow certain models of religious behavior. There are what I would call the "quasi-religious" groups which straddle the line from the point of view of living within established order. They would like to benefit from the legal advantages that accrue to those groups which define themselves and are recognized as religious, and, at the same time, they want to be able to apply their beliefs to everyone, so that they are really secular in their universal impact.

The most noted characteristic of participants in such groups is what I would call their desire for social change through personal transformation. Two elements that are the sine qua non of participation are the desire to see some kind of social change and the belief that social change can best be achieved through some form of personal transformation: for example, if the world is to change, let that change begin with me. I am describing a large array of groups that have assumed form and structure in the mid-nineteenth century, for example, Christian Science, Spiritualism, Mormonism, Unity, New Thought, and so on. My own data indicate that approximately 20 million Americans are involved in such movements (Zaretsky and Levine 1974). Others estimate that approximately 13 percent of the population is involved, an even larger number than my data would reveal, and there is some indication, as we get better statistical information, that the population may be even greater.

The present renascence and preoccupation with religious movements seems to have had its beginning with the economic affluence of young people in the 1960s. There was a large amount of public education funds for scholarships and fellowships, there was freedom to travel cheaply by airline, and there was a vogue of inexpensive clothing and food-consumption patterns. The movement has continued into the present time, but the economic situation has changed. The cost of living has risen, inflation seems unchecked, educational funds have been decreasing, and more and more people need professional skills to find an economic niche within society.

The role of the family in this economic situation has changed. With inflation and the change in economic conditions, the family is called upon to aid young people much more today than a decade ago. Concurrently, the nuclear family is losing control over its children in terms of the greater personal liberties and freedoms that young people have, supported by the general ethos that encourages individuals to develop at their own rate and in their own direction. This increase in personal freedom and expression of personal liberties has created a major tension with regard to alternate life-styles: the creation of communes, the substitution of a social family for a biological family, and the need to recreate a parental group based on affinity and compatibility as opposed to biological relationship. In a sense, we have moved from status to contract, into a period in which we are involved in voluntary associations. Along with these phenomena, we have observed the beginning of what I would call a "portable ecclesia," a movable church that essentially allows individuals to associate with one another on the basis of choice and to create a religious or quasi-religious association whenever they find themselves so inclined.

We have also been confronted with phenomena new to our Western civilization: reversible rites of passage. In the past, through religious initiation, or through secular intitiation, rites of passage had a unilinear evolutionary trend in which an individual moved progressively from one status to another. In terms of our overall societal outlook, such movement would be one directional, toward progress, growth, maturity, and aging.

We have come to a point at which, both individually and socially, rites of passage may be reversible. For example, an individual who converts from one faith to another was considered to have undertaken a unilinear conversion which man cannot undo. But today we find social groups who, in fact, can divest an individual of his status, or attempt to do so, depending on their need. We are also witnessing trends which are alarming to some and refreshing to others: the deprogramming phenomenon. Ascending generations, very concerned about the choices that individuals—especially young people—make in terms of their secular and religious life, attempt forcibly to reverse the rite of passage to a previous or natal tradition.

In 1964, from the viewpoint of anthropology, I undertook a city-wide study of the branches of one denomination of spiritualism in Central California. Observing the population and the behavior, I began at that time to see an increase in participation in alternative religious styles. Later I collected some comparative data in the Midwest, the Middle-Atlantic states, and finally, New England. Based on that work, I moved on to consider not only spiritualism but also other religious groups which provided alternative ways of studying the questions of how people utilize their personal goals in the process of group formation and institution building, how they confront a society which is often hostile to such alternatives (Zaretsky and Levine 1974).

Religious dissent in the United States has existed since the days of settlement; here we begin about 1835, with the work of Phineas Quimby in the corridor between Portland, Maine, and Boston, Massachusetts (Judah 1967). The interest at that time, emerging from the influence of Germany and France, was in the power of mind over body: the ability of an individual through thought processes and cognitive abilities to control or to affect what is happening in a biological or physiological sense. Mary Baker Eddy spent about twenty years with Quimby, at the end of which time (Dresser 1919) she acquired his diaries. In these diaries, the terms ''science'' and ''health'' were first used, and some have claimed that the first publication of her book (Eddy 1916) in 1864 was overindebted to the Quimby manuscripts. In upstate New York and in New England were the roots of the nineteenth-century religious revival. It was followed by Christian Science, Mormonism, New Thought, and, in 1893, the Chicago Parliament of World Religions. In the West there was a rise of religious communes and fundamentalist Bible colleges; by the 1920s, 1930s, and 1940s, a variety of religious groups became organized around charismatic leaders who offered their participants a solution to personal life problems.

What began in the nineteenth century was a renewal of the individual's access to the supernatural and the individual's ability to become his own theologian and his own therapist. Today this phenomenon is increasing so that individuals coming to a group may do so to find help in personal decision making, daily-life problem resolution, and achieving some new status through certifications and accreditations (sometimes marginal) in order to be better able to enter the competitive marketplace. From this very broad picture we can see that there is nothing new about religious movements in America today. These religious movements have a strong and important tradition, one that is really responsible for developing our notions of the free exercise of religious ideas.

But religious groups have to be defined in terms of a continuum. In the nineteenth century we saw more of the phenomenon of families joining groups. For example, the spiritualistic camps in Maine, Indiana, Pennsylvania, and Michigan were essentially enterprises which families joined as a unit. It was expected that children would be brought up in that tradition, and in fact they were. It was there that the lyceum movement (Davis 1952) began to service entire families.

The area of contemporary religious movements is the last frontier for the American entrepreneur. The spirit of conquering the new West, the spirit of adventure in the land of opportunity, is most vividly shown by individuals who were not able to receive education but had an ability to translate their talents into a marketable commodity and thus enter the world as entrepreneurs. Theories that try to describe young people's involvement with religious groups as fitting the model of social deprivation, the dominance of one group over another, are not necessarily valid. It is important not to view religious groups from the model of social disorganization or to view their members as deviant or defective individuals. My work and that of most anthropologists begins with a premise that there is nothing inherent in religious activity that would allow us to label it as pathological. Perhaps our attention is called to certain variations in the style of religious worship or some of the tenets of belief. But when we discuss degrees of difference, we have to keep in mind that a distinctive religiosity is not in and of itself pathology.

The Psychotherapy of Religious Groups

We tend to think of religious movements as happening only in the last decade, but there is a rich historical American experience in marginal religious movements that is endemic to our democratic institutions. As a social scientist working with such groups, one sees that in the last decade more and more young people have entered this realm of experience. Very frequently today, youngsters from the age of twelve or thirteen may come into a group, sometimes with parental consent. They either attend the group in person or they acquire techniques such as meditation and bring it into their lives.

Individuals who join, whether in their teenage years or later, usually join groups or practice these religious beliefs as individuals. One of the most important findings in my research was that married people enter the group more as individuals than as couples. Conversion is very much an isolating experience.

The phenomenon of death and rebirth is a continuing theme in these movements. Individuals can die several times and be reborn several times, not in a reincarnating sense, but in social terms of individual identity. Similarly, with the definition of the child, there is a growing distrust toward and alienation from the parental generation. Younger people increasingly demand identification and self-recognition as autonomous adults.

An example will illustrate how some of these groups work and their impact on young people: the spiritualist churches of the mid-nineteenth century represented a kind of religiosity that we find today; spiritualism is in reality the prototype of that religiosity. It is composed of individuals who believe that there is no death. They believe that individuals simply go on to another realm of being and continue to care about us, communicate with us, and inform us about daily-life decisions that we have to make. The church is organized through mediums and healers. Healers are really in charge of the laying on of hands; mediums are charged with giving information about life problems. Individuals come to a church anonymously and will simply write their question on a piece of paper. The medium will try to answer that question. At other times the medium will simply go into the audience and bring back a message from a loved one on the other side.

The church is organized hierarchically in the sense that there are students learning to become mediums, healers, licentiates, and ministers. Each one of these positions provides a kind of legal status to perform marriages and burials, to give aid and comfort to individuals in institutions such as hospitals and prisons, and to help their members receive insurance benefits for those services. Essentially, individuals come to the church to receive answers to questions that are regarded as imperative. They will usually describe their question in metaphoric terms and will receive the answer in code.

These groups strive toward harmonizing family relationships. In many cases, especially in those groups that are noncommunal in nature, the effort is to try to resolve problems between parents and children. The communal groups try to substitute for the family and to provide a screen between the individual and the family.

For the most part, individuals go from one religious group to another asking the same questions, getting similar answers, and being very reluctant to rid themselves of the problem or the question. It seems to become a life-style called "seeking." As a psychological type, it is perhaps the one thread of continuity from the nineteenth century. There are people who do not regard that quest as a transition zone but as a lifelong occupation. They couple this with a notion that everyone is a student of life and religiosity. In that sense, one always brings problems to the church because it is through such exercise that one excels in his or her studies.

Conclusions

Contemporary religious trends, then, are an American phenomenon, usually conceptualized as religious dissent, dating back from the days of settlement. After the Reformation, every man could be his own priest, but today every man can be his own theologian and therapist. A great many individuals came to these religious movements by virtue of the worldliness of leaders and their ability to render services under the guise of religious work.

Problem definition for those individuals attracted to contemporary religious movements is of keenest consideration. If you deal with movement individuals in or outside of a university setting, you must first recognize that the language that you are hearing is a learned language. It is not necessarily personally generated. Their experiences have taught them to present themselves in a particular way that requires the use of a special language. The language being used provides a grammar through which to participate in religious life. One must be able to deal with a patient as an actor in a religious setting as well as an individual who comes for therapy. You cannot strip an individual of his religious identity and expect to be offered the empirical data you need in order to offer competent psychotherapy.

Psychotherapists have to remain our ultimate anthropologists. In social science, and especially religious research, we know very little about the longitudinal effect of this kind of religious participation. It is essential that longitudinal studies be carried out on young people that will allow us to respond best to the psychological problems, the legal problems, and the societal response to these ultimate religious traditions. In the long run, what we learn will determine whether we are hospitable to these forms of experimentations.

REFERENCES

Davis, A. J. 1952. *The Great Harmonia*. Boston: Sanborn, Carter & Bazin.

Dresser, H. W. 1919. *A History of New Thought Movement*. New York: Crowell.

Eddy, M. B. 1916. *Science and Health*. Boston: Stewart.

Judah, J. S. 1967. *The History and Philosophy of the Metaphysical Movements in America*. Philadelphia: Westminster.

Zaretsky, I. I., and Levine, M. P. 1974. *Religious Movements in Contemporary America*. Princeton, N.J.: Princeton University Press.

23 CONTEMPORARY YOUTH CONSCIOUSNESS: EMERGENT THEMES IN RECENT AMERICAN FICTION

JOHN CAWELTI

In part, we interpret literature in terms of life, but we also process life in some ways through those story plots we carry around in our heads. Art imitates nature but, as Oscar Wilde reminds us, nature imitates art. We tend to read the fiction of our own time as if it addressed itself particularly to those social or psychological concerns that are uppermost in our minds, and, in turn, we apply symbols and metaphors gleaned from our favorite stories to what is going on around us. Thus, in analyzing some of the basic themes of contemporary fiction, I cannot claim to be giving an account of the causes of contemporary youth consciousness. But, insofar as I am correct, I will be describing literary patterns which are correlated with that consciousness. The nature of that correlation I must leave to those with different skills than literary analysis.

In general, the period of the late 1960s and early 1970s was one of major generic and mythical shifts. Types of literature which had been popular for a long time seemed to wither away and be replaced by new genres. This was particularly noticeable in two cases: the decline of the western and the increasing importance of science fiction, and the atrophy of the traditional detective story and the expansion of the spy thriller.

After over a hundred years as one of America's most important literary and dramatic genres, the western seems on the verge of extinction, at least in its traditional form. Since the canceling of the television shows "Gunsmoke" and "Bonanza" and John Wayne's last hurrah as a western hero in the early 1970s, few important westerns have been produced, and most of these have been burlesques or ironic transformations of the form, like Mel Brooks's *Blazing Saddles* or Arthur Penn's *Little Big Man* and *The Missouri*

Breaks. One interesting exception was Clint Eastwood's 1975 film, *The Outlaw Josey Wales,* which had a considerable success at the box office. However, this was such a traditional western that it harked back beyond Eastwood's own grotesquely powerful spaghetti westerns of the early 1960s to the simpler good guy versus bad guy epics of an earlier period. As such, it was more a gesture of nostalgia than of renewed vitality in a popular form. The traditional western adventure novel has probably been moribund for an even longer time. The remaining fans must depend largely on reprints of westerns written in the twenties, thirties, and forties by writers like Zane Grey, Max Brand, and Luke Short, or by contemporary imitators of these writers like Lewis Patten and Wayne Overholser. Only one writer of traditional westerns, Louis L'Amour, has a very wide public following, and I do not believe he is read by many young people.

It is too simple to say that in the last fifteen years the frontiers of space have replaced the Great Plains as the most vital imaginary landscape for young people, but there is enough truth in this observation to make it worth refining. Since the inception of science-fiction magazines in the 1920s, there has existed a dedicated and highly articulate core of science-fiction readers among the young. Thus, the shift in interest from western to science-fiction adventure is not by any means total, because a significant number of young science-fiction fans already existed. However, it does seem true that during the 1960s this basic core of science-fiction readership was joined by a large and diverse group of young people who would probably not have read science fiction before. In addition, this increase in readership was accompanied by certain changes in the character of science fiction, also beginning in the early 1960s. These new trends in science-fiction writing reflect the influence of a younger generation of writers, such as Harlan Ellison, Samuel Delany, Ursula LeGuin, Frank Herbert, and Larry Niven. A number of these writers have sometimes spoken of themselves as constituting a ''new wave'' in science fiction and have gathered their work together in anthologies with titles like *Dangerous Visions.* The difference between this new-wave writing and traditional science fiction will be one basis for my analysis of emergent themes in recent fiction.

Another important generic change that began during the 1960s and has continued to the present day is the proliferation of the international intrigue thriller. The decline of the western and the flourishing of science fiction parallels the rise of the intrigue thriller at the expense of the traditional detective story. Certain kinds of spy thrillers have existed alongside the traditional detective story throughout most of the twentieth century, but until the post–World War II era, the detective story was unquestionably the dominant form. In the 1960s, however, novels of intrigue proliferated into a variety of different types which had hardly existed before: the assassination thriller, the terrorist thriller, the imaginary coup d'état, and now the Watergate thriller. A number of recent political figures—among them Spiro Agnew, John Erlichmann, John Lindsay, and William F. Buckley, Jr.—have chosen to write their own intrigue thrillers. *Time* magazine has given its imprimatur to the spy story in the form of a cover essay on John Le Carré, probably the best contemporary writer in this genre. On the other hand, very few younger writers have chosen to work in the detective-story format. Though still popular, its best sellers are reprints of stories by writers like Agatha Christie, Erle Stanley Gardner, Ngaio Marsh, and Ellery Queen, most of which were written at an earlier time. Even the hard-boiled detective story has taken on a nostalgic ironic cast with films like *Chinatown* and *The Long Goodbye* and writers like Andrew Bergman, Stuart Kaminsky, and Richard Brautigan. The intrigue thriller is less distinctively a literature of young people than the new wave in science fiction, but as the currently dominant form of mystery writing, it is probably read widely by them. Many of the most successful movies of the last decade have been in this area.

The third major generic trend is harder to characterize, and I feel less certain of my ground here. It is what I perceive as an increasing importance of fantasy on the cultural scene. Of course, there is a sense in which all types of popular literature—spy thrillers, westerns, detective stories, etc.—can be characterized as fantasies, in that they tend to follow certain "unreal" plot conventions in order to portray the solution of mysteries, the victory of good guys, the happy ending. But I wish to refer here to a more limited conception of fantasy, which not only distinguishes a certain type of story from other kinds of popular literature, but also from much science fiction. The sort of fantasy I have in mind is exemplified by Tolkien's highly influential works, *The Hobbit* and *The Lord of the Rings,* and by the phenomenally successful recent film, *Star Wars.* These are only the two most prominent examples of a prolific subliterature which includes such phenomena as the *Marvel Comics'* superhero sagas and the work of writers like Robert Howard, Andre Norton, and Roger Zelazny.

This type of fantasy was highly popular with college students in the 1960s and remains so today. It is characterized by premises that are frankly counternaturalistic, that is, "impossible" in terms of the conventional modern view of reality and history. There are various ways in which an impossible premise can be manifested: Tolkien invented a whole historic time and space (Middle Earth) which, according to our modern view of world history, did not and could not exist. In addition, he peopled this world with both humans and other conscious beings (hobbits, elves, dwarves, etc.), and postulated the operation of certain occult and magical forces. It seems certain that Tolkien's work paved the way for the creation and the enormous success of *Star Wars*, which also represented human beings in an impossible space-time ("many years ago in a galaxy far away") with other conscious beings and occult powers (the "force"). *Marvel Comics'* superheroes differ from the traditional Superman and Batman in the cosmic setting of their actions. Where Superman and Batman were fantastic extensions of the traditional detective and gangbuster heroes of an earlier period, the new superheroes not only span the cosmos, but move between alternate universes where incredibly vast moral forces clash together.

It is difficult to define a precise boundary between this kind of fantasy and science fiction. Indeed, certain tendencies in new-wave science fiction make it increasingly like fantasy. However, we can distinguish between fantasy and two different but related literary types: extrapolative science fiction and the fantastic. The fantastic has been lucidly defined by the structuralist critic Todorov as a type of story in which the relationship of the experience narrated to ordinary reality remains in question either to the character who experiences it or to the reader. Was it a dream or did it really happen? Was that really a ghost I saw or something else? This is the sort of question raised by the fantastic. Todorov suggests, rightly I think, that this kind of literary experience was particularly associated with the later nineteenth and early twentieth centuries in Western culture, and that it reflected deeply ambiguous feelings connected with the transition between traditional religious and modern scientific world views. Extrapolative writing does not generally raise the problems of the fantastic because it presents a frankly imagined reality. However, there is always an important linkage between the imagined reality and our present world, and this linkage is very much a part of the story. Much traditional science fiction is extrapolative in this sense, presenting stories which center around imagined worlds based on new technologies or on a future historical evolution which can be seen as a possible development out of present technology, science, or society. Often, these imagined worlds function as criticisms of the present world. So H. G. Wells criticized the complacency and class divisions of *fin-de-siècle* Britain with his imagined Martian invasion and travels into the future.

Fantasy, however, is neither fantastic nor extrapolative. It simply sets forth a different reality and ignores its linkage to the ordinary world. In *Star Wars* or *Lord of the Rings*, there is no question of relation to the present world, no sense that the *Star Wars* galaxy or Middle Earth are developments out of our society. Indeed, it is characteristic of this type of fantasy that it takes place in a mythical past rather than an imagined future.

There have always been fantasies of this sort, but in the past it was common for this kind of literature to be allegorical—that is, there was a system of interpretation by means of which the fantasy events and characters could be related to concepts or events of the ordinary world. This was the case, for example, with the science fantasy of C. S. Lewis's *Perelandra* trilogy, which presented a traditional Christian mythos in terms of science-fiction conventions. There are certain allegorical elements in *Star Wars* and *Lord of the Rings,* but there does not appear to be any consistent system of symbolization in these works by means of which we are encouraged to relate them to a present system of thought. On the contrary, we seem to value these fantasies because they set forth a different reality.

Different as they are, the two most popular fantasies of our time share one basic pattern. Both *Star Wars* and *Lord of the Rings* postulate a universe in which great moral forces are at work; they tell a story in which a relatively weak and insignificant person (the young man Luke Skywalker and the Hobbitt Frodo Baggins) becomes a channel of the occult force for good and brings about an apocalyptic destruction of evil. This Manichean quality is by no means unique to contemporary fantasy and is to a certain extent a tendency of the genre. Nonetheless, if we look at some of the fantasies of past eras, we can see that there are very different directions which writers of fantasy can take. In *Alice in Wonderland,* for instance, the fantasy world is, if anything, more ambiguous and morally quirky than the ordinary world. Some of this is, of course, intended as satire—a *reductio ad absurdum* of the ordinary world—but it is also the case that the ordinary world is implicitly portrayed in Carroll's work as a place of security and order in contrast to the world of Alice's dream. It is true that *Alice in Wonderland* is a different type of fantasy than *Lord of the Rings* and *Star Wars,* but there are also earlier cosmic fantasies, such as David Linday's *A Voyage to Arcturus,* in which the fantasy world is a realm of murky uncertainty and the hero's quest a very ambiguous enterprise. On the contrary, the sense of contemporary popular fantasies is that only in an impossible world are there clear moral alternatives and virtuous choices which can lead to the defeat of evil. This becomes particularly significant, I think, when we set the world of fantasy over against the world of the international intrigue thriller which is conventionally a representation of our world or something very close to it. In the contemporary thriller, there is a little that is morally clear. The opposing forces are rarely

292

simple manifestations of good versus evil, as they were in the traditional spy thriller. Moreover, the protagonist is usually more anti-heroic than an epitome of courage and goodness, and, in the action, the protagonist is as often betrayed from within his own organization as he is stymied by enemy action. The basic point I wish to make is that in terms of the popular genres of the present we have a distinct antithesis in the way the moral nature of reality is presented. Those genres which deal with the ordinary world set forth a society of moral uncertainty and ambiguity in which the moral nature of opposing forces is obscured and the protagonist's actions are dubiously related to the fight against evil. On the other hand, it is only in an impossible or fantasy world that readers are apparently prepared to accept stories which depend on a clear opposition between good and evil forces with heroes who can tap the power of good to defeat evil.

This is almost antithetical to the popular literature of an earlier generation. Genres like the detective story, the gangster saga, the western, and earlier forms of the spy thriller represented the clash of good and evil and the triumph of justice in the world of the present or immediate past. After the Depression and World War II, there were increasing ambiguities in these popular syntheses of reality and morality. By the 1960s, most traditional genres were becoming increasingly ambivalent in their version of the quest for justice. Only romance has remained a fairly stable and even expanding traditional style, though this may be another indication of the present tendency to imagine the triumph of good only in an impossible or fantastic world. For one of the central themes of modern popular romance is the contrast between the real or ordinary world and the unchanged world of true love, a world that is usually set apart either in time or space from the reader's ordinary present. One indication of this is the development of the whole new formula of so-called Regency romances. Somewhat like imitations of Jane Austen's *Pride and Prejudice*, these novels present tales of true love overcoming social and psychological obstacles in Regency England. The growing popularity of this type suggests that readers are able to participate vicariously in the happy simplicities of a true and permanent love only in the fantasy world of an imagined past. When love stories are set in the ordinary present, it seems more appropriate for the heroine to die of leukemia, as in Erich Segal's *Love Story*.

These generic shifts and the changes in existing genres associated with them reflect an interest on the part of writers and their audience to explore certain themes which can be more effectively presented in these newer generic patterns. As we shall see, these same themes have become increasingly significant in the work of important nongeneric writers like Thomas Pynchon, giving us further grounds for thinking that they are an important part of our current imaginative landscape.

The Sense of Cosmic Vertigo

In one of Isaac Asimov's cleverest stories, "Nightfall," a civilization on the imaginary planet Lagash goes through a curious cycle. Since this planet is part of a solar system with six suns, darkness descends only once every 2,000 years, when a combination of eclipses temporarily blocks out the light from all these suns. At this time the world of Lagash falls into chaos. Mass lunacy seizes upon everyone and the whole civilization is destroyed. It turns out that it is not the fear of darkness that causes this terrible catastrophe, but the sudden and totally unexpected discovery of the stars and the shattering realization of the immense empty spaces they imply.

Such a sense of immensity both in space and in time is one of the primary emotional dimensions of modern experience, and one of the things which, I think, makes science fiction both possible and necessary. In a sense, this view of the universe has been a part of the experience of Western civilization since the Copernican revolution. Indeed, Asimov's story is sometimes interpreted as a kind of allegory of the profound transformation in man's understanding of his situation in the cosmos. However, the testimony of literature suggests that the full impact of the Copernican revolution was not felt by most people until the mid-twentieth century. For literature retained its basic orientation toward man as the center of the universe. Lyric poetry, novels, and plays dealt primarily with the feelings and fates of individual people in relation to other individuals or to society. Even the rather pessimistic naturalism of writers like Zola, Dreiser, Crane, and Norris was most concerned with the deterministic impact of biological and social forces on individual lives. It did not express the same sense of man's relation to an unimaginably vast space-time that has become a commonplace in contemporary science fiction.

Evidently, certain major scientific events of the second half of the twentieth century, such as the atomic bomb, the landing of astronauts on the moon, and the sending of probes into deep space, have opened us up imaginatively to the vastness of the universe in a new way. One sign of this is the number of science-fiction works which represent some version of the end of man, the earth, and even in a few instances, the universe. Significantly, William Faulkner announced in his Nobel Prize speech that he declined to accept the end of man. However, for science-fiction writers like Arthur C. Clarke, Isaac Asimov, Samuel Delany, and Ursula LeGuin, the replacement, transformation, or destruction of man is an often-imagined drama. The vastness of their canvas in works like the *Foundation* trilogy, *Childhood's End, 2001, The Einstein Intersection, Babel 17,* and *The Dispossessed* places man in a larger context of cosmic space and history. In order to deal with immense settings in space and time writers have widely adapted a number of highly dubious scientific extrapolations: faster-than-light travel, space-time warps, instantaneous communication over cosmic distances, and various forms of time travel. These are all stratagems to enable stories to take place over cosmic distances in time and space, and, in spite of their having little support in current scientific theory, they have become basic conventions in the literature.

Though it probably does reflect a new kind of imaginative insecurity, the sense of cosmic vertigo is by no means always portrayed in dark or pessimistic terms. Indeed, it is difficult to find in contemporary science fiction a vision as bleak and hopeless as the time traveler's final experience of a dying sun at the end of H. G. Wells's *The Time Machine.* On the contrary, what was for Wells the ultimate horror and meaninglessness of a universe running down becomes in much contemporary science fiction an ambiguous expression of hope. This is particularly clear in the writings of Arthur C. Clarke, where entropy can become a kind of ironic comedy (as in ''The Nine Billion Names of God'') and the transformation of man into cosmic mind may be the salvation of the universe. In *Childhood's End* and *2001,* the transcendence of technological man by a new transcendental consciousness is represented as the only way in which man can be prevented from destroying his world in an atomic holocaust. Works like Isaac Asminov's *Foundation* trilogy and Frank Herbert's *Dune* trilogy, strikingly different in many respects, share a vision of mystical mental powers emerging as the way to prevent eons of galactic chaos. The cosmic view may lead to a recognition that entropy and catastrophe are the universal fate, but this realization seems to result less in despair than in a rekindling of hope for some new kind of mystical transcendence. Thus, it is not surprising that much contemporary science fiction blurs into the mythical and the occult, or that the increased popularity of a literature which is associated with science is also accompanied by a resurgence of pseudosciences, or that scientology, one of the currently prospering mystical cults, was founded by a former writer of science fiction.

The Concept of the Alien as Redeemer

Fascination with the alien is nothing new, but one distinctive aspect of recent science fiction and fantasy is the quest for the alien as a solution to human problems. The fantasy of the sympathetic, benevolent alien who uses his mysterious powers to prevent human catastrophe is a significant departure from the treatment of aliens in earlier twentieth-century science fiction. Until the 1950s, aliens were most commonly represented as terrifying potential enemies, more likely to invade earth and conquer the human race than to help man deal with his own inadequacies. This was the view of alien creatures reflected in H. G. Wells's monstrous Martians from *The War of the Worlds,* and this fantasy was still powerful enough on the eve of World War II to send millions of Americans into a state of hysteria when a younger Welles brought the Martian invaders to American radio. There were a few instances of more sympathetic treatment of alien creatures prior to World War II, such as Stanley Weinbaum's *A Martian Odyssey* of 1933, which is often noted by historians of science fiction as the first portrayal of alien creatures without diabolical or monstrous overtones. However, beginning in the 1950s, the representation of alien creatures changed considerably. In films like *The Day the Earth Stood Still* and novels like *Childhood's End,* powerful alien creatures appear on earth in response to the threat of nuclear holocaust, using their greater powers to bring a new reign of peace and prosperity on earth. Significantly, Arthur Clarke's alien controller Karellen had the physical characteristics commonly ascribed by human beings to the devil, but this was a transformed devil whose mission was to prevent man from destroying himself and to create the conditions for a new transcendent consciousness.

The theme of the sympathetic alien was important in the novels of Kurt Vonnegut, Jr., one of the cult writers of the 1960s, and in most of the science-fiction works of that period which achieved exceptional popularity, such as Robert Heinlein's *Stranger in a Strange Land.* Vonnegut's use of aliens in *The Sirens of Titan, Slaughterhouse-Five,* and *Breakfast of Champions* was especially fascinating, mixing irony, seriousness, and satire in a unique blend. His Tralfamadorians, philosophical robots from a distant planet, have achieved perfect happiness through their recognition of the multiplicity of time and their ability to focus their lives around nothing but the best and most fulfilling moments. They are not, like human beings, bound to an irreversible time sequence which can lead only to death. In effect, they have found the secret of reversing entropy. Their technology is magnificent, and they have the capacity to span the cosmic vertigo. Their relationship to human beings is one of bemused indifference mixed with quirky curiosity. In *The Sirens of Titan* it turns out that the whole course of human history has been controlled by the Tralfamadorians in order to send trivial messages across space to one of the emissaries, while in *Slaughterhouse-Five* Billy Pilgrim is taken to Tralfamadore in a flying saucer and kept there in a zoo with the beautiful Montana Wildhack. Yet, there is no sense in these curious fantasies that the Tralfamadorians are evil. Instead, the human race is portrayed by Vonnegut as so ridiculous and absurd it seems appropriate for man to be treated as an inferior species by the Tralfamadorians.

Heinlein's version of the sympathetic alien is more simplistic, though it evidently had a powerful impact on many young people. The Martian protagonist of *Stranger in a Strange Land* brings to earth a message of polymorphous loving union between individual beings. The invented vocabulary with which Heinlein expressed this state—terms like "grokking" and "water brotherhood"—became cult words for a time in the later 1960s. Like all Messiahs, Heinlein's Martian finally realized that he could only impress his message on mankind by a willing sacrifice of himself. Thus, at the climax of the novel he courts a martyrdom obviously intended by the author to be read in Christian terms. Heinlein's portrayal of the sympathetic alien as a Christ figure was the most extreme treatment of this theme yet presented, but its large popularity was indicative of the degree to which the alien had been transformed from a figure of diabolical fear into a hope for salvation.

This treatment of the alien-encounter in science fiction and fantasy is obviously related to those cultural phenomena which cluster around the sighting of unidentified flying objects and the study of ancient astronauts. While some of the concern about UFOs reflects the traditional fear of the alien, it is striking how many of the recent legends of rides in spaceships stress not the fearsomeness but the courtesy and kindness of the alien creatures. Similarly, the theory of ancient astronauts seems to fascinate people at least in part because it implies the presence in the universe of greater powers which are concerned with the doings of man. The underlying hope that leads many people to grasp eagerly at the highly speculative "evidence" set forth by the ancient astronaut's exponents may well be a yearning for their return. It is this feeling of yearning for contact with unbelievably powerful alien creatures that seems to be the dominant element in the increasing importance of this theme. Significantly, the film arousing the greatest public excitement during the Christmas season of 1977 was *Close Encounters of the Third Kind*, a striking embodiment of the alien theme.

Fascination with Conspiracy or Paranoia as Norm

In the previous discussion, I noted the motif of control as an aspect of the theme of the quest for alien contact. One recurrent fantasy, expressed in its most extreme form in Vonnegut's *The Sirens of Titan,* is that human events, institutions, or persons have become controlled or taken over by a hidden force. This motif is, I think, the common element in the contemporary popularity both of certain kinds of science fiction and of the intrigue thriller. For the theme of conspiratorial control is the very essence of the current thriller. Like most of the themes we have looked at, the motif of conspiracy did not suddenly make its appearance in the wake of the Vietnam War. There have been many widespread conspiracy fantasies in modern European and American history, and these have been, to some extent, reflected in the literature of the times. Anti-Semitism fed by the sensational forgery of the *Protocols of the Learned Elders of Zion* and by false accusations in the Dreyfus case stimulated many early-twentieth-century Europeans to imagine a secret Jewish conspiracy controlling the world. More recently, fantasies about an omnipotent communist or Mafia conspiracy have proliferated. Here is an example of the kind of rhetoric which is often employed to express these visions of conspiracy:

A treasure of billions is at the disposal of members of the inner council of the Mafia, men who have come up through the ranks of crime. The high priests of the Mafia are, without exception, Sicilian or of Sicilian origin. Every continent on earth has a governing board of Mafia members who rule all *organized* criminals, listen to their arguments and dispense justice, which may take the form of a grant of money or a sentence of death. The power of the Mafia is not entirely in its wealth, but in its ability to kill anyone, anywhere, at any time. [Reid 1964]

But at the present time, there seems to be not only a greater proliferation of the sense of conspiracy, but also a difference in its attribution. Most earlier conspiracy fantasies were primarily directed against an imagined enemy subversion. They expressed the fear that an enemy country—Russia, Germany, or Zionist Israel—had established an espionage system or revolutionary organization which threatened to take over key positions of power in the nation. While these enemy groups were often able to disguise themselves as native citizens, they remained outsiders who could be exposed, expelled, or destroyed. This type of conspiracy fantasy often represented a fear of change, which was symbolized by the influence of ideas associated with a foreign country. Thus, American fantasies about a communist conspiracy probably reflected anxieties about social changes associated with radical ideas and the influence of Soviet Russia. Typically, this kind of conspiracy theme was most often expressed by conservatives and reactionaries and rejected or denounced by liberals.

The fictional world of the contemporary intrigue thriller is quite different from the traditional thriller of enemy subversion exposed by a dashing and gallant agent. First of all, instead of a single enemy conspiracy, the newer thrillers present a world of multiple or total conspiracy in which everyone seems involved. It is no longer easy to tell the friendly forces from the enemy conspirators because one's own secret service is likely to be run by enemy agents or by ambitious men more concerned with the expansion of their own power than with the defeat of enemy plots. Even the most dedicated and selfless of friendly agents is subject to the subtle corruptions of the system and may become a betrayer of the good without intending it or even knowing that he is doing it. At the end of John Le Carré's *The Honourable Schoolboy* (1977), Le Carré's hero, George Smiley, writes a letter to his wife in which he expresses the sense of inescapable conspiracy which pervades the imaginative world of the contemporary thriller: "I honestly do wonder, without wishing to be morbid, how I reached this present pass. So far as I can ever remember of my youth, I chose the secret road because it seemed to lead straightest and furthest toward my country's goal. The enemy in those days was someone we could point at and read about in the papers. Today, all I know is that I have learned to interpret the whole of life in terms of conspiracy. That is the sword I shall die by as well." This despairing confession is more articulate than those of most thriller writers about the vision of total conspiracy, but it is a dominant note in the satires of assassination, terrorism, and Watergate-like cover-ups which pour from the presses and the movie and television screens. A striking number of recent Republican politicians—ranging from conservatives Spiro Agnew and William F. Buckley, Jr., through Nixonite John Erlichman to liberal John Lindsay—have expressed themselves through the conspiracy thriller, for the fantasy of total conspiracy no longer belongs to a particular ideology but has become the property of liberals, conservatives, and radicals alike.

One could pick illustrations of this theme almost at random, but I will draw on a recent thriller film, the Charles Bronson vehicle *Telefon*. Here Bronson, the hero, plays a soviet agent (!!!) whose mission is to disrupt the plans of a now crazed former Russian agent to unleash a massive sabotage campaign in America by giving a cuing signal to a number of Americans hypnotically programmed to carry out their tasks of destruction. He is aided in his attempt to stop these unintentional saboteurs by a variety of other characters who are involved in their own plots. In a world where a foreign agent tries to prevent a number of American citizens from unintentionally playing their roles in a conspiracy of destruction because the foreign country has changed the direction of its own conspiracy, we should perhaps not be too surprised if paranoia begins to seem the ultimate form of sanity.

Thomas Pynchon's novels richly develop the themes of cosmic vertigo, universal conspiracy, and the quest for transcendence. In addition, he gives a deeper and more complex presentation of the cultural context and significance of these themes than any other novelist. His representation of contemporary experience as it reflects the shambles of the past, the catastrophe of war and violence, and the cosmic civilization shows man poised on the edge of history. The final scene of *Gravity's Rainbow* (Pynchon 1974) depicts an audience gathered in a decaying movie theater waiting for a show which will never go on. Instead, there comes a rocket, recaptured by the force of gravity: "And it is just here, just at this dark and silent frame, that the pointed tip of the rocket, falling nearly a mile per second, absolutely and forever without sound, reaches its last unmeasurable gap above the roof of this old theatre, the last delta-t." This, the final moment of Pynchon's novel, expresses perhaps better than any other passage in contemporary fiction the sense of contemporary experience which is reflected in the emergent themes of our literature.

REFERENCES

LeCarré, J. 1977. *The Honourable Schoolboy*. New York: Knopf.
Pynchon, T. 1974. *Gravity's Rainbow*. New York: Bantam.
Reid, E. 1964. *Mafia*. New York: New American Library.

GERALD L. KLERMAN

Common elements in the theories of depression and adaptation are particularly relevent to the study of the transition period from youth to young adulthood. The purpose of this chapter is threefold. One is to describe some of the empirical findings from clinical studies of depression within a conceptual framework. This approach regards depression, particularly the emotion and symptom, as an attempt on the part of human beings to adapt to a changing environment. It simultaneously explores concepts of depression and adaptation. The second purpose is to try to link these concepts to Erikson's ideas about developmental life stages (Erikson 1950). The third purpose is to bring to bear the combined developmental-adaptational approach to understanding the transition from youth into young adulthood.

Age of Melancholy

It is part of the pastime of historians to divide life into various ages. Probably the most successful instance of this was the poem by W. H. Auden (1947) which seems to have captured the emergence of an age of widespread anxiety. Many people, particularly Lifton (1976), related it to man's awareness of the potential power of destruction of the whole species with the advent of nuclear capability.

In the 1960s there began to be speculation as to whether or not anxiety was giving way to depression and despair as a dominant mood. How good is the evidence indicating an actual increase in epidemiologic rates of depression? Some of it is valid and some is not. For instance, more articles are written about depression than ever before, there is an increase in the prescription of the antidepressant drugs, yet there is also an increase in the prescription of the antianxiety drugs. A slight increase in the diagnosis of depression is seen also in nationwide data. But the fact that more people are being diagnosed as depressed in general hospitals, community mental health centers, and clinic settings may be an artifact of more attention to the problem and of increased insurance coverage. It is nicer to call someone depressed than schizophrenic or paranoid.

There are worldwide data indicating a rise in suicide attempts (Weissman, Paykel, French, Mark, Fox, and Prusoff 1973). The suicide-attempt rate has increased dramatically, almost tenfold, mostly among adolescents and young adults. Women have higher rates than men, with the highest prevalence under age thirty, and the most common technique is pill ingestion, perhaps a tribute to our new technologies. Other findings, less well documented, show also that the median age of depressed patients is dropping.

There is no doubt that the depressive phenomenon is well known throughout the history of Western civilization. There are excellent descriptions in the Bible, particularly of Saul's depression which was treated by David with some success. There are also excellent clinical descriptions in the Egyptian, Greek, and Roman literature from which a modern clinician has no difficulty in recognizing the symptoms of depression.

To what extent the literary writers reflect epidemiologic trends is difficult to know. It is tempting to think that we are in an age of melancholy as a transition after an age of anxiety. This is a period in which rising expectations, generated after World War II, have come up against harsh realities of population explosion and doomsday prophecies. One of the situations that psychologically predisposes individuals to depression is the presence of a gap between expectations and actuality. One experiences feelings of despair not so much when a situation is actually bad as when one has given up hope.

Adaptation and Depression

In addition to looking at depression clinically and developmentally, it is useful to consider depression as an evolutionary phenomenon for our species and for most mammalian species. Emotional states like depression, anxiety, fear, and anger have a function in the lives of humans in that they promote adaptation of the organism to the environment. That idea was first enunciated by Darwin (1965), who proposed in his study of the expression of emotions in animals that not only are morphologic structures adapted by natural se-lection but that there is also an evolutionary sequence to emotional states which he calls mental and expressive capacities.

Many of Darwin's ideas and observations lay dormant until after World War II, when a remarkable upsurge of interest and study of the biology of behavior occurred. Lorenz (Lorenz and Leyhausen 1973) and Tinbergen (1951) are the best known for their ethological studies of behavior, and Harlow, McKinney, and their colleagues have gone one step further from natural observations and experimentally induced various emotional states by separating primate (Rhesus monkey) offspring from their mothers and from their peers (McKinney, Suomi, and Harlow 1973). This is an experimental induction of various psychopathologic states, most prominently that of depres-sion.

The first stage of behavioral response as described by the authors is that of protest. There is an increase in motor activity, an increase in vocalization, and the animals run around seeking to reestablish contact. In the second stage—the despair stage—the infant huddles in the corner, the mother turns away, there is a general reduction of all motor activity, and again the facial expressions are empathically identifiable. There are similar observations by Jane Lawick-Goodall (1971) of chimpanzees separated from each other.

The capacity to become depressed is not exclusively a human one. It has been part of our evolutionary heritage and has played a biologically adaptive function. It performs a "signal" function, to use Engel's (1962) term, by alerting the social group, particularly the parental mothering group, that one of its precious offspring is in some danger. This is based in part on two facts about mammalian species in general and primates and humans in particular. One is that we produce very few offspring compared with fish or insects, and second that our offspring are born biologically immature and truly helpless. Adults may at times feel helpless and wish to be taken care of but are for the most part capable of biological survival. This is not true of human infants or other mammalian infants, which are born truly helpless and incomplete. In order for the species to have survived as long as we have, mechanisms had to develop to nurture and protect the helpless offspring. According to this view, the depressive experience as reflected by the cry or the facial expression is a signal to the adult members of the primate or mammalian group that one of its precious offspring is in danger and that it is necessary to come to its assistance.

Turning to humans, the general thesis from these points of view is that the affective state of depression is a specific response to the disruption of at-tachment bonds. Attachment bonds have been essential and useful to the survival and development of our species. There is biological apparatus developed through the centuries that we humans have inherited from our mammalian ancestors, particularly the primates and others. One interesting aspect of this apparatus is that we resist with great biological force any disruption of attachment bonding. We do not give up our attachment bonding without great psychological and physiological anguish. The wisdom of the body is such that it fights against the disruption (Klerman and Izen 1977).

Developmental Aspects

How is this evidence regarding the effects of life stresses related to the kinds of phenomena seen clinically in adolescents? It is appropriate here to apply Eriksonian concepts to developmental stages (Erikson 1950). Young individuals in our society in particular are involved in a number of developmental tasks, the most important of which includes leaving the parental home and establishing independence. As part of modern life we give a value to independence. This goes against a certain amount of our biological heritage.

As I have already indicated, we human beings do not give up our attachment bonds easily. We do so at an emotional and physiologic price. Yet, in a modern industrial society such as the one in which we live, we go from one place to another—to school, to take a job, and from that job to another. We send our children to summer camp, to pajama parties, to weekend events. We purposefully train our children to anticipate the disruption of attachment bonding and to be able to cope with the uncomfortable sense of separation and anxiety it brings. We expect them purposely to move, to leave the attachment of the primary family. In fact, if they stay too long with the primary family we consider them dependent and not moving properly in the developmental cycle. More significantly, we see this movement as an opportunity for growth and development. In the Eriksonian scheme, the outcome is the achievement of the capacity for intimacy—namely, to make new forms of attachment bonding, most importantly with members of the opposite sex. With this is a commitment to some sense of enduring responsibility and capacity to share in emotional give and take. I would propose that this is a relatively new experience in the history of our species. Most of the social support systems which our forebears have dealt with have emphasized some degree of stability.

The three most common social support systems, at least in the past 10,000 years, have been: (1) the family, (2) the church, and (3) the immediate neighborhood. Ever since the introduction of urban life we have relied upon these support systems to buttress against emotional states, including depression, fear, and anger. It is a characteristic of the times in which we now live that all three of these social support systems are in various degrees of disarray or disrepute.

Limits of Loss Theory

There is a limit, however, to the extent to which the phenomena one sees in a research clinic, a child guidance clinic, or, more importantly, in a college health service can be explained in terms of loss and separation. It is tempting theoretically to subsume all or most of depressive phenomena under the rubric of loss, separation, or disruption of bonding. Many theorists and textbook writers have emphasized one aspect or another of these phenomena as a necessary condition to understanding depression, whether as a normal mood, a symptom, or a syndrome.

Data indicate the limits of loss theory. First of all, loss and separation are not the universal antecedent events in all clinical depressions. In one group of depressives (Klerman and Izen 1977) we could find a discernible loss or separation in only about 25 percent of the patients who were clinically depressed, although there was a predominance of exits or separations within the group.

Second, not all individuals who are exposed to loss, separation, or disruption of attachment bonds become depressed. The majority of individuals do in fact cope with things like going to college, being drafted, or going to summer camp. Most even cope with as profound a disruption as the death of a parent or a child. There have been some prospective studies of individuals in the bereavement situation (Clayton 1978; Parkes 1970; and Parkes and Brown 1972). Evidence from these studies and others (Maddison and Viola 1968) indicates that the majority of individuals who are widowed and bereaved do in fact go through a period of emotional distress, with increased susceptibility to physical illness and increased use of the health-care system. However, by the end of one year about 85 percent of people are back to normal. That still leaves 15 percent clinically symptomatic at the need of one year (Clayton 1978). Whether these individuals will continue to have symptoms and be more vulnerable to psychosomatic disorder or clinical depression has been speculated upon by clinical observers such as Engel (1962) and Lindemann (1944) but has not yet been fully substantiated by prospective controlled studies. Most people cope because of either inner resources or some combination of available social support systems.

The third point that limits loss, separation, and disruption as a theoretical concept is that these events are not specific to depression. They have been described as the precipitating events for a wide variety of clinical conditions, not only psychiatric but also medical, such as coronary artery disease, peptic ulcer, rheumatoid arthritis, and automobile accidents.

Loss and separation and disruption of attachment bonding thus seem to result in a general propensity to a variety of illnesses—perhaps more so to depression, but evidence for this has not yet been exclusively determined. I come to the conclusion that environmental stress, particularly loss and separation and disruption of bonding, by itself cannot explain the clinical phenomena. One must look to other aspects of the lives of the individuals or their social support systems to give an explanation, let alone a prediction, of why certain individuals adapt and others do not.

A number of factors can easily be predicated as to what makes the difference. Some of these may be genetic, others may be early life experiences in which the individual became sensitive to loss, which has been a major theme in clinical theory. Another factor is any circumstance which lowers the self-esteem of the individual. This may be particularly a problem for college students if they attend a competitive institution. Other factors are changes in the social support system, the absence of the extended family, and the failure to be able to make friends or to participate in developing group supports. Zeiss, Lewinsohn, and Munoz (1978) define one of the propensities to depression as the absence of a social repertoire. They write that one of the things that characterizes normal people is the capacity to elicit positive social reinforcements from those around them. They speculate that the depressed individual is lacking in that set of social skills from impairment of early development or failure of learning, and the depressive-prone individual is unable to elicit from the social environment the kinds of social supports that are so important for the maintenance of self-esteem.

Conclusions

The thesis described in this chapter attempts to relate the clinical phenomena of depression to two concepts—an adaptive one and a developmental one. It is increasingly clear from recent research on the biology of emotional states that all mammalian species, particularly humans and other primates, have benefited from attachment bonding. It is essential to protect the individual. Nonverbal, depressive behavioral phenomena, such as the voice, the facial expression, the posture, and movements have been a powerful social and physiologic mechanism through the millennia to alert the parental group and the extended social group that the organism is in danger.

As we mature from the state of actual biological helplessness of our infancy, we become less dependent for biological survival upon our attachments, particularly parents. In the developmental process, psychosocial and interpersonal attachments to human beings acquire a new importance in our adaptation. They are not as important as they have been in the biological past of our species for survival, but they become important for our sense of self-worth, for our identity, and for the meaning and value we give to ourselves. Thus the attachments provide a central focus around which our cognitive sense of self, or inner representations, to use the psychodynamic concept, are integrated.

It is a thesis of many who have studied these phenomena that the biological function of depressive affect of a species changes as the maturity of the organism unfolds. Nevertheless the psychophysiological and biological apparatus that we were born with and that we have inherited through the millennia has not been modified. We still resist with great protest any disruption of attachment bonding. What has changed are the stimuli and environmental circumstances that initiate or terminate these profound reactions. In modern life, the main forces that initiate these depressive responses are more often threats to the psychosocial integrity of the individual, such as sense of self and worth, as well as the disruption of more important bonds which reinforce this self-esteem, rather than the survival per se as individuals.

REFERENCES

Auden, W. H. 1947. *The Age of Anxiety*. New York: Random House.
Clayton, P. J. 1978. The sequelae and nonsequelae of bereavement. Paper presented at the annual meeting of the American Psychiatric Association, May 8–12, 1978, Atlanta, Ga.
Darwin, C. 1965. *The Expression of the Emotions in Man and Animals*. Chicago: University of Chicago Press.
Engel, G. L. 1962. *Psychological Development in Health and Disease*. Philadelphia: Saunders.
Erikson, E. H. 1950. *Childhood and Society*. New York: Norton.

Klerman, G. L., and Izen, J. E. 1977. The effects of bereavement and grief on physical health and general well-being. *Psychosomatic Medicine* 9:63–104.

Lawick-Goodall, J. 1971. *In the Shadow of Man*. Boston: Houghton Mifflin.

Lifton, R. J. 1976. *The Life of the Self: Toward a New Psychology*. New York: Simon & Schuster.

Lindemann, E. 1944. Symptomatology and management of acute grief. *American Journal of Psychiatry* 101:141–148.

Lorenz, K., and Leyhausen, P. 1973. *Motivation of Human and Animal Behavior: An Ethological View*. New York: Van Nostrand Reinhold.

McKinney, W. T.; Suomi, S. J.; and Harlow, H. F. 1973. New models of separation and depression in Rhesus monkeys. In J. P. Scott and E. C. Senay, eds. *Separation and Depression*. Washington, D.C.: American Association for the Advancement of Science.

Maddison, D., and Viola, A. 1968. The health of widows in the year following bereavement. *Journal of Psychosomatic Research* 12:297–306.

Parkes, C. M. 1970. The first year of bereavement: a longitudinal study of the reaction of London widows to the death of their husbands. *Psychiatry* 33:444–467.

Tinbergen, N. 1951. *The Study of Instinct*. London: Oxford University Press.

Weissman, M. M.; Payfel, E. S.; French, N.; Mark, H.; Fox, K.; and Prusoff, B. 1973. Suicide attempts in an urban community, 1955 and 1970. *Social Psychiatry* 8:82–91.

Zeiss, A. M.; Lewinsohn, P. M.; and Munoz, R. F. 1978. Nonspecific improvement effects in depression using interpersonal, cognitive, and pleasant events focused treatments. Paper presented at the Western Psychological Association meeting, April 21, San Francisco.

PHILIP S. HOLZMAN

The theme struck by contributors to this special section is that human attachments are required for growth, for maturation, and for well-being. If attachments are weakened, one is in trouble. This trouble can be both an antecedent and a consequence of diminished attachment. All authors seem to agree that we are seeing an increase in psychopathology during adolescence and therefore of weakened attachments. We have learned that there are personal and environmental factors that interfere with attachment bonds, and the focus is on the nature of factors that have made for the loosening of these attachments. Three perspectives attempt to establish the phenomenon of detachment or of loosening attachments as a real social phenomenon. Other chapters focus on the impact of detachment on the individual, psychological views from inside and outside the person.

Philip N. Hauser speaks as an expert demographer. He brings evidence that there has been a very rapid change in the social order that followed the baby boom just after World War II. He states that people born after 1946 have had more schooling and have been exposed to more television than those born prior to 1946. But the schools have been terribly hard pressed to accommodate the then mushrooming population, and therefore educational quality has been inferior to that to which the previous cohort of youth had been exposed. Hauser points to the undeniably high unemployment rates, which are especially and appallingly high for blacks, and to the instability of marriage as inferred from increasing divorce rates and the number of unmarried couples living together. What he does not say, but implies is that, at least in white middle-class culture, there is something more to interpersonal attachments among married people than simply living together. He does, however, make the point that this may not have been necessarily so for white middle-class culture in the latter part of the nineteenth century, but there are fewer stabilizing influences for today's youth, in terms of traditions, norms, and ideologies.

I think that Hauser has made a very interesting case for inferring that today's youth have cut their moorings (or perhaps their moorings have been cut for them) to the past, to the present, to people, and to things. Evidence is that the number of ceremonies that people engage in seems to have decreased. As Erikson (1950) pointed out, ceremonies are extremely important because they bring the generations together.

Another observation is that there is rapid change in our society and technology and a huge increase in what it is that we have to learn. The effect of these rapid changes seems to be the greatest on those people who can comprehend most and yet are most immature, that is, adolescents. Although certainly the effects of rapid change would be apparent throughout the life cycle, the effects are probably not the same on all age groups.

There is no single effect of stress. The same stressful event can have many meanings to different people. Stressful events have to be interpreted, worked over, and responded to, and therefore responses to stress are not generally predictable. But we can say that if stresses impinge on an immature organism—one that is going through rapid bodily changes and whose period on this earth has not yet endowed him or her with the wisdom to look at stress with reflectiveness or with ironic detachment—stresses can lead to untoward changes in that vulnerable organism.

What might those outcomes be? First, I think we would be on firm ground to say that this rapid change has not produced any increase in schizophrenia. As measured by almost any demographic statistic, schizophrenia does not seem to have increased significantly. There is, however, a clear increase in suicide attempts, delinquency, and divorce. And this is what Hauser has documented. A question that one can raise about these facts is, Have these changes produced an increase in the depressive syndrome itself? The answer is that we do not have any good evidence one way or the other.

I want to make one personal observation with respect to Hauser's account of the violence to which we are exposed daily. With all of the violence that television directs our way, with the fact that there are mass murderers and multiple murderers afoot, it is too easy to believe that we are living in an increasingly lawless society and that aggression and hostility are on the increase. But I think that one can make a good case for the fact that we are actually becoming a more lawful society; we are becoming more tamed and more socialized. If, for example, one compares the West as it was before the turn of the century with contemporary society in our western states, the kinds of murderers that we now read about in the paper and that shock us occurred much more frequently then. The fact that we are very much concerned about reducing nuclear proliferation, that we are more socially minded, and that we are thinking about what happens to less advantaged people in other parts of the world indicates that things may not be as bad as we sometimes paint them. However, despite the increasing taming of aggressivity, there is an alarming increase among adolescents in suicides, attacks, marauding bands, and so on.

From his anthropological perspective, Irving I. Zaretsky presents a unique view of youth's search for faith and community through contemporary quasi-religious groups. I am impressed by the characteristics these groups have in common. I wonder how independent these characteristics are from each other. Furthermore, I am struck by the probability that all of these people—many of them young people—who enter these groups are seekers after contact. The difference between the nineteenth-century healing movements which had been very prevalent and those Zaretsky describes is that the contemporary groups emphasize touching, physical contact, and making sure that people are welcomed. These contemporary movements seem to be extended to those people who feel extruded from society and who seem to have lost their moorings. Many people who gravitate to these movements are unhappy, and, as Zaretsky mentions, they look to these organizations to given them a reprieve from sexual pressures and from demands on their social, intellectual, and occupational competence. In these groups they can be absorbed. In these respects, Zaretsky, like Hauser, documents the issue of youth's loss of ties, of attachments.

From the perspective of literature, John Cawelti seems to be saying that the more things change the more they seem to be the same. He is able to show that the fictional themes that have emerged fit into the perspective of detachments. He isolates three themes. One is the sense of cosmic vertigo, man's relation to the unimaginably vast space as depicted in *Star Wars* and *Close Encounters of the Third Kind*—the end of the earth, and the end of the universe. This is an emergent theme from the western and the detective story, new versions of which have all but disappeared. Both the western and the detective story share a cosmic vision of reality, reassuring us that in the end we are safe, things do seem to come out well. Thus, in Cawelti's view these books, which emphasize the sense of cosmic vertigo, are ways of mastering anxiety about the unknown.

The second theme concerns the appearance of the alien as redeemer. This theme also appears in *Close Encounters of the Third Kind* and in a number of other romances that emphasize the yearning for contact with powerful

311

people, evidently reflecting our own sense of loneliness and of being cut loose from our moorings. This theme has the same kind of romantic thrust found in many nineteenth-century novels and operas, for example, Wagnerian opera, whch focused on romantically religious quests for something higher than oneself and emphasized the theme that one can be redeemed, no matter how badly one may have behaved in the past, through merging with this mystical power.

The third theme, the most malignant of the three, is the fascination with conspiracy, or paranoia as the norm. Here the emphasis is on the experience of cosmic emptiness which seems to be a kind of weltanschauung. For example, in the movie, *Three Days of the Condor,* the viewer really doesn't know what is happening or who's on whose side. Who is the enemy and who is the friend? What is depicted here is rapid change, too rapid to grasp rationally.

This theme is probably not completely new. At the end of the nineteenth century we began to see changes in the way people saw the world. For example, in French impressionaism literal representation of figures gave way to how one sees and interprets objects at a particular moment; in Joyce's novels syntax and grammar were stretched beyond their usual usage; Schoenberg stretched music beyond tonality; and Picasso stretched visual form beyond representability. Yet it seems to me that although all of these people may have adopted an alien style, the content of their work still emphasized attachment. I understand Cawelti to be saying that today there is the loss of a very clear dialectic and, therefore, we are faced with moral uncertainties. In the past our inner fantasies were projected into literature; today it seems as if we do not know what is inside and which is outside. Is Pogo's dictum that "we have met the enemy and he is us" a representation of the evil that we seem to be battling within ourselves? Is it too unclear? Is our world too uncertain? Today our youth cannot see clearly what is happening. Although conflict seems to be the norm, they sense that they are without redeemers.

Gerald L. Klerman documents the increasing prevalence of depressions, particularly in younger persons. What can account for these events? Klerman underscores the role of attachment in depression. In humans attachments are not given up easily, and he views depression in terms of an adaptive point of view.

I found this to be a particularly fruitful aproach to a theory of depression. This would fit with the Freudian adaptive view of anxiety and George Klein's (1976) view of pleasure. Just as anxiety has been thought of as a signal indicating danger and mobilizing the person to defensive efforts, and pleasure has been thought of as a signal to approach, mobilizing the person to sustain contact, so depression can be thought of as a signal of impending or actual detachment. In this instance, what one could call "signal depression" is an experience in which there is a loss of some life-sustaining support that may not necessarily be a current danger to the person's personal or biological life, although earlier such a loss might have been life threatening. This anticipation of loss brings with it corresponding feelings of emptiness and longing. The adaptive quality of this signal depression emerges when one considers that the depressed person appears forlorn and thus mobilizes the environment to approach him. When, however, depression continues chronically, the depressed person tends to become a nuisance. Anyone who has had the experience of trying to treat a chronically depressed person with psychotherapy realizes that after a while the countertransference becomes a formidable obstacle to treatment.

It would thus seem that the interruption of attachments is a crucial variable in understanding the rise of depressions among young people. Adolescence requires separation and a beginning detachment from one's biological nuclear family. Add to this necessary, phase-specific detachment the decay of our social support systems—the family, the church, and the neighborhood. We may then ask, Is it because those institutions are in disarray that they are now unable to ease the vulnerable adolescent's transition into adult independence, thereby contributing to the apparent epidemic of depression among youth?

Attachments, Klerman emphasizes, are important for a sense of worth and value. He offers a multifactorial model of depression, or perhaps an additive model, that included five factors. The first is loss and separation, particularly during early life experiences. It is true that loss and separation are not universal antecedent events of depression. They do, however, seem to contribute to an increasing risk of later depression. It is also true that not all persons who suffer losses and separations get depressed. And losses and separations are not specific to depressions. That is to say, separations can be antecedent conditions in a number of other syndromes as well as depressions. The second factor is genetic predisposition. The third factor is personality attributes, particularly those that predispose a person toward excessive feelings of guilt. The fourth is an inadequate repertoire of social and interpersonal skills. The fifth is the presence or absence of social supports and nurturance.

Conclusions

The main theme of this section is a multifactorial view of vulnerable youth. All of the views seem to be important, and one cannot be an advocate of one

313

over the other. One question we can ask is, Where can we intervene so that we can have the most effectiveness in helping vulnerable young people? But I think, before that, we must establish what, in our population, is the effect of these rapid changes that are taking place. Is there in fact an increase in depressive disorders? What has been documented is that young people today face many crises and are exposed to many more pressures than previous generations. They are generally vulnerable because of social, intellectual, and biological immaturity. The social environment today may indeed be imposing unbearable burdens on the more vulnerable members of this generation.

REFERENCES

Erikson, E. H. 1950. *Childhood and Society*. New York: Norton.
Klein, G. 1976. *Psychoanalytic Theory*. New York: International Universities Press.

PART III

PSYCHOPATHOLOGICAL ASPECTS OF ADOLESCENT DEVELOPMENT

EDITORS' INTRODUCTION

Adequate understanding of the psychopathological aspects of adolescence is based on the solid knowledge of adolescent development when viewed from the perspective of maladaptation due to both ego defects and constitutional deficits. Psychodynamic knowledge, however, is incomplete without an appreciation of cultural, social, biological, and genetic influences on personality.

Discovery of the genetic roots of bipolar affective illness and its response to lithium carbonate requires that we develop skills to detect the earliest stages of the disorder. The rising divorce rate has resulted in a proliferation of literature on the subject with ambiguous conclusions as to its effects on children and adolescents. The liberalization of sexual attitudes has brought about a drastic increase in teen pregnancies, with a large number of the young women keeping their babies while declining options of abortion or adoption. Furthermore, the more open attitudes toward homosexuality is bringing gay youngsters into treatment at an earlier age. Although many adolescent therapists resist the urge to pull out their own hair, hair-pulling as a symptom of adolescent conflict provides a fascinating means of studying many of the psychodynamic issues characteristic of this stage of development.

Aaron H. Esman approaches adolescent psychopathology through study of Margaret Mahler's early developmental theories. Emphasizing evolution of self- and object representations, Mahler has described early development as a separation-individuation phase with four subphases: differentiation, practicing, rapprochement, and attainment of object constancy. Esman analogizes these stages to adolescent development and focuses on the rapprochement subphase as a period of great vulnerability for the child and eventually for the adolescent.

Sherman C. Feinstein reviews the evidence for the presence of bipolar affective disorder in children and adolescents. He hypothesizes that manic-depressive illness appears early in life in the form of equivalent behavior which is the precursor of the cyclothymic personality and manic-depressive states of adulthood. A psychiatric case study of Virginia Woolf is presented which views, from a developmental point of view, manifestations of manic-depressive illness in childhood, during puberty and adolescence, at the onset of adulthood, and ending in its subsequent cyclic, bipolar end state with her suicide. Feinstein concludes that a history of affective instability in childhood along with severe affective reaction during adolescence should be considered an early manifestation of manic-depressive illness.

Clarice J. Kestenbaum reviews the growing literature on adolescents at risk for manic-depressive illness, particularly the evidence for a genetic hypothesis for affective disorders, and presents three clinical vignettes. She found that genetic factors play a role in the etiology of major affective disorders, symptom clusters emphasizing dysphoria and fluctuations in mood are present, and psychological evidence of lowered performance scores and right hemispheric dysfunction are suggestive. Kestenbaum believes that true mania in childhood is extremely rare and is probably masked by developmental issues. She recommends, however, early diagnosis and awareness of the premorbid state of manic-depressive illness, particularly where there is a family history of affective disorder.

Sidney Berman attends to parental reactions to adolescent depression. He reviews the complementary parental responses to adolescent development and views the parenting responses as a psychological task within adulthood. In a mild transitory depression the parents, with help and guidance, are able to bear with the adolescent's discomfort. With more severe depressions, parents react with characteristic responses, depending on the etiology of the reaction. Berman views the parental response as transactional and multidetermined, with the quality of the response dependent on the character structure of the parents.

Allan Z. Schwartzberg notes the accelerating divorce rate, the large numbers of children and adolescents living in the single-parent family, and the specific dynamic interactions of the young person with the remaining parent and how this relationship may affect future mental health. He studied middle-class adolescents, seen in private practice, who represented a wide range of diagnostic categories. The predominant mood was depression or, its equivalent, acting out. Schwartzberg recorded the adolescents' reactions to the event, the nature of parental relationships, and determined there were three clusters of adolescents: those with exacerbation of preexisting psychopathology, those with temporary regression, and those who made premature attempts at mastery. Symptoms persisted longer than expected, acting out was extensive, and there was a positive correlation between effective parenting by the custodial parent and good adaptation and coping in the adolescent.

Susan M. Fisher and Kathleen Rudd Scharf believe that we now have in the United States an epidemic, not of teenage pregnancy but of teenage baby keeping. In their overview of the problem from anthropological, sociological, and psychological considerations they describe three groups: girls for whom a baby fills a deep narcissistic need related to faulty self-concept; a better-integrated group attempting an oedipal resolution through pregnancy; and another group for whom pregnancy represents an attempt at maturation, a rite de passage, kin ties, economic-skill utilization, or a tradition of their social group. Programs utilizing an understanding of developmental factors are described which can make a contribution to future growth, provide a "second chance," and perhaps help the young person to be better able to hand down newly discovered experiences to her offspring.

Carlos Salguero, Edilma Yearwood, Elizabeth Phillips, and Nancy Schlesinger report studies of pregnancy and parenthood in adolescent girls who live in an inner-city neighborhood. They found that large numbers were pregnant, that a substantial percentage of child-abuse and neglect cases had adolescent mothers, and that pregnant adolescents did not use prenatal care facilities. They were concerned about the psychological trauma of pregnancy on the adolescent as well as the child and report a program developed to protect the fragile mother-infant bond through the evaluation of infant-at-risk criteria.

Lillian H. Robinson approaches the developmental aspects of adolescent homosexuality and the relationship of early object experiences with psychosexual development. She discusses factors which predispose to homosexuality. These may be found in defective child-parent relationships, early traumatic sexual experiences, as well as cultural and developmental influences. Treatment philosophies are considered along with diagnostic psychopathological issues. Robinson believes that homosexuality should be considered from a developmental point of view and that adolescents with homosexual conflicts benefit from therapy.

Arthur D. Sorosky and Marlis B. Sticher consider an ancient disease entity: trichotillomania, an irresistible urge to pull out bodily hair. Hair-pulling is not a distinct clinical entity but rather a symptom which may be associated with a variety of psychiatric disorders. The case examples of two adolescent girls are described. Treatment consisted of an uncovering of repressed incestual and aggressive strivings in individual psychotherapy as well as an adolescent group-therapy experience which enabled the patients to push toward adolescence and to counter the regressive pull to the pregenital fixation points.

AARON H. ESMAN

The process of human psychological development can be likened to a house
with many windows; one's view will depend on the particular opening through
which one looks. Thus, to the Piagetian, development is a succession of
cognitive stages in orderly and invariant sequence; to the classical Freudian
it is a complex progression through a series of overlapping psychosexual
phases; Erikson sees it as a passage through a sequence of psychosocial crises;
while the behaviorist observes a gradual accretion of learned responses and
competences.

Over the past twenty-five years, another approach to the understanding of,
at least, the early stages of psychological development has been propounded
in the work of Mahler and her associates.[1] The window through which Mahler
views the process is that of the evolution of self and object representations,
and with them, of mental life itself. In this chapter I propose to explore the
application of Mahler's ideas and, in particular, her thoughts about the crucial
role of what she calls the "rapprochement" subphase to the study of adolescence and the clinical care of disturbed adolescents.

It was Blos (1968) who first described adolescence as a "second individuation" phase. Granted, of course, that we cannot speak of the normal
latency or preadolescent child and his parents as being involved in a symbiotic
state akin to that of the first few months of life, it remains true that there are
distinct behavioral parallels between the adolescent process (in our culture,
at least) and the normal separation-individuation phase and its several subphases, as Mahler has described them.

The early adolescent can be said to be involved in a massive "hatching"
or differentiation process, as he—in part defensively, no doubt—seeks to
establish psychological distance from the primary objects of his preoedipal
and oedipal longings. The first motor efforts of the infant that initiate and

accompany his emergence from the symbiotic dual-unity can readily be analogized to the beginning gestures of independence and self-assertion displayed by the pubertal or postpubertal youngster. As he becomes more comfortable with his new body image, his increased muscular strength, and the enhancement of his cognitive capacities through the development of operational thought (Piaget 1969), the young adolescent moves, like the junior toddler, into a "practicing" period in which he tests out his newly won powers and his greater range of freedom—always assuming, of course, that his parents grant him both adequate scope and adequate protection for such explorations of autonomy and individuation.

Much of the rebelliousness and experimentalism of this period has a quality analogous to the "love affair with the world" that Mahler (citing Greenacre) ascribes to the practicing toddler as he seeks to probe the limits of his world. Similarly, the "low keyedness" which Mahler and her associates (p. 92) have observed in the later practicing toddler as he senses the mother's absence is frequently mirrored by the early adolescent's oft-described moodiness and irritability, as he seeks to deal with the relative objectlessness and self-depletion that result from his efforts at detachment.

Periodically, therefore, we see the young and even the mid adolescent turning back for security and support to the parents from whom he is ostensibly—and often noisily—seeking to remove himself. As with the toddler, however, such closeness to the parent may evoke fears of regressive engulfment and dedifferentiation, leading to renewed assertions of autonomy and individuation or desperate searches for substitute attachment objects. This rapprochement-like phenomenon, tinged with ambivalence (or, in Mahler's terms, "ambitendency") and frequently marred by turmoil, seems distinctly similar to that described by Mahler for the toddler. In both cases one can recognize the anxiety and insecurity generated by the process of distancing. This is all the more true for the young adolescent because the unconscious conflicts around the reactivated oedipal and preoedipal wishes have not yet been resolved and truly integrated, and realistic mental representations of the self and of the parents, devoid of idealizations or defensive denigrations, have yet to be consolidated.

By late adolescence, however, this last work is normally well under way. Just as with the establishment of an at least relative self- and object constancy in the three-year-old, its completion allows for a genuine, nonconflictual separation from parents, for the consolidation of character organization (Blos 1968), and for the undertaking of the age-appropriate work and object relations that characterize youth, on the one hand, and nursery and primary school life on the other.

It is true that, as Schafer (1973) has reminded us, symbiosis and separation-individuation concepts have as their referents mental representations rather than overt behaviors. Further, he points out that "only an already highly individuated person is capable of giving up his infantile relations to others (actually, of modifying these relations greatly)" (p. 43). It must be clear, then, that we are speaking here of analogies, rather than identities. Even so, it is possible, I believe, to use this schema as a framework for understanding certain clinical phenomena in adolescence. Blos (1968), in his discussion of the "second individuation process," points up the dialectic tension between ego growth in adolescence and the pull toward regression to more primitive, less differentiated modes of behavior. It is his view that the capacity to tolerate and master such regressive episodes is a central feature of normal adolescent development. While, like Gradolph (1978) I question the ubiquity or necessity of major ego regressions in normal adolescence, it is surely true, unfortunately, that massive regressions to earlier levels of mental and behavioral function characterize much of adolescent psychopathology, especially in its severe forms. Differentiation between these grave disorders and the regressive shifts Blos describes sometimes represents a serious diagnostic challenge, although one must bear in mind Masterson's (1968) observation that the burden of proof is on the psychiatrist, who suggests in such cases that one deals with "normal turmoil" rather than psychopathology.

I believe that Mahler's schema proves to be of great value in meeting this challenge, in helping to conceptualize the nature of the pathology, and in formulating a therapeutic program. Mahler and her associates suggest that "islands of developmental failure might lead to borderline symptomatology in . . . adolescence," but note that they "deliberately have not dealt with these vicissitudes in detail" (p. 229). I should like to do precisely that in the following case illustrations:

Case 1

Gladys is a sixteen-year-old girl of mixed Chinese and Puerto Rican ancestry admitted to a residential treatment center. She was sent there because of her long history of truancy and street activity dating back to age fourteen. According to Gladys, she had been extensively involved with alcohol, drugs, and sexual promiscuity.

Gladys was born when her mother was seventeen. The father, an alcoholic, abandoned them when Gladys was two, after the birth of her younger brother.

The mother then returned to Puerto Rico where the maternal grandmother increasingly assumed the care of the children because the mother had lost interest in them and finally abandoned them when Gladys was four. Grandmother was a rigid, fanatical, fundamentalist Christian who regarded all sensual indulgence as sinful. Gladys clung to her grandmother and was extremely compliant and submissive at home throughout her childhood, indeed, even while leading an active, rebellious street life for the two years prior to admission. Gladys explained, "I used to pick up men on the streets because of feeling lonely and because I wanted affection." Drugs and alcohol were clearly related to profound depressive feelings.

In the treatment center Gladys replicated this pattern. She was initially compliant, cooperative, and well behaved. Gradually, however, she became increasingly angry and aggressive, at first with peers and then with adults. She became especially agitated on weekends when the child-care staff was depleted and when her therapist, to whom she became intensely attached, was absent. Unwilling or unable to attend school, she was at times left to wander aimlessly about the campus during the day, feeling detached, isolated, and abandoned to the destructive power of her own impulses and fantasies. In the absence of clear-cut structure and formal programming, she felt lost and helpless and her primitive affects and wishes asserted themselves. She began to bring a rubber rabbit to her therapeutic sessions as a combination alter ego and transitional object. Gradually she became more disorganized and fragmented, with suicidal and homicidal thoughts and impulses, until it became clear that hospitalization was required. In the hospital, she recovered quickly and was able to return to the treatment center, where she did well for a time. Weekend visits, however, with her grandmother led to increasingly sharp regressions culminating in a suicide attempt which was followed by violent assaults on staff. This necessitated her discharge into her grandmother's custody, who thereupon took her to Puerto Rico, and contact with Gladys was lost.

This case is complex and Gladys's pathology multiply determined. Nonetheless, I believe that she demonstrates a developmental failure during separation-individuation at the level of the rapprochement subphase. In the absence of an adequate developmental history, there is some reason to think that her early symbiotic phase was fairly well established. Her intense, somewhat hypomanic street activity evokes images of the practicing period, during which the child tests out the possibilities and limits of his environment and of his own resources—tinged, no doubt, by an intense need for emotional refueling through human contact. What seemed unbearable to Gladys, however, was the absence of dependable, protective, and nurturing figures in her

323

life space. Under these conditions, she would lapse into primitive, regressive fantasies of symbiotic fusion and/or effusions of intense unmodulated aggression. One can reconstruct that Gladys experienced the psychological loss of the mother at the time of rapprochement—around two or so—due first to the birth of her sibling and then to the immature, narcissistic mother's growing emotional and physical detachment and ultimate abandonment. Gladys was left with no secure sense of the availability of a protective object (her father having abandoned her, too) and no possibility to develop object constancy. The absence of her therapist meant to her total abandonment, with rage, panic, and disorganized hyperactivity as the only recourse—that, or a regressive restitution of symbiotic fusion with her grandmother, who had served, however inadequately, as a substitute for the lost primary object.

It seemed clear, therefore, that a rational treatment plan for this girl would include the more-or-less constant availability of nurturing objects and a structured program that left no gaps in which she could feel abandoned to the power of her own impulses. A rapprochement-like situation had to be feasible for her at all times, to avert disorganizing panic and self-destructive behavior and to prevent her from acting out in order to obtain affection. In the absence of such a structure, her decompensation was inevitable, probably resulting in those permanent characterological fixations characteristic of borderline personality organization.

Case 2

Jane was a twenty-year-old college dropout when she came to me, her fifth therapist. She had been in treatment more or less continuously since age fourteen, when she began seeing a male therapist primarily because of severe behavioral and learning difficulties in school. At that time she was overactive, distractible, and assumed the role of the class clown. She had had social problems for years; usually she had one good friend, but was regarded by many of her peers as somewhat odd. At home, she was frequently in conflict with her mother, an unstable, impulsive woman who was alternately intensely possessive and harshly critical. The father, apparently something of a successful con man, had left the family when Jane was eleven. There had been only sporadic contact since, though he seemed to have provided adequately for them financially during Jane's early adolescence.

Over the years that had elapsed since her initial entry into therapy, Jane had had three more therapists—two women and one man—before coming to me. With none of them had any major changes in her behavior occurred, though she retained a tender affection for one of the women, who had been very supportive and maternal toward her and provided her with much intellectual insight. She acknowledged that little of substance had resulted from their work beyond what might be expected of normal maturation.

Jane presented herself as a pathetically appealing, attractive, somewhat disorganized young woman who described herself as barely able to concentrate on anything related to school or work; she had lost a number of jobs because of her distractibility and erratic performance. She complained bitterly and intensely of a "talking problem" in which people who were speaking, such as lecturers, actors, or even social acquaintances, would appear to her to have distorted mouths and their words would seem similarly distorted and incomprehensible.

Her primary preoccupation, however, was her relationship with Jim, a young man who, she said, was cruel, unaffectionate, and manipulative, but on whom she felt totally dependent and whom she could not give up. She had idealized him for years and regarded her involvement with him as a triumph, since she had never really had a boyfriend before. She felt incapable of doing virtually anything for herself, relying on him, her roommate, her best friends, or, of course, her mother for help with many of the practical aspects of her life. She maintained a divided existence, spending some nights in her own apartment and some in her mother's—the latter rationalized on the ground that it was more convenient for her to come to her early-morning treatment hours from her mother's home than from her own. She was beset with fears that her mother might die at any time and she would be left alone and helpless, and she had numerous rituals designed to ward off such thoughts. With her two-year-younger sister she had a distant relationship; the latter figured little in her associations except as a sometimes rival.

Much of the early work in treatment focused on her conflict about "breaking up" with Jim. Previous therapists had suggested she do so, but she could not. "Having him is like magic-country," she said. "I don't know what would happen if I were alone—I'd probably be spaced out all the time." "My mother says I should hold on to him because it's terrible not to have a boyfriend." Her problems with concentration were in large measure the consequence of her immersion in fantasies about Jim or other idealized men. Jane's desperate clinging mirrored in many respects her relationship with her mother. Her profound separation fears represented the residues of unresolved ambivalent conflicts. She described her mother as cold, critical, and unaffectionate, just as she did Jim. Her barely repressed rage at her mother seemed to me to be the legacy of her disappointment in the rapprochement period, when her efforts at establishing contact were met with rebuff or criticism. This served to intensify her feelings of helplessness and desperate need. It was as though she were involved in a continuous effort to establish a rapprochement position, from which she could move out into the world for brief periods, only to return for more support to the maternal object—mother, friend, roommate, therapist, boyfriend.

In maintaining her attachment, she was able to cling to an illusion of magical, omnipotent control, without which she felt like a helpless, incompetent toddler. From the therapist she expected magical intervention requiring no active efforts toward change on her part, even to the extent of taking prescribed medication, which she usually forgot to do. Recurrently she accused me of acts of negligence or attitudes of disinterest or indifference, seemingly reactivating in the transference what she had experienced as her mother's affective unavailability in the rapprochement period. It emerged that she had a long-standing fantasy of being placed in a hospital, where she would be given extensive therapy—that is, where she would be totally cared for.

Jane's "talking problem" remains an obscure and puzzling symptom which, although it suggested a thought disorder, was encapsulated and did not appear to be part of a manifest psychosis. It is a fact, however, that the development of speech is central to the separation-individuation process (Busch 1978) and is roughly coincident with the rapprochement subphase; indeed, speech is one of the primary means through which the process of rapprochement and its resolution—what McDevitt (1975) has called the "rapprochement crisis"—is carried on. In her quasi-hallucinatory distortions of both the visual and auditory aspects of speech, it seems possible that she might be projectively reproducing the experienced distortions of her own and her mother's speech in the angry, tormented exchanges of the rapprochement period. Such a reconstruction is unverifiable, at least at this time, but it has, for me at least, a measure of plausibility. It is certain that, as Sander (1978) has pointed out, the fate of the entire symbolic process is founded on the events of this early period; it is striking how for this borderline adolescent it is precisely the symbolic functions that are most grossly impaired.

Mahler (1971) has stated that there is not always a direct line from the deductive use of borderline phenomena to substantive findings in observational research. As I have suggested earlier, we deal here largely with analogies, rather than identities. The borderline adolescent reveals in his mental organization—or lack of organization—a bewildering range of regressions, fixations, developmental arrests, precocities, and islands of normality that bespeak a developmental process which, however skewed, makes him a far different organism from the "junior toddler" of Mahler's observations. Meissner's (1978) recent penetrating review of the literature on the borderline syndrome defines both the gains and the losses in considering it from the developmental (and other) perspectives.

It will be apparent that much of what I have discussed here is congruent in some respects with ideas presented by others—notably, Masterson (1973, 1977), Masterson and Rinsley (1975), and, most recently, Shapiro (1978), whose review of the borderline syndrome merits careful study. Masterson and Rinsley (1975) have delineated what they consider to be a characteristic mode of mother-child interaction in the borderline syndrome: "The borderline child has a mother with whom there is a unique and uninterrupted interaction with a specific relational focus, i.e., reward for regression, withdrawal for separation-individuation . . . the mother's withdrawal of her libidinal availability in the face of her child's efforts towards separation-individuation creates the leitmotif of the borderline child . . . the mother is available if the child clings and behaves regressively, but withdraws if he attempts to separate and individuate" (p. 167).

In my view, this picture comes dangerously close to what I have called "mother-baiting." The mother emerges as the unvarnished villain of the piece in this work, rewarding clinging submission, punishing separation-individuation, immersed in the satisfaction of her own narcissistic needs. That this may at times be a fair portrait cannot be denied, but case 2 is typical of a group of borderline adolescents whose histories strongly suggest significant intrinsic deviations in the range of minimal cerebral dysfunction that have contributed substantially to the disturbed mother-child interactions. Jane is a virtual nonreader, a grown-up dyslexic (confirmed by psychological testing). This represents another aspect of the disturbance in her symbolic functions.

Winnicott (1965) speaks of the normal infant's capacity, often in the face of massive traumatization, to derive enough "goodness" from the mother-child relationship to develop coherent self- and object images. This capacity, it would appear, Jane lacked; she could not extract from her mother's erratic behavior those elements of goodness that might have countered her own intrinsic tendencies toward object splitting, unresolved ambivalence, and self-fragmentation. It is the child's experience (Escalona 1963) of his interactions with the mother, not the mother's actual behavior, that is crucial for the laying down of self- and object representations in the separation-individuation phase. It is this process, not a person, as Masterson and Rinsley (1975) would seem to suggest, that miscarries in the pathogenesis of borderline disorders.

Kaplan (1980) and Mahler and Kaplan (1977) have sought to counter the tendency, explicit in Masterson's (1977) work, to identify specific diagnostic entities with specific subphase deviations. To quote Masterson, "If the arrest occurs in the symbiotic phase, self- and object representations are fused . . . ego defenses are those of the psychotic . . . the clinical diagnosis is schizophrenia. If the arrest occurs in the separation-individuation phase, the self- and object representations are separate but split . . . the ego defenses are still primitive . . . the clinical diagnosis is borderline personality organization. If the arrest occurs late in the on-the-way-to-constancy phase or in the early phallic oedipal phase, the self- and object representations are separate and whole . . . ego defenses are more mature . . . the clinical diagnosis is psychoneurosis" (Masterson 1977, p. 477).

In challenging this categorical linkage of the borderline syndrome with the resolution of the separation-individuation phase in general and the "rapprochement crisis" in particular, Mahler and Kaplan emphasize the need to consider "subphase adequacy" on all levels. Kaplan seeks to relate subphase disturbances to Spitz's (1959) classic definition of "psychic organizers," and proposes to extend his concept beyond the three which he proposed—differentiation of self and object, recognition of the mother as a specific object, and the development of speech—to a fourth, the Oedipus complex, which, she contends, has crucial developmental impact on the formation of all human personalities, including the borderline.

One cannot, I acknowledge, seriously quarrel with these formulations or differ with Mahler and Kaplan's wish to avoid oversimplifications, dogmatic and simplistic one-to-one correlations, and exaggerated emphases. Nonetheless, we have long been familiar with the concepts, imported into psychoanalytic developmental theory from embryology, of epigenesis and critical periods. The idea that earlier subphase inadequacy will modify the evolution of later subphases and will cast a shadow on the oedipal configuration is, in essence, a restatement of the concept of epigenesis and, though a salutary reminder, adds nothing new to what is already known. That the oedipal crisis is central to psychic development is, of course, an article of psychoanalytic faith, and deserves restatement at a time when separate developmental lines and separate psychologies of the self are being advanced in some quarters and preoedipal development is, pendulum-fashion, being accorded what may be disproportionate attention. But we have long been accustomed to associate specific pathological formations with fixations at or regressions to particular developmental phases in the psychosexual line—for example, obsessional disorders with anal fixations—and have, therefore, come to view certain phase developments as *critical* ones. It does not, therefore, seem either artificial or grossly oversimplifying to propose as a heuristic hypothesis that the separation-individuation phase, and, specifically, the rapprochement subphase, may be such a critical period for the development—or transcendence—of borderline pathology, recognizing that on the one hand the transactions of this subphase will in part be shaped by the experience of earlier subphases, and that, on the other, they will color the child's manner and timing of entry into, experience of, and emergence from the Oedipus complex. A growing body of clinical data such as those presented here would seem to lend support to this proposition.

Conclusions

The formulations offered here demonstrate, I believe, the value of Mahler's conceptual framework for the psychiatric study and care of adolescents. Particularly in those cases of severe pathology with major elements of preoedipal fixation and regression, the specificity of her scheme of separation-individuation subphases often allows for a precise delineation of the locus of trauma and for a detailed prescription of object-related remedial intervention. It is through the processes she has so graphically described—differentiation, practicing, rapproachement, development of object constancy—that the psychological birth of the human infant occurs. Adolescence offers, as Eissler (1958, p. 250) has said, a "second chance" to rework some of the unfinished business not only of the oedipal conflicts but of some of these earlier developmental issues as well.

One must note a disposition in some quarters to designate such object-related conceptualizations as social psychology, reserving the accolade of true depth psychology to formulations concerning the organization and experience of a self system. Such dismissals do not, I think, do justice to the richness and subtlety of Mahler's elaboration of the representational world of the child, or to the solid grounding of her observational research in hypotheses derived from clinical psychoanalysis. In any event, it is only through open clinical inquiry that we can ultimately assess these questions.

NOTE

1. Except where otherwise indicated, all references to Mahler's work are to Mahler, Pine, and Bergman (1975).

REFERENCES

Blos, P. 1968. Character formation in adolescence. *Psychoanalytic Study of the Child* 23:245–263.

Busch, F. 1978. The silent patient: issues of separation-individuation and its relationship to speech development. *International Revue of Psychoanalysis* 5:491–500.

Eissler, K. R. 1958. Notes on problems of technique in the psychoanalytic psychotherapy of adolescents. *Psychoanalytic Study of the Child* 13:223–254.

Escalona, P. 1963. Patterns of infantile experience and the development process. *Psychoanalytic Study of the Child* 18:197–203.

Gradolph, P. 1978. Developmental vicissitudes of the self and ego-ideal during adolescence. Paper presented at the Fall Meeting, American Psychoanalytic Association, New York, December 1978.

Kaplan, L. 1980. Rapprochement, organization and transformations: relevance for the understanding of borderline phenomena in childhood, adolescence and adulthood. In R. Lax, ed. *Rapprochement*. New York: Aronson.

McDevitt, J. 1975. Separation-individuation and object constancy. *Journal of the American Psychoanalytic Association* 23:713–742.

Mahler, M. 1971. A study of the separation-individuation process and its possible application to borderline phenomena in the psychoanalytic situation. *Psychoanalytic Study of the Child* 26:403–424.

Mahler, M., and Kaplan, L. 1977. Developmental aspects in the assessment of narcissistic and so-called borderline personalities. In P. Hartocollis, ed. *Borderline Personality Disorders*. New York: International Universities Press.

Mahler, M.; Pine, F.; and Bergman, A. 1975. *The Psychological Birth of the Human Infant*. New York: Basic.

Masterson, J. 1968. The psychiatric significance of adolescent turmoil. In A. H. Esman, ed. *The Psychology of Adolescence*. New York: International Universities Press, 1975.

Masterson, J. 1973. The borderline adolescent. *Adolescent Psychiatry* 2:240–268.

Masterson, J. 1977. Primary anorexia nervosa in the borderline adolescent: an object-relations view. In P. Hartocollis, ed. *Borderline Personality Disorders*. New York: International Universities Press.

Masterson, J., and Rinsley, D. 1975. The borderline syndrome: the role of the mother in the genesis and structure of the borderline personality. *International Journal of Psychoanalysis* 56:163–177.

Meissner, W. 1978. Theoretical assumptions of concepts of the borderline personality. *Journal of the American Psychoanalytic Association* 26:559–598.

Piaget, J. 1969. The intellectual development of the adolescent. In G. Caplan and S. Lebovici, eds. *Adolescence: Psychosocial Perspectives*. New York: Basic.

Sander, L. 1978. New perspectives in early development: behavioral analysis twenty years later. Given as the David M. Levy Memorial Lecture of the Association for Psychoanalytic Medicine, New York, October 3.

Schafer, R. 1973. Concepts of self and identity and the experience of separation-individuation in adolescence. *Psychoanalytic Quarterly* 42:42–59.

Shapiro, E. 1978. The psychodynamics and developmental psychology of the borderline patient: a review of the literature. *American Journal of Psychiatry* 135:1305–1315.

Spitz, R. A. 1959. *A Genetic Field Theory of Ego Formation*. New York: International Universities Press.

Winnicott, D. W. 1965. The effect of psychotic parents on the emotional development of the child. In *The Family and Individual Development*. New York: Basic.

27 WHY THEY WERE AFRAID OF VIRGINIA WOOLF: PERSPECTIVES ON JUVENILE MANIC-DEPRESSIVE ILLNESS

SHERMAN C. FEINSTEIN

While the normal individual is generally aware that he is subject to variations in mood, he rarely perceives that rhythmic changes also affect his biological and emotional patterns over a long period of time. Natural rhythms are such a basic part of our lives that they are usually not noticed, although daily or circadian rhythms affect all our activities (Feinstein 1973).

At birth and for the first sixteen weeks of life the infant's biological rhythms of sleep and other physiological functions deviate from the twenty-four-hour rhythm of the adults caring for him. The maternal care provides a stimulus barrier for the still vulnerable newborn, and slowly the infant begins to exhibit activity and feeding patterns consonant with those of his family and the world around him.

During early childhood, from seven to eighteen months of age, Mahler (1972) points out that phenomena of mood are of great importance. Most children demonstrate major periods of exhilaration or relative elation alternating with their being "low-keyed" when they become aware that mother is absent from the room. At these times gestural and performance motility are reduced, interest in their surroundings diminishes, and they seem preoccupied, with inwardly concentrated attention. This low-keyed state becomes evident when: (1) comfort from another person may cause the child to burst into tears, and (2) the state disappears with the return of the absent mother. Mahler compares this toned-down state to a miniature anaclitic depression and believes that during this time the child is attempting to hold onto the memory of the mother by "imaging" (Rubenfine 1961). This is an early stage of the subsequently developed object constancy during which the introjected memory of the mother can be easily maintained.

Do people who eventually develop manic-depressive illness actually have a dyssynchronization in this area of development? The early histories of many manic-depressive patients clearly indicate an interference with the capacity to dampen down, a developmental milestone which should be accomplished by two years of age. Is this the result of incompatibility in the mother-child relationship or some genetic-physiological impairment in the switching mechanisms, as described by Bunney, Goodwin, Davis, and Fawcett (1968) and Bunney, Goodwin, and Murphy (1972), in which rapid and reversible changes from mania to depression and vice versa involve neurotransmitter (i.e., biogenic amine) function at the adrenergic nerve endings or some instability of the neuronal membrane?

My hypothesis is that bipolar affective disorder manifesting a manic-depressive pattern may show specific equivalent behavior in childhood which is the precursor of the cyclothymic personality and manic-depressive states of adulthood and that, in increasing incidence, manic-depressive illness can be recognized in childhood and adolescence as well as adulthood. The affective system of patients with manic-depressive illness may have a basic vulnerability which, when overstimulated, begins a discharge pattern that does not easily lend itself to autonomous emotional control. Some biological variation (probably on a genetic basis) leaves the affective system with a specific vulnerability to affective stress. The typical bipolar cyclic states of adulthood, therefore, are considered far advanced illness patterns rather than minimal criteria for diagnosis (Feinstein 1973; Feinstein and Wolpert 1973).

Childhood and Manic-Depression

Arieti (1959) and Cohen, Baker, Cohen, Fromm-Reichman, and Weigert (1954) both described early childhood patterns of manic-depressive adults and saw them as repressed children dominated by strong but changeable parents. Anthony and Scott (1960) questioned whether manic-depressive illness ever occurred in a clinically recognizable form in the younger child but were "prepared to admit . . . that certain 'embryonic' features may make a transient appearance in the very early years." They believed that there was a "manic-depressive tendency" that was latent in the susceptible individual and existed in an internalized form.

This manic-depressive tendency is quite common historically in the child, adolescent, and adult manic-depressives that I have evaluated. An early developmental and behavioral profile usually consists of all or most of the following characteristics:

1. Early evidence of affective instability. As early as one year of age parents recognize a pattern of affective extremes.

2. Difficulty with early stages of separation-individuation. The child may have impaired ability to dampen down or achieve a low-keyed state. Separations usually lead to exaggerated reactions to loss.

3. Dilatation of the ego with persistence of grandiose and idealizing self-structures owing to failure of normal transformation of narcissism. This may manifest itself as an outgoing, dramatic quality with a theatrical flair. Many histories reveal early interest in acting and an easy willingness to perform. One mother reported she could always depend upon her daughter to do a "soft-shoe routine" on meeting new people.

4. Infantile circadian patterns tending to persist with reactions governed by inner, affective impulses rather than shifting to the environmental patterns of the family. Bizarre eating and sleeping patterns may continue in spite of all efforts to enforce normal daily rhythms.

5. There is very frequently a family history of affective disorder. In addition to the presence of bipolar and unipolar patterns, equivalent states such as alcoholism or compulsive gambling may be elicited.

The diagnosis of manic-depressive illness has been considered in children only rarely, but specific results from the use of lithium make it important to determine the childhood nature of the disease. In addition to possible genetic factors, early manifestations of severe psychic illness interfere with emotional growth and development and result in fixations and deviant character formation. The so-called actual neurosis of Freud (1923), a physiological illness with psychological consequences (Wolpert 1975), results in partially developed emotional growth now recognized as borderline personality organization.

Adolescence and Manic-Depressive Illness

The longitudinal, observational approach has confirmed the etiological importance of early infantile development, the oedipal period, and latency to psychic growth. Adolescence as a developmental stage is now considered to have the same degree of significance as an etiological precursor of later development. This developmental work, which has been described by Blos (1967) as a recapitulation of the separation-individuation tasks, makes the adolescent vulnerable not only to normal everyday stress but also to unresolved conflicts from infancy and childhood. Other descriptions of the developmental work during adolescence include a liquefaction of the ego (Eissler 1958) and partial regression of the ego to the stage of undifferentiated object relationships at the service of ego mastery (Freud 1958; Geleerd 1961). This major reworking of the ego defenses at the service of character synthesis renders the pubertal adolescent susceptible to a breakdown of defenses and an emergence of symptoms.

The emergence of symptomatic manic-depressive illness is more common during adolescence than during childhood. Again, the early manifestations of the affect-based illness do not conform to the traditional descriptions, but rather reflect the developmental level and the particular vicissitudes with which an adolescent is dealing. In addition, the amount of bipolar affective instability may be dependent on the genetic configuration and the quality of early character development.

Manic-depressive illness may emerge during puberty and adolescence, manifesting some of the following symptoms of intense adolescent turmoil:

1. Severe adolescent rebellion manifested by exaggerated self-esteem, overconfidence, and an insistence on well-being.

2. Grandiose conceptions of physical, mental, and moral powers with overcommitment to adolescent tasks.

3. Exaggeration of motor activity manifested by restlessness, hyperactivity, and in some examples by the compulsive hyperactivity of anorexia nervosa. Several patients with anorexia nervosa were later discovered to have manic-depressive illness, and this should be thought of and ruled out in every case of anorexia.

4. Exaggeration of libidinal impulses may surface as a sudden change from an inhibited child to an aggressive, sexually acting-out adolescent. Puberty, particularly in girls, may be seen as a great threat to the body image. In one case a period of amenorrhea after menarche eventuated into a manic-depressive breakdown with delusions of being pregnant.

5. Gradual emergence of a cyclic, bipolar pattern of affect disorder but often manifesting itself as marked instability, with short periods of depression and mania rather than the longer periods typical of adult manic-depression.

Diagnostic Aspects of Manic-Depressive Illness

The criteria usually utilized for the diagnosis of manic-depressive illness are still deeply influenced by the earlier descriptive studies of Kraeplin (1921).

335

This tends to obscure the developmental process which is interfered with by the presence of affective instability. The diagnostic requirement that there should be a distinct and marked phasic disturbance of affect (Redlich and Freedman 1966) and evidence of a state approximating the classical clinical description (Anthony and Scott 1960) frequently delays the diagnosis for many years.

Schizophrenia in adolescents is frequently a difficult diagnosis to make and, as Masterson (1967) points out, only in 25 percent of seriously disturbed adolescents can the diagnosis be made at the onset; the long-term picture of the disease process emerges slowly during the diagnostic and therapeutic process. Stone (1971) discusses the difficulties of making a definite diagnosis of manic-depressive illness and the present tendency to call a patient "schizophrenic till proven otherwise." The diagnosis of manic-depressive illness in adolescents is a particularly difficult diagnosis to make, but keeping in mind adolescent behavioral equivalents of the classical end results of a bipolar affective disorder will facilitate the diagnostic process.

Psychiatric Case Study of Virginia Woolf [1]

Virginia Woolf was born on January 25, 1882, in London, the third of four children of her father's second marriage. She came from an unusual family, the Stephens, where "there was scarcely a one who did not publish and never a generation which did not add something to the literary achievements of the family." She was described as an "unusual child" who did not talk "properly" until she was three years old. When she began to talk, words became her chosen weapons, although she was not above using her nails against her siblings (Bell 1972).

From the first she was felt to be erratic, eccentric, and accident-prone. She could say things and experience misadventures which earned her the nickname of "the goat," a name which stuck to her for many years. But it was not by words alone that Virginia could vent her displeasure. She was able to create an atmosphere of "thunderous and oppressive gloom," a winter of discontent. Her siblings were made to feel that she had raised a cloud above them, and frequently she turned "purple with rage." At other times she appeared to be dilated and excited, manifesting behavior that amused the grown-ups and made them laugh.

Virginia was enormously sensitive to criticism, and her excitement could become unbearable. She was also susceptible to depressions, and following

336

an attack of pertussis at age six, she recovered slowly, lost a great deal of weight, and seemed to become a different kind of person, more thoughtful and more speculative.

Her biographer notes that she was exposed early to "madness, death, and disaster." At age thirteen she was approached by her half-brother, who exposed himself. This made a deep impression and was described in a later novel, *The Years* (1937). Her half-sister Laura was described as "mad" and eventually was placed in an asylum. Her first cousin began manifesting symptoms of "madness" following a mild head injury. "He was in a state of high euphoria and painted away like a man possessed."

Although her parents were felt to have an unusually good marriage, her mother was required to devote an enormous amount of energy to being supportive of her temperamental and insecure father. An editor, who wrote the *Dictionary of National Biography*, Leslie Stephen described himself as a "skinless man" who required his wife's continuing protection and indulgence during his episodes of insomnia and anxiety. Her mother Julia, a beautiful woman, became increasingly worn and harassed. She was obsessed by time, was always in a hurry, and was ever anxious that others be spared. Following an attack of influenza, she reportedly developed rheumatic fever and died when Virginia was thirteen years of age.

"Her death," said Virginia, "was the greatest disaster that could happen." While her father went into a period of deep mourning, Virginia reacted intensely to the loss. She developed severe anxiety, became painfully excitable, and eventually intolerably depressed. She became terrified of people, blushed deeply if spoken to, and was unable to face a stranger in the street. Eventually she began to experience hallucinations and spoke of "those horrible voices." She went through a period of morbid self-criticism during which she accused herself of being vain and egotistical. She condemned herself as inferior to her sister, Vanessa, and was intensely irritable. This episode lasted about a year.

After the death of her mother and following recovery from the depression, Virginia's literary interests began to manifest themselves. At the age of fifteen, however, she again experienced a period of "irritability and nervousness" and was terrified of the simplest journey through the streets. This occurred at the time of the illness of her half-sister, Stella, who died that same year.

Another, more serious episode began with the death of her father when she was twenty-two. Virginia denied his chronic depressions, hypochondriasis, and extreme dependency and became convinced that he had wanted to live and that the "true and happy relationship between him and his children

337

was only just beginning.'' She felt guilty and dreamed nightly that he was alive again and she could say all the things she had meant to say.

While this produced at first a sadness and grief reaction, she again began to mainfest a feeling of "profound irritation.'' She became irritated by the letters of condolence, by the obituaries, by her relatives, and by herself. Her grief became "feverish," something which made her feel isolated and afraid. She began to have headaches, cardiac palpitations, and an awareness that something was wrong with her mind. Her activities attained frenetic intensity. She began to mistrust her sister and her grief became maniacal. She heard voices telling her to commit bizarre acts. She believed that this might be due to overeating and began to starve herself, developing what seems to have been an atypical anorexia nervosa.

This led to her first suicide attempt, in which she jumped out of a window. However, the window was near the ground and little harm was done. She spent the rest of the summer hallucinating "birds singing in Greek and imagining that King Edward VII lurked in the azaleas using the foulest possible language.'' This episode lasted about six months following which she was able to write, "You can't think what an exquisite joy every minute of life is to me now. . . . I . . . emerge less selfish and cocksure . . . and with greater understanding of the troubles of others" (Bell 1972). Her physician, Dr. Savage, pronounced her completely cured and able to return to Bloomsbury.

Virginia's behavior could best be described as volatile. She might be in "one of her fantastic moods" one day and explode the next. She was at war with herself, "a state of delight and of rage" which went on for months and years. Her imagination was described as being "furnished with an accelerator and no brakes; it flew rapidly ahead, parting company with reality, and, when reality happened to be a human being, the result could be appalling. . . .''

Physically she complained of acute nervous tensions, headaches (numbness in the head), insomnia, and a strong impulse to reject food. While she was unable to stop her excessive concern with these symptoms, she was at the same time self-confident, elated, and excited about the future and looked forward to fame and marriage.

At the age of thirty-three, Virginia began to have cycles of manic behavior (manifested by garrulousness and eventually gibberish leading to coma) and alternating periods of depression (usually languid, sometimes violent, more often quietly suicidal). Usually it was hard to believe that there was anything wrong, but exposure to ordinary pressures might precipitate headaches and sleepness nights which would be cured only by long periods of rest and seclusion. The shifts of mood were "unusually abrupt and the impression unusually deep and lasting."

In spite of the remarkable limitations imposed by her illness, Virginia's moments of depression were followed by moments of creativity. She usually found it impossible to follow the prescribed rest treatment and continuously wrote books, a great deal of journalism, letters, and kept an extensive diary. By 1936, her literary abilities began to pay the toll for her frequent periods of psychosis. She began to have obsessive fears of impoverishment and remarkable ambivalence about her writing, interspersed with euphoric intervals.

On March 28, 1941, she wrote, "I feel certain I am going mad again. I feel we can't go through another of those terrible times." She made her way to the river, forced a stone into the pocket of her coat, and went to her death.

Discussion

The psychiatric history of Virginia Woolf is of interest because of the vast amount of biographical material available in her novels, letters, and diaries along with an unusual biography written by a famous relative, Quentin Bell (1972). We are presented with a classical case of manic-depressive illness which fulfills every criterion and, because no definitive treatment was available at the time, was allowed to run its course to an eventual suicide at the age of fifty-nine.

In a clinical sense one can view Woolf's life from a developmental point of view and see the manifestations of manic-depressive illness in childhood, during puberty and adolescence, at the onset of adulthood, and in its subsequent classical, cyclic, bipolar end state. This end state, until recently, was considered the disease process itself. In current terms, with the availability of diagnostic and therapeutic modalities, the achievement of the classical state might be considered a neglect syndrome in the sense that one rarely sees hybephrenia or catatonia since phenothiazine therapy has been introduced into the treatment of schizophrenia.

Virginia was an unplanned child, but seemed to have been well accepted in a family that was considered to be in the lower division of the upper middle class. Raised in a home with seven servants for four small children, she formed intense attachments to her two older siblings and they remained, as long as they lived, passionately fond of each other. In spite of this history of good object relationships, she is described as having had a profound effect on the family from the onset. Her biographer raised the question as to whether these attacks indicated "any seed of madness" or "were the symptom of some psychic malady" (Bell 1972). At the age of six, after an attack of pertussis, she appears to have experienced a depression.

At that point in Woolf's childhood it would be rather difficult to make a definitive diagnosis of manic-depressive illness. One can at best conclude that marked affective instability exists which is beyond developmental expectations of immaturity of mood controls. Klein (1934) contended that "the child in his early development goes through a transitory manic-depressive state," which she considered a defense against early infantile depression and was inferred when a feeling of omnipotence and control over objects became evident. By the age of two, however, this natural affective overreaction should have disappeared with the introjection of early ego derivatives from successful working through of the separation-individuation process. The persistence of an early state of mood extremes must be considered an indication of a tendency toward manic-depressive illness. A family history of manic-depressive illness and the persistence of alternating affective states, particularly of dilated, hypomanic behavior, could be considered presumptive for development of an affective disorder.

Davis (1979) described what he calls a specific manic-depressive variant syndrome of childhood which requires the presence of: major disruptive affective storms; a family history of significant affective dysfunction; mental, physical, or verbal hyperactivity and upheaval (but less than the prolonged grandiosity of adults); seriously troubled interpersonal relationships; and the absence of psychotic thought disorder in children who respond well to lithium carbonate.

Virginia's first clear psychotic breakdown occurred at the age of thirteen following the death of her mother. Mother's death, however, was unexpected, and Virginia reacted by becoming alternately agitated and depressed. Virginia was now subject to severe anxieties, excitability, and hyperactivity. She became phobic and withdrawn, and later wrote of experiencing hallucinations. Virginia was also approached sexually by her half-brother, following the death of their mother. She wrote that he had "spoiled her life before it had begun"—sexuality became associated with frozen and defensive panic.

In her subsequent writings she focused on the physical aspects of this period of upset, but she realized that "she had been mad and might be mad again." This adolescent episode lasted a year, during which time she stopped schooling and was prescribed a simple life and outdoor exercise. She lost the desire to write, read feverishly, and went through a period of "morbid self-criticism," blaming herself for being vain and egotistical. She was described as being intensely irritable. She slowly recovered but remained nervous, irritable, and severely phobic.

The frequency of breakdown in manic-depressive illness increases with the development of puberty and the onset of adolescence. Again, the reaction is age appropriate and emphasizes those defenses which are critical at a particular stage of life.

The question of the timing of the breakdown is of great interest. The loss of a mother and the transition from childhood to adolescence are both considered major demands on the gradually emerging adolescent ego. Mourning and the progression through transitional developmental states require the capacity to utilize ego defenses in the mastery of the loss of loved objects (mother, childhood). A fundamental defect in the affect system, probably genetically determined, overwhelms the ego defenses and the resultant affective reactions may be characterized as manic-depressive, essentially indicating exaggerated or blocked capacities to deal with the normal affective response to the perception of a loss. If the intensity of the affective stimulation is too great, or the environmental supports are sadomasochistic rather than accepting and supportive, an alteration of consciousness may result, manifested by psychotic thinking or behavior.

Anthony and Scott (1960) explain that a genetic clock is operative in an individual who is genetically predisposed or environmentally handicapped. Compensatory fantasies preserve an inner omnipotence but are threatened by a real situation. This may result in extraversion of these inner fantasies in an attempt to deny reality. I differ from them in that they believed that juvenile bipolar affective disorder was a very rare occurrence, whereas I speculate that manic-depressive illness, a physiological illness with psychological consequences, is more common than was previously thought.

Conclusions

The diagnosis of juvenile manic-depressive illness in Virginia Woolf might still be a difficult one today. However, the history of affective instability in childhood along with a severe affective reaction characterized by profound regression during adolescence should be considered in any diagnostic evaluation as an early manifestation of a bipolar affective disorder.

1. This case report was abstracted from Quentin Bell's study, *Virginia Woolf: A Biography,* with the collaboration of Janet Hoffman, M.S.W.

REFERENCES

Anthony, E. J., and Scott, P. 1960. Manic-depressive psychosis in childhood. *Journal of Child Psychology and Psychiatry* 1:53–72.

Arieti, S. 1959. Manic-depressive psychosis. In S. Arieti, ed. *American Handbook of Psychiatry.* New York: Basic.

Bell, Q. 1972. *Virginia Woolf: A Biography.* New York: Harcourt Brace Jovanovich.

Blos, P. 1967. The second individuation process of adolescence. *Psychoanalytic Study of the Child* 22:162–186.

Bunney, W. E., Jr.; Goodwin, F. K.; Davis, J. M.; and Fawcett, J. A. 1968. A behavioral-biochemical study of lithium treatment. *American Journal of Psychiatry* 125(4): 499–512.

Bunney, W. E., Jr.; Goodwin, F. K.; and Murphy, D. L. 1972. The "switch process" in manic-depressive illness. III. Theoretical implications. *Archives of General Psychiatry* 27(3): 312–317.

Cohen, M. D.; Baker, G.; Cohen, R. A.; Fromm-Reichmann, F.; and Weigert, E. V. 1954. An intensive study of twelve cases of manic-depressive psychosis. *Psychiatry* 17:103–137.

Davis, R. E. 1979. Manic-depressive variant syndrome of childhood. *American Journal of Psychiatry* 136(5): 702–705.

Eissler, K. R. 1958. Notes on problems of technique in the psychoanalytic treatment of adolescents. *Psychoanalytic Study of the Child* 13:233–254.

Feinstein, S. C. 1973. Diagnostic and therapeutic aspects of manic-depressive illness in early childhood. *Early Child Development and Care* 3:1–12.

Feinstein, S., and Wolpert, E. 1973. Juvenile manic-depressive illness: clinical and therapeutic considerations. *Journal of the American Academy of Child Psychiatry* 12:123–136.

Freud, A. 1958. Adolescence. *Psychoanalytic Study of the Child* 13:255–278.

Freud, S. 1923. The ego and the id. *Standard Edition* 19:13–66. London: Hogarth, 1961.

Geleerd, E. R. 1961. Some aspects of ego vicissitudes in adolescence. *Journal of the American Psychoanalytic Association* 9:394–405.

Klein, M. 1934. The psychogenesis of manic-depressive states. *Contributions to Psycho-Analysis*. London: Hogarth.

Kraeplin, E. 1921. *Manic-Depressive Insanity and Paranoia*. Edinburgh: Livingston.

Mahler, M. 1972. On the first three subphases of the separation-individuation process. *International Journal of Psycho-Analysis* 53:333–338.

Masterson, J. F. 1967. The *Psychiatric Dilemma of Adolescence*. Boston: Little, Brown.

Perris, C. 1969. The separation of bipolar (manic-depressive) from unipolar recurrent depressive psychosis. *Behavioral Neuropsychiatry* 1(8): 17–24.

Redlich, F., and Freedman, D. 1966. *The Theory and Practice of Psychiatry*. New York: Basic.

Rubenfine, D. L. 1961. Perception, reality testing, and symbolism. *Psychoanalytic Study of the Child* 16:73–89.

Stone, M. H. 1971. Mania: a guide for the perplexed. *Psychotherapy and Social Science Revue* 5(10): 14–18.

Wolpert, E. 1975. Manic-depressive illness as an actual neurosis. In E. J. Anthony and T. Benedek, eds. *Depression and Human Existence*. Boston: Little, Brown.

CLARICE J. KESTENBAUM

Recent advances in the study of individuals at risk for affective disorder point to the finding that serious forms of depression in childhood and adolescence not only exist but are commonly encountered. Several systems for classifying depressive disorders of childhood have been proposed. Cytryn and McKnew (1972) describe two types of depression: (*a*) *pure depression* with predominant features of sad affect, social withdrawal, psychomotor retardation, anxiety, school failure, sleep disturbance, feelings of hopelessness, helplessness, and suicidal preoccupation; (*b*) *masked depression,* characterized by hyperactivity, aggressive behavior, hypochondriasis, psychosomatic complaints, and delinquency. Weinberg, Rutman, Sullivan, Penick, and Dietz (1975) found that childhood depression was a common condition in children doing poorly in school; his ten diagnostic criteria included, along with many noted by Cytryn and McKnew, self-deprecatory ideation and a change in attitude toward school.

Other investigators (Petti 1978; Poznansky, Krahenbuhl, and Zrull 1976) have described depressed children with similar symptoms. All of the investigators noted that while depressive symptoms were common, mania in childhood was extremely rare. In fact, it has long been believed that manic-depressive illness similar to the adult disorder did not occur in childhood. Recent genetic studies, however, have demonstrated that a first episode of bipolar illness in adolescence is not uncommon. Winokur, Clayton, and Reich (1969) in a study of sixty-one bipolar probands noted that one-third had a first episode occurring between ten and nineteen years of age; Perris (1966) reported that 40 percent of his cases first became ill between fifteen and twenty-four years of age.

Loranger and Levine (1978) confirmed these findings in a study of 200 rigorously diagnosed bipolar in-patients and determined that one third were hospitalized before their twenty-fifth birthday while one fifth had been symptomatic since adolescence. Despite these findings, a psychotic episode in an adolescent is often given a schizophrenic label; frequently it is not until a second or third hospitalization that an affective illness is recognized as the primary disturbance. Carlson and Strober (1978) described six cases of adolescents initially diagnosed as schizophrenic who were, at a later admission, rediagnosed manic-depressive. They wondered whether developmental issues masked the affective disorder. The patients exhibited the symptoms of thought disorder (blocking and flight of ideas), mania, euphoria, verbosity, expansiveness, hypersexuality, irritability, aggressiveness, sleep loss, and hyperactivity in the manic phase; in the depressive phase, lowered mood, psychomotor retardation, social withdrawal, loss of concentration, and guilt feelings were predominant. The authors called into question the disproportionate prevalence of schizophrenic diagnoses in young psychotic patients, along with "adjustment reaction" for less disturbed adolescents. They suggested that "stereotyped notions of diagnostic practice may, in some instances, lead clinicians to be unduly hesitant in inferring the presence of manic-depressive illness from an adolescent's expressions of behavioral maladjustment. Stone (1971) also discussed the present tendency to label young patients schizophrenic "until proven otherwise."

The subject of a juvenile form of manic-depressive illness was discussed by Harms (1952), who questioned how similar or dissimilar symptoms occurring in childhood or adult life had to be in order to warrant giving individuals in both age groups the same diagnosis.

In a landmark review of manic-depressive psychosis in childhood, Anthony and Scott (1960) suggested ten criteria to be considered in arriving at a diagnosis. (1) Evidence of an abnormal psychiatric state at some time of the illness approximating the classical clinical description as given by Kraepelin, Bleuler, Meyer, and others. (2) Evidence of a positive family history suggesting a manic-depressive diathesis. (3) Evidence of an early tendency to a manic-depressive type of reaction as manifested in (a) a cyclothymic tendency with gradually increasing amplitude and length of the oscillations and (b) delirious manic or depressive outbursts occurring during pyrexial illness. (4) Evidence of a recurrent or periodic illness. This entails the observation of at least two episodes, separated by a period of time (gauged in months or years), and regarded as clinically similar. There should be diagnostic agreement by different clinical judges on the nature of any one episode and diagnostic agreement by different clinical judges on the identity of different episodes. (5) Evidence of a diphasic illness showing swings of pathological dimension from states of elation to states of depression and vice versa. (6)

Evidence of endogenous illness indicating that the phases of the illness alternate with minimal reference to environmental events. (7) Evidence of a severe illness as indicated by a need for in-patient treatment, heavy sedation, and electro-convulsive therapy. (8) Evidence of an abnormal underlying personality of an extroverted type, as demonstrated by objective test procedures. (9) An absence of features that might indicate other abnormal conditions such as schizophrenia, organic states (alcoholic delirium, G.P.I., hysteria, etc.). (10) The evidence of current, not retrospective, assessments.

In a review of the literature from 1896 to 1960, twenty-eight reports of "juvenile" (age twelve and under) manic-depressive cases were found; only three cases (all were eleven years of age) fulfilled at least five of their ten criteria for a manic-depressive psychosis. Anthony and Scott concluded that manic-depressive illness in childhood is extremely rare; that the early variety may be due to heavy genetic loading and intense environmental experience (as in the one case presented by the authors themselves). They stated that the tendency is "latent in the susceptible individual; that it occurs in an internalized psychodynamic form in early life; that it may be transiently manifested during childhood under strong physical or psychological pressure, and that, eventually, at a certain moment in history, for reasons that are sometimes apparent, it undergoes extraversion and becomes clinically recognized as a psychosis" (p. 68).

Youngerman and Canino (1978) in a review of 190 cases of lithium carbonate use in children and adolescents found twenty reports of rather typical cases of manic-depressive illness (two in childhood and eighteen in adolescence) successfully treated with lithium carbonate. "These cases can be broadly characterized as mood disturbances with and without periodic swings, frequently with family histories of bipolar illness" (p. 221). A wide spectrum of other symptoms was reported, including anorexia, enuresis, epilepsy, auditory hallucinations, cyclic increments, and decrements in academic performance. In retrospect, they state, ". . . many adolescent manic-depressives have histories of behavior and mood disorders often dating back to early childhood. Affective symptoms are mixed and masked in childhood, and it is hard to elicit reports of sustained mood swings" (p. 223).

Single, periodic cases of manic-depressive illness in children have appeared in the recent literature. Feinstein and Wolpert (1973) presented a case of a girl first seen at three with a periodic alternating affective disorder; the subsequent affective attacks seemed to have been precipitated by an overwhelming reaction to loss. They speculated that adult manic-depressive patients may show specific and equivalent behavior in childhood "which is the precursor of the cyclothymic personality and depressive states of the adult, and in some cases, manifest a juvenile version of the illness" (p. 124).

346

Annell (1969) described twelve children with various symptom complexes including a family history of positive bipolar illness, sleep disorder, and night terrors.

Berg, Hullin, Allsopp, O'Brien, and MacDonald (1974) reported a case of manic-depressive psychosis in early adolescence. A fourteen-year-old girl who presented symptoms of school refusal, suicidal preoccupation, and a twenty-pound weight loss was initially diagnosed as having anorexia nervosa. Given a trial of amitriptyline she became elated. Her father had experienced severe depressions as well as manic episodes. The daughter responded to lithium carbonate during her second hospitalization when the diagnosis was changed to manic-depressive psychosis. She required three times the usual dose (as did her father).

McKnew, Cytryn, and White (1974) described a hypomanic eight-year-old who exhibited excessive familiarity, jocularity, grandiosity, rage attacks, and socially inappropriate behavior.

Davis (1979) has proposed that there is an identifiable syndrome which he calls *manic-depressive variant syndrome* of childhood (MDV) characterized by the following features: a family history of affective dysfunction, hyper-activity, affective storms (disruptive temper outbursts), and impairment in personal relationships. Secondary symptoms may include sleep disturbance, short attention span, enuresis, and some evidence of neuropathology.

The underlying question linking all the clinical studies thus far presented is, what are the indications that a child with behavior disorder, hyperactivity, or mood disturbances may be at risk for future manic-depressive illness, may be exhibiting a manic-depressive variant, or that the symptoms are evidence of manic-depressive illness already in full force? Furthermore, which individuals are vulnerable to manic-depressive disorder and which premorbid characteristics indicate vulnerability to a subsequent episode? Since recent advances in the study of affective disorders point to a hereditary factor, the final question under discussion is, What role does the genetic component play? Is the "hereditary taint" (as Kraepelin [1921] called it) in and of itself sufficient for a manic-depressive breakdown to occur in later life, or is a particular kind of environmental stress necessary to precipitate the illness?

Genetic Hypothesis for Affective Disorders

Kraepelin in 1896 classified manic-depressive psychosis as a unitary form of mental illness distinct from schizophrenia. He noted (1921) that the strength of the hereditary factor was 75 percent, that 70 percent of his cases were women, and that 25 percent of his male manic-depressive patients were alcoholic. Pooled data from studies done in the 1920s and 1930s (Slater 1953) suggested that bipolar manic-depressive psychosis occurred in 0.5 percent of the population contrasted with the 0.85 percent worldwide incidence of schizophrenia.

There is little doubt that there is a high rate of lifetime prevalence of affective disorders in the first- and second-degree relatives of patients with primary affective disorders as compared with the general population (6–24 percent vs. 1–2 percent according to Rosenthal [1970]).

Rosenthal also summarized data on manic-depressive psychosis in the first-degree relatives of manic-depressive index cases from eleven studies from the years 1921 to 1953. He found the median morbidity risk were (*a*) parents— 7.8 percent; (*b*) siblings—8.8 percent; (*c*) children—11.2 percent.

A genetic hypothesis in manic-depressive illness has been given further support by evidence from twin studies. Six major twin studies have been reviewed by Zerbin-Rudin (1972). She found that the overall concordance rates for monozygotic twins were consistently higher than for dizygotic twins (74 percent vs. 19 percent).

Bertelson, Harvald, and Hauge (1977) in a recent Danish twin study of manic-depressive disorder obtained similar results. From a total population of 11,000 same-sexed twin pairs born in 1870–1920, sixty-nine monozygotic probands with manic-depressive illness were studied; forty-six twins were found to have manic-depressive disorder as well. Using strict diagnostic criteria they determined that the concordance rate was 67 percent while the corresponding dizygotic twin concordance was 20 percent (the difference is significant at $P<.001$).

The twin studies have given support to the proponents of a genetic hypothesis for the transmission of primary affective disorder. Environmental factors, however, seem to play an important role in protecting some predisposed individuals from becoming ill; if this were not the case concordance rates for monozygotic twins would be still higher. The relative contributions of heredity and environment are difficult to identify, however, when twins are reared together. A few case reports of monozygotic twins separated early in life and reared apart have been reported.

The most carefully documented report is the study of Rosanoff, Handy, and Plesset (1935) of monozygotic twin brothers who were separated at age two months. Both had manic psychotic episodes at age twenty-one and repeated hospitalizations throughout their lives. The case has been reexamined by Farber (1980) and adds much weight to the genetic hypothesis.

Several studies of the adopted-away offspring of manic-depressive parents who were reared by normal parents have been reported, which adds further evidence that a genetic factor exists. Cadoret (1978) found that the incidence of depression was significantly higher in the affect-disordered parent adoptees than in adoptees whose biological parents had other psychiatric conditions or were apparently psychiatrically well.

The findings of Mendlewicz and Rainer (1977) in a Belgian adoption study point to a similar conclusion. Adoptive and biological parents of manic-depressive adoptees were compared with (a) the parents of manic-depressives who were not adoptees, (b) the adoptive and biological parents of normal adoptees, (c) the parents of individuals who had contracted poliomyelitis during childhood. The results indicated that psychopathology in the biological parents was in excess of that found in the adoptive parents of the same manic-depressive offspring. Thirty-one percent of the biological parents of bipolar adoptees had affective spectrum illness (i.e., bipolar, unipolar, schizoaffective, cyclothymic) compared with 2 percent of the biological parents of normal adoptees.

Family studies have led some investigators to conclude that unipolar and bipolar illnesses are genetically different entities (Angst and Perris 1968; Leonhard, Korff, and Schulz 1962). Many researchers had confirmed Kraepelin's view that there was a female preponderance in manic-depressive psychosis. Rosanoff et al. (1935) believed that the mode of transmission involved two "factors"—one was autosomal, predisposing to cyclothymia; the other, an "activating" factor presumably on the X chromosome. When Angst and Perris differentiated their affective subgroups into bipolar and unipolar types, the overall female 2:1 ratio was fractionable into a 2:1 excess of females with unipolar depression, whereas in the smaller bipolar group an evenly divided sex ratio of 1:1 was noted. Cadoret and Winokur (1975) and Mendlewicz, Rainer, and Fleiss (1975) have postulated an X-linked gene as fundamental to bipolar illness, which is, they believe, genetically distinct from unipolar illness. An association with red-green color blindness and X_g^a blood-type antigen was found as well.

Genetic heterogeneity has been postulated by Price (1972). Gershon, Baron, and Leckman (1975) described a multiple-threshold model. A variable liability to a disorder is postulated, to which genetic and independent factors may contribute. If the net liability crosses a threshold, the disorder becomes manifest. Gershon et al. believe that unipolar and bipolar illnesses represent positions on a continuum of liability. Greater liability tends to manifest itself as a bipolar, lesser liability as a unipolar, disorder. He believes, furthermore

(Gershon, Dunner, and Goodwin 1971), that the individual with manic-depressive illness had "an inherited vulnerability to loss, with increased likelihood of development of pathological loss reactions."

Winokur (1979) has noted both the genetic and clinical differences between bipolar and unipolar illness. Bipolar probands had a higher suicide rate, peptic ulcer, earlier age of onset; and bipolar females had heightened vulnerability to postpartum psychosis. Unipolar disorders tend to begin later (forty-three vs. thirty-one years), are more frequently female, are less severe, and rarely have a family history of mania. There are significant neurophysical and biochemical differences reported as well—subdivisions other than mania and depression have been suggested. Those individuals who have been hospitalized for depression only but experience hypomanic episodes have been designated "Bipolar II" by Dunner, Fleiss, and Fieve (1976). Winokur (1979) and Winokur, Cadoret, Baker, and Dorzab (1975) have suggested depressive disorder be divided into autonomous subtypes based on family history: (*a*) depressive spectrum disease in an individual with a first-degree family history of alcoholism or antisocial personality; and (*b*) pure depressive illness in an individual without similarly affected relatives.

The At-Risk Child: Possible Predictors

It appears evident that genetic factors play a role in the etiology of major affective disorders; how large a role is still in question.

Gershon et al. (1971) state, "The relative contribution of genetic and nongenetic factors in accounting for the probability of an individual's developing affective illness during his lifetime may be referred to as the heritability of affective illness." It seems probable that some children of manic-depressive parents will develop an affective illness. Several recent studies of the children of affectively ill parents have appeared in the literature. Welner, Welner, McGrary, and Leonard (1977) reported that 25 percent of twenty parents hospitalized for depression had children who exhibited episodes of depression. McKnew, Cytryn, Efron, Gershon, and Bunney (1979) studied the children of fourteen parents with an affective disorder. There was a high incidence of depressive symptoms in the offspring of adults with depression. What is not at all evident is which particular individuals might be identified early as being vulnerable to subsequent affective illness.

The number of at-risk studies although small, is increasing (Dyson and Barcai 1970). There are relatively few studies, however, of the children of bipolar manic-depressive parents. Clinical descriptions from actual examination rather than from parents' reports together with psychological test scores are sparse. Kestenbaum (1979) has described thirteen children with a family history of bipolar manic-depressive disorder. Six of the children exhibited the following features: (1) family history positive for bipolar illness; (2) specific clinical symptomatology including temper tantrums, compulsive rituals, dysphoria, lability, obsessional preoccupation, learning disability, hyperactivity, impulsivity; (3) specific patterns in psychological test scores (WISC) revealing verbal achievement significantly greater than performance, with considerable subtest scatter.

Of the remaining seven, three had psychological test scores that did not follow the pattern described above; four were not given psychological tests. The presenting symptoms of these seven children were depressed mood ($N = 5$) and behavior problems ($N = 2$). The presenting symptoms of the six children exhibiting the triad of features of the triad mentioned above were learning problems with depressed mood ($N = 5$) and hyperactivity with behavior problems ($N = 1$).

Weintraub has corroborated the psychological test findings.[1] In his study of the offspring of schizophrenic and manic-depressive probands he found that the offspring of the bipolar parents had the highest mean verbal IQ and constituted the only group in which verbal IQ was greater than the performance (see table 1).

TABLE 1

	N	Verbal IQ	Performance IQ
Offspring of schizophrenics	56	85.2	98.35
Unipolars	87	89.95	90.95
Bipolars	76	105.35	99.95
Controls	134	101.7	103.25

The following three vignettes are illustrative. All patients are from Hollingshed-Redlich Socioeconomic classes I or II and were treated for at least two years with psychodynamically oriented psychotherapy, with follow up of three to ten years.

CLINICAL VIGNETTE 1

Robert M, an eighteen-year-old undergraduate, was referred for emergency psychiatric treatment by the admitting psychiatrist of a university hospital.

He had appeared in the emergency room the previous evening, agitated and tearful. "I can't function in school and I don't want to live anymore," he announced. His girl friend of six months had left him two weeks before. Robert had lost his appetite, was unable to sleep, and found it impossible to be alone. He was referred to me for long-term psychotherapy on a twice-weekly basis.

Robert's father, a fifty-year-old accountant, was described as hard working and even tempered. There was no family history of mental illness. Robert's mother, however, was a "nervous, highly emotional" woman whose brother had been hospitalized twice for bipolar manic-depressive illness. One sibling, Robert's sixteen-year-old sister, was reportedly "somewhat moody."

Robert described his childhood as troubled. He recalled having multiple fears, frequent temper tantrums when he did not get his way, and numerous fights with his sister and schoolmates. In his own words, "I was hyperactive, unable to catch a ball or tie my shoelaces. My spelling and handwriting were atrocious because I was switched from left to right hand in first grade." Although Robert was very bright, in the seventh grade he was changed from public to private school where, his parents felt, he could receive more personal attention. He was graduated from high school with honors and was accepted at several highly regarded colleges. Robert's first attempt to live away from home was marred by a recurrence of fears (of the dark, of being alone) which abated only in the presence of his girl friend. The symptoms reappeared when she ended the relationship. Obsessional thoughts of suicide also occurred at the time of the breakup.

Psychological tests revealed a twenty-seven-point discrepancy in the WISC. The verbal IQ was 124 while the performance IQ was only ninety-seven with a wide intratest scatter. The very superior vocabulary contrasted with low scores on alternating timed tests (digit symbol and block design). His object assembly was in the defective range. The psychologist noted the poor eye-hand coordination and pointed out that Robert exhibited a definite laterality problem. He had difficulty with planning and organization as well. Projective tests revealed inordinately low self-esteem and phobic preoccupation.

Psychotherapy was begun on a twice-weekly basis. This led to prompt relief of symptoms. Robert made a sticky attachment to me and used the sessions as a stabilizing force in his life. He spent many hours describing his mood swings and perceptions about himself. One day he could feel as "lowly as a worm" or as a "worthless child," while the next day he felt himself to be a super figure, whom no one understood. His secret world was polarized into feelings either of adoration for a few admired friends or teachers or of loathing and contempt for those who stood in his way. He recalled as a young adolescent lying awake at night, thoughts racing, wondering whether to be like Caesar or Christ. He also described numerous compulsive daily rituals which interfered with his work.

Six months after treatment was instituted Robert was better able to concentrate on his studies, was less phobic (although he had to sleep with a night light and occasionally called me in a panic), and made friends. Treatment continued two and a half years. Following graduation with honors, Robert was accepted in graduate school in another city and plans were made to terminate with me. His depression, however, became more pronounced and was accompanied by a resurgence of suicidal thoughts. He became so agitated following his moving to the new campus that he had to be hospitalized briefly. Antidepressant medication was prescribed at this time.

I saw Robert on occasion during the next ten years and followed his course. He did brilliant work in graduate school and became a college teacher soon after completing his thesis. He still had difficulty with separation and deep insecurities in his social life. Nonetheless he met and married another graduate student and for the first time felt his life was happy. When Robert was twenty-four his uncle, who had been hospitalized for a second manic episode, committed suicide while on a weekend pass from a hospital. Robert's mother, then fifty-three, had a first episode of mania following her brother's death. She went on a "shopping binge" and spent $50,000 on clothes in one day. Robert's new therapist wrote me that he considered Robert to be a manic-depressive (bipolar-type II) at this point, but felt the antidepressant medication was sufficient to keep him symptom free.

Robert, at age thirty, discussed with me, at length, his own understanding of his manic-depressive tendency. He felt as if something within himself caused him to react more intensely to life experiences than did other people. A slight criticism from a colleague could set him into deep despair, while an evocative scene from a novel or film could cause him to weep unabashedly before strangers. At other times he became wildly enthusiastic about a planned trip or business venture and could not sleep for days. "My palate has more colors," he ventured. "When the mood takes over, however, and I think the feelings are getting out of control, I know it's time to call the doctor and go back on the medication." The years of therapy, he added, taught him how to recognize the difference between feelings which could add depth to his life experience and those which could interfere with his functioning and hamper his intellectual and emotional growth. His treatment also taught him how to live with his particular temperament and when to call for help.

CLINICAL VIGNETTE 2

Marcy W was a thirteen-year-old girl who reluctantly agreed to have a psychiatric evaluation when she was threatened with suspension from school for truancy and smoking marijuana. "She was a beautiful, precocious child, somewhat of a tomboy," her mother informed me, "until last summer when she went to summer camp a little girl and came home a woman." Violently antagonistic to her mother, adoring of her father, Marcy was considered wild by her teachers and counselors. She was popular with girls and had several close friends. Her father told me "she attracts boys like flies, but they soon drop her because of her constant irritating telephone calls and protestations of love." She seemed bright and had done well academically until the seventh grade, when her school performance became extremely inconsistent.

Family background was significant in that there was a strong family history of mental illness on both sides. Marcy's maternal grandfather had been chronically depressed and was hospitalized once. Mrs. W, an explosive, volatile woman, had been treated for depression with psychotherapy and antidepressant medication for many years. One of her brothers had been hospitalized on numerous occasions for alcoholism, antisocial behavior, and suicide attempts. Mr. W had a sister who committed suicide at the age of twenty-five following hospitalization for "mental breakdown." Her diagnosis remains uncertain. Marcy's sixteen-year-old brother had been a hyperactive child treated with amphetamines from age six to twelve. His lack of judgment resulted in getting caught for stealing from classmates, truancy, and other delinquent acts which lead to expulsion from school.

Marcy's early history was uneventful. She was described as happy and outgoing until age twelve, when "overnight" she became sullen and rebellious. Sibling rivalry, always present, became intense. Marcy habitually told her parents she hated her brother and wished he were dead.

Psychological tests revealed a fourteen-point discrepancy between the verbal and performance WISC (114 vs. 100). The lowered performance score was due to inattentiveness to objective detail on the picture-completion test and coding. Projective tests revealed a projective tendency, distrust of authority figures, rage, and an underlying depressive trend.

Marcy began psychotherapy on a twice-weekly basis. The treatment course was stormy. Marcy attempted to control the sessions. She was manipulative in her efforts to "divide and conquer" by playing one against one or another parent, or at times, both parents. She was labile both during sessions and reportedly at home, her moods shifting from ebullience to despair in a matter of hours. Her dreams were often frightening or filled with gloom. For example, "I dreamed I was dead; I went to my own funeral and saw myself lying in a coffin." At other times she was overexcited and could talk nonstop for an hour if not interrupted.

On several occasions Marcy responded to me with a modicum of trust, bringing in poems and stories. She was a talented writer, and her stories were creative and imaginative. After several such encouraging sessions, however, her tendency was not to come at all or to berate me for not understanding or helping her. She had frequent temper tantrums in the office and had difficulty controlling her impulses.

Marcy's school work continued to deteriorate. She had difficulty concentrating and was often truant. Finally she was caught smoking marijuana during school recess and was expelled from school. Her reaction to the marijuana (probably mixed with a hallucinogenic agent) was severe. She experienced visual hallucinations and became terrified and disorganized. Feelings of depersonalization persisted for two weeks despite phenothiazine medication. Following the episode she refused further treatment with me.

During the next three years Marcy attended three separate boarding schools which were suitable for adolescents with emotional problems. In each school, after an initial good adjustment she became rebellious, refused to obey the rules, and had to be expelled. She ran away in a "borrowed" car and was sexually promiscuous with boys ("one night stands are better—that way you don't get involved"). She refused psychiatric treatment although one consultant diagnosed her as having "emotionally unstable character disorder" and recommended lithium management.

At age seventeen Marcy received home tutoring, and obtained her high school equivalency. Her mood swings continued unabated, and a psychiatrist consultant recommended hospitalization for manic-depressive illness with appropriate medication and psychotherapy following the hospital course.

CASE VIGNETTE 3

Milo was thirteen when his parents first consulted me because of poor academic work in the eighth grade and "failure to live up to his potential." His family had been living abroad for several years but returned to the United States the previous summer. Milo had not adjusted to the change, missed his friends in France, and had not made friends in the new school.

The family history was significant in that many members of the father's family had documented, bipolar manic-depressive illness. Mr. R was a forty-five-year-old lawyer with an international firm. He was very successful but highly competitive and "driven," according to his wife. He had been under care for recurrent depression but had never been hospitalized. His own father had been "an explosive, temperamental artist" prone to impulsive fits of behavior. This grandfather had married a woman twenty years his junior who had a diagnosed manic-depressive illness herself, with her first depressive episode requiring hospitalization following her husband's death. She had four hospitalizations for manic episodes, the last one responding well to lithium carbonate. Several of the grandfather's siblings have had manic-depressive illness resulting in hospitalization.

Mrs. R was forty-two. A former teacher, she had no history of psychopathology. The R's had two other sons: the eldest, aged fifteen, was considered gifted, was a brilliant student, but was prone to feelings of shyness and insecurity; his ten-year-old brother had dyslexia and other learning problems, and had received special remedial help.

Milo's past history was unusual in that the family moved several times during the first year of his life and Milo was left in the care of nursemaids on frequent occasions. When he was eight months old his father reappeared on the scene after a seven-week absence, and Milo reportedly "shrieked and screamed in fear" when his father tried to pick him up. His mother became aware of his extreme sensitivity to noise (e.g., trains, fire engines) and to strangers—behavior which lasted until he was two. When Milo was fifteen months old Mrs. R delivered a stillborn child and was depressed for several months. Milo became very attached to his nursemaids and, at age six, wept when the family moved away, leaving the nursemaids behind.

Milo's school performance was always problematic. He was asked to leave his French nursery school at three and a half for being too active and independent, lacking social skills, and being too excited. In second grade he was constantly in the principal's office for "pulling the fire bell, throwing spit balls, and just being full of beans," according to his mother. At home he was loving and affectionate with family members and his pet dogs, but he developed a series of fears—of the dark, of imaginary monsters, and of being alone. In fact, Mrs. R noted, Milo, at age nine, seemed to believe in the Easter Bunny or Tooth Fairy longer than her other children had. Despite parental warnings, he threw rocks and fired B-B guns at passing cars and once caused a driver to swerve and hit a tree. Such examples of thoughtless behavior were commonplace. Milo would appear remorseful but would repeat a similar piece of behavior the next week. He would then cry and promise not to do it again. "I don't know why I do it," he acknowledged.

The family moved to a third European country when Milo was ten. Milo was again in trouble academically. He was constantly losing his books and his papers and was always in trouble for fighting or cursing. He did well with special tutorial help but could not seem to work alone. The final move to the United States resulted in the last change of schools and the subsequent consultation.

When I first met Milo he was a thin, pale boy, attractive and well coordinated, who looked immature for thirteen years. He gazed at his shoes most of the time, and his eyes filled with tears when he thought of his friends in Europe. "I wish I could get A's in school like my brothers and my parents—they were both straight-A students—but I always mess up. I forget to do my homework, I lose my notebooks—I only do well in sports. . . . The kids here are all crumbs. One day they like you and the next day they don't talk to you. I am a great disappointment to my family." Milo noted other problems: "I do things I know are bad, but I can't stop myself—like telling lies to teachers or taking things from other kids." He also described feeling frightened when alone in his room in the dark. He imagined monsters of every shape about to attack him. He described a series of rituals he performed nightly to make himself feel better: touching things twice, placing his shoes under the bed at "just the right angle, but I still feel scared." He sometimes wished he had not been born and often wished he were dead.

Psychological tests were obtained because of Milo's academic performance. His IQ was in the superior range. It was felt his learning inhibition was not only the result of changing schools but was related to Milo's giving up a task when he could not grasp it immediately. He could not remain with an activity because frustration resulted in his avoiding the task altogether. His full-scale IQ (WISC) was 120 with verbal 128 and performance 107. The lowest score was on Coding, the other scores were average to superior. The psychologist felt that the lower score was due to slower timing rather than visual-perceptual or motor performance. The Bender-Gestalt reproductions were good. Because of the lack of appropriate school-age skills, remedial education was recommended along with psychoanalytic psychotherapy.

Milo eagerly grasped for help. He spent many sessions describing his anxieties and his inability to fall asleep. "I just toss and turn and think of all the ways I'm a failure." His mood fluctuated between black despair and euphoria. When he was "down" even his choice of colors was gloomy. "I wanted to have my room painted black. Black is like the underdog. I wanted to give black a chance." When his mood was "up" his speech became pressured and his language overinclusive. He described his analysis of a thematic aperception test card: "It was about Beethoven. His mother made him practice but he really didn't have time to study. Maybe he had a lousy teacher, maybe he was sick or paralyzed and couldn't hold the pencil,

357

maybe he had a headache, maybe he was an alcoholic or a drug addict, maybe he got no pleasure in anything, maybe he didn't believe in himself.''

Milo hated to study his assigned texts but was fascinated by science fiction. ''I can go into a secret world of my own and be king.'' He spent hours in such fantasy, winning all the games and taking all the honors.

As Milo began to obtain some relief from the sessions, he became more outgoing in school, but not in ways conducive to academic success. He made friends with some of the local delinquents in school and became involved in incidents of minor vandalism, writing obscenities on the blackboard and tossing books around the room. He was suspended from school for several days. His friends rarely got caught.

He admitted that he often acted on impulse, getting in more trouble than any of his friends. ''I'm just sick of feeling low, and when I get happy for once my parents scream at me and I get suspended.'' He was, indeed, much happier according to his parents, but, ''in a childish way—dancing on door stoops, acting like a six-year-old and clowning,'' they complained. Milo became overexcited in the office on occasion, giggling and telling jokes. He became interested in a girl at school and began discussing sexual feelings. He was frightened by his masturbatory wishes but highly stimulated as well. He began to reveal intensely sadomasochistic fantasies and dreams of being tied up and tortured, much like characters he had read about in *Lord of the Flies*. When he saw *Jaws* he identified with the shark.

At the semester's end Milo was doing somewhat better academically with the aid of a tutor. Family relationships, however, were still troubled. Milo continued to be clinging, childish, quarrelsome, and belligerent. Mr. R was enraged and punitive most of the time. The therapy, which had proceeded in relatively smooth fashion for six months, was interrupted for the summer.

All did not go well during the vacation. Milo ran away from the family's summer house for several days following a fight with his uncle over the ''unfair'' demand to mow the lawn. A second emergency occurred the following month when the police called the family. Milo and several other boys had stolen ten cases of wine from a local bar. Milo did not call me himself; when his family brought him to see me, he was detached and expressed the wish to terminate treatment. ''Why should I call you when I'm in trouble? You don't help.'' His participation in the escapade had been impulsive, and he had acted as a ''follower,'' he reported. ''Since that is all in the past,'' he argued, ''I don't want to think about it. You're just trying to upset me.'' The family was in turmoil. Mr. R had become so upset with Milo's behavior that in a fit of pique he ''nearly wrapped the family car around a tree.'' Mrs.

R tended to forgive and infantilize. Treatment was resumed. Milo admitted that he felt abandoned by me, just as he had been by his beloved nursemaids long before; he had hoped that somehow, as if by magic, I could work miracles and make his problems disappear.

During the next six months Milo began discussing deep feelings of inadequacy, particularly in school. He felt stupid, unable to learn, and helpless in the real world of insurmountable obstacles. He began describing murderous fantasies about eighth graders he "hated." He recalled hospital experiences of being jabbed by needles and described detailed fantasies of revenge by torturing his enemies. Milo was no longer the depressed, quiet loner of the previous semester. He became involved in several school fights and acquired the reputation of being a bully. He became extremely successful in athletics. Tall and husky by now, he was selected to be on the varsity basketball team, an honor rarely awarded to a freshman. His fantasies about being a basketball player, a detective, a shark fisherman infiltrated his homework time. He felt so helpless in real life his fantasied omnipotence enabled him to shut out the reality of his precarious academic situation. His new success in sports led to dreams such as the following: "I was the worst criminal in the world. I was caught and handcuffed. I knew I had special powers and could remove the handcuffs. I did so and ran away."

Milo made friends with another aggressive boy who got into fights and enjoyed gambling and other exciting activities. Milo began to emulate him in every way. He began to miss sessions saying "I forgot." That month he was nearly expelled from school for impulsively striking a boy in the face and breaking his jaw. Following this incident Milo refused to come for sessions, professing a hatred of me, of the sessions, of being forced to come to the office, which was like "jail." He later admitted that all adults, including me, had let him down by not helping him with his confused feelings or magically helping him control himself when he lost control. The second year of treatment ended with an improvement in grades and an award for high achievement in sports.

The following summer Milo did call me during the long vacation when, again, he was about to run away from home after an altercation with a cousin. He was able to settle the dispute without having to leave home.

Mrs. R reported that her husband's temper had become more violent and that he was generally enraged at Milo. Milo became depressed, silent, and sullen in sessions. He said he was "hopeless—nothing can help, even you. You're just a stupid lady who can't change things." Indeed, in my office Milo did have insight into his own behavior, fear of his father, displacement of his rage toward siblings and peers, his wish to "make everything O.K." by magic, his belief that women were weak and helpless. He could not, however, control his impulses or plan any action more than minutes away.

He made efforts to "hold the line" with his tutor and did improve in most of his subjects. He even wrote an essay describing the effects of psychotherapy on a hypothetical boy: "His getting into trouble was due to the fact that he would act on impulse no matter what the consequences were instead of thinking over the actions and then deciding whether or not they were prudent."

Milo was now fifteen. Toward the end of the second semester it became obvious that boarding school was the best solution to the school and home problem—Milo very much wanted to leave and only regretted not being able to continue treatment. He intended to come home every month to at least continue our talks. He was still extremely moody, despondent one day, overexcited the next. I encouraged the family to consult a psychopharmacologist for possible future medication, particularly in view of the fact that Milo would be away at school. Before an appointment was arranged, however, Milo became involved in an incident which necessitated emergency measures. One of his teammates called him a name during a hockey game. Milo reached for a stick and struck the boy, fracturing his leg. He was immediately suspended from school.

In the following session with me Milo confessed, "I don't remember what happened. It's as if my mind went blank—I just went crazy mad when he cursed me out and that's all I remember until I saw the stick in my hand and the guy on the ground." The consultant who saw Milo on an emergency basis recommended a trial of lithium. Milo was allowed to complete his semester with the understanding he would remain on the drug.

Milo spent the summer with his family, but this time reports were very different. There were no altercations with family members or strangers. Milo felt capable of being with his family—even his father—without exploding. I had asked him to keep a "mood-diary" of his feelings during the past year. Two months after starting therapy, instead of jagged peaks and deep pits with explanatory inscriptions written above the red line he used to measure his mood swings, there was a gently curved or flat line with the comment "feeling O.K."

Milo's two years in boarding school were successful academically and socially as long as he remained on lithium. After the first year he decided to stop taking the drug and within three months had relapsed, becoming grandiose and unrealistic. Suspended once again, Milo had a psychotic episode. He ran away from school to join the Yankee team and was hospitalized briefly before therapy was reinstated. There was no further problem and he completed his second year, graduating with high marks and numerous sports awards.

Milo continued to visit me from time to time. "I realize now that the lithium helps me when my feelings get out of control. All those things you used to tell me—I believed you, but I couldn't stop myself from doing bad things. Now I don't get such violent reactions to everything. When I get blue, I tell myself it's not the end of the world. I'm just like everyone else now—everyone gets blue sometimes."

Discussion

Some fundamental questions raised in the introduction ask which individuals are vulnerable to manic-depressive disorder and which premorbid characteristics indicate vulnerability to subsequent episodes. The three vignettes highlight many of the important features and share many elements in common: all subjects have a family history positive for manic-depressive illness.

All three patients exhibited at various times dysphoria and marked fluctuations in mood. All had a history of temper tantrums, impulsivity, and low frustration tolerance. Two were called hyperactive in childhood. All three were considered bright, creative, and imaginative. Dreams and fantasies were either gloomy and preoccupied with suicide and death or filled with grandiose and omnipotent wishes. Childhood fears, magical thinking, and obsessive rituals persisted for a longer duration than is usual for young children. Behavior problems and school failure were prominent manifestations of Milo's and Marcy's disorder, as were distractibility, short attention span, and lack of judgment.

If these three individuals had been examined in childhood they might have been given a variety of diagnostic labels. None would have fit the symptom picture of pure depression, but some clinicians might have considered masked depression an appropriate diagnosis. The significance of such symptom clusters in childhood has often been overlooked, as though the symptoms are unimportant and will disappear by adolescence.

The interesting psychometric finding was the similarity in WISC scores. All three patients demonstrated superior verbal IQ with significantly lower performance scores, a finding Anthony and Scott (1960) noted. There are obvious similarities in their WISC performance scores with wide scatter among the six performance subtests. Low scores on the visuo-constructive tests are reminiscent of the scores obtained by children with certain types of minimal brain damage, according to Gardner (1979). Appreciation of spatial relationships is considered to be primarily a function of the right cerebral hemisphere, as is the processing of complex nonverbal sensory input (Gazzaniga 1970). Right-hemispheric dysfunction could interfere with the ability to perform well on block design, picture arrangement, picture completion, object assembly, and maze subtests (Russell, Neuringer, and Goldstein 1970).

Bemporard (1978) has noted that some children who have a family history positive for manic-depressive illness may have a greater right- than left-hemisphere deficit. Moreover, they may have high incidence of disinhibition syndrome which could be the result of subtle frontal brain systems dysfunction. She believes that this syndrome may be similar to some descriptions of hyperkinetic disorder.

Flor-Henry (1978) has formulated a similar hypothesis for adults with manic-depressive disorder. The findings suggest the possibility of a fundamental genetic liability—the lack of some central inhibitory regulating mechanism—which may lead to a manic-depressive illness in later life.

The three patients described seem to have a genetic vulnerability to manic-depressive illness. The precipitating event in Robert's case was object loss, as in Feinstein and Wolpert's case (1973), and fits the pattern of extreme sensitivity to loss described by Gershon, Dunner, and Goodwin (1971). The younger adolescents did not seem to have one particular precipitating stress. The onset of puberty with the physiological and psychological stresses—increased sexual and aggressive drives—may have been enough to cause a gradual breakdown of control mechanisms.

As Carlson and Strober (1978) pointed out, true mania in childhood is extremely rare and is probably masked by developmental issues. Bunney, Goodwin, and Murphy (1972) conceptualized the change from depression to mania as a "switch process" which, they believe, is genetically transmitted and has physiological and social concomitants. The manic state may be brought on by bereavement or other stressful life events in constitutionally vulnerable individuals. The adult in the manic phase is bombarded by stimuli he cannot sort out (i.e., flight of ideas, pressured speech, clang associations). He can be verbose, hyperactive, expansive, grandiose, hypersexual, hyperaggressive, and elated. Eventually there is breakdown of reality-testing functions and he can become delusional. The child so constitutionally prone may also exhibit similar features early in life. He can exhibit extreme silliness, hyperactivity, sleep disturbance, pressured speech, and increased magical thinking as an attempt to deny social or academic problems.

The issue of control becomes paramount. Milo, for example, described his state of mind during an examination week: "I feel as if I have a powerful

Cadillac engine all revved up to go, but the body is only a Model T Ford. I can barely hold it down and if I lose control for a minute, it'll go off on its own and I'll never be able to stop.''

The necessity of early diagnosis and awareness of the premorbid state in a vulnerable individual is of major importance. Every child exhibiting the symptoms described in a family where there is a history of affective disorder should have psychometric tests ordered even if academic work is satisfactory. Yearly examination by a child psychiatrist could help determine whether psychiatric intervention is indicated.

Conclusions

The question of early intervention and treatment is beyond the scope of this chapter. Psychotherapy, parental counseling regarding management, and appropriate school selection is always useful for an initial approach. When psychotherapy has proceeded for six months without diminution of symptoms, psychopharmacological treatment is indicated. It is not recommended that lithium carbonate be used indiscriminately in cases where a manic component seems prominent (Youngerman and Canino 1978). In certain individual cases, however, where diagnostic criteria can be established, lithium may indeed be the drug of choice. Further investigation on the effects of lithium on children and adolescents is necessary before it can be recommended for more general use. Psychotherapy is not useful during a psychotic state but can be of benefit, as in the cases of Robert and Milo, in helping the patient modify his behavior and understand his illness.

In order to answer more fully the questions posed, it is necessary that prospective, controlled studies be undertaken of children at risk for manic-depressive illness, such as those involving children at risk for schizophrenia (Erlenmeyer-Kimling 1975). Psychiatric, psychological, neurophysiological, and neuropsychological investigation may lead to more accurate diagnosis and earlier intervention through enhanced awareness of the premorbid state.

NOTE

1. S. Weintraub, personal communication, 1979.

Annall, A. 1969. Lithium in the treatment of children and adolescents. *Acta Psychiatrica Scandinavia* 207:19–30.

Anthony, E. J., and Scott, P. 1960. Manic-depressive psychosis in childhood. *Journal of Child Psychology and Psychiatry* 1:53–72.

Angst, J., and Perris, C. 1968. Zur Nosologie endogener Depressionen. *Archiv für Psychiatrie und Gesamte Neurologie* 210:373–386.

Bemporad, B. 1978. A neuropsychological study of children of bipolar parents. Master's thesis, City College of New York.

Berg, I.; Hullin, R.; Allsopp, M.; O'Brien, P.; and MacDonald, R. 1974. Bipolar manic-depressive psychosis in early adolescence—a case report. *British Journal of Psychiatry* 125:416–417.

Bertelsen, A.; Harvald, B.; and Hauge, M. 1977. A Danish twin-study of manic-depressive disorder. *British Journal of Psychiatry* 130:330–357.

Bunney, W. E.; Goodwin, F. K.; and Murphy, D. L. 1972. The "switch process" in manic-depressive illness, III. Theoretical implications. *Archives of General Psychiatry* 27:312–319.

Cadoret, R. J. 1978. Evidence for genetic inheritance of primary affective disorder in adoptees. *American Journal of Psychiatry* 135:463–466.

Cadoret, R. J., and Winokur, G. 1975. X-linkage in manic-depressive illness. *Annual Review of Medicine* 26:21–25.

Carlson, G. A., and Stober, M. 1978. Manic-depressive illness in early adolescence. *Journal of the American Academy of Child Psychiatry* 17(1): 138–153.

Cytryn, L., and McKnew, D. H. 1972. Proposed classification of childhood depression. *American Journal of Psychiatry* 129:149–155.

Davis, R. E. 1979. Manic-depressive variant syndrome of childhood: a preliminary report. *American Journal of Psychiatry* 136:702–704.

Dunner, D.; Fleiss, J. L.; and Fieve, R. C. 1976. The course of development of mania in patients with recurrent depression. *American Journal of Psychiatry* 133:905–908.

Dyson, W. L., and Barcai, A. 1970. Treatment of children of lithium-responding parents. *Current Therapeutic Research* 12:286–290.

Erlenmeyer-Kimling, L. 1975. A prospective study of children at-risk for schizophrenia. In R. Wirt, G. Winokur, and M. Roff, eds. *Life History Research in Psychopathology*. Minneapolis: University of Minnesota Press.

Farber, S. 1980. *Identical Twins Reared Apart: A Reanalysis*. New York: Basic.

Feinstein, S. C., and Wolpert, E. A. 1973. Juvenile manic-depressive illness: clinical and therapeutic considerations. *Journal of the American Academy of Child Psychiatry* 12:123–136.

Flor-Henry, P. 1978. On certain aspects of the localization of the cerebral systems regulating and determining emotions. Paper presented at the meeting of the American Association for Biological Psychiatry, Atlanta, October 7.

Gardner, R. A. 1979. *The Objective Diagnosis of Minimal Brain Dysfunction.* Cresskill, N.J.: Creative Therapeutics.

Gazzaniga, M. S. 1970. *The Bijected Brain.* New York: Appleton-Century-Crofts.

Gershon, E. S.; Barron, M.; and Leckman, F. 1975. Genetic models of the transmission of affective disorders. *Journal of Psychiatric Research* 12:301–317.

Gershon, E. S.; Dunner, D. L.; and Goodwin, F. K. 1971. Toward a biology of affective disorders. *Archives of General Psychiatry* 25:1–15.

Harms, E. 1952. Differential pattern of manic-depressive disease in childhood. *Nervous Child* 9:326–356.

Kestenbaum, C. J. 1979. Children at-risk for manic-depressive illness: possible predictors. *American Journal of Psychiatry* 136:1206–1208.

Kraepelin, E. 1921. *Manic-Depressive Insanity and Paranoia.* Edinburgh: Livingston.

Leonhard, K.; Korff, I.; and Schulz, H. 1962. Die Temperamente in den Familien der monopolaren und bipolaren phasischen Psychosen. *Psychiatrische Neurologie* 143:416–434.

Loranger, A., and Levine, P. 1978. Age of onset of bipolar affective illness. *Archives of General Psychiatry* 35:1345–1348.

McKnew D. H.; Cytryn, L.; Efron, A. M.; Gershon, E. S.; and Bunney, W. E. 1979. Offspring of patients with affective disorders. *British Journal of Psychiatry* 134:148–152.

McKnew, D. H.; Cytryn, L.; and White, I. 1974. Clinical and biochemical correlates of hypomania in a child. *Journal of Child Psychiatry* 13:576–585.

Mendlewicz, J., and Rainer, J. 1977. Adoption study supporting genetic transmission in manic depressive illness. *Nature* 268:327–329.

Mendlewicz, J.; Rainer, J. D.; and Fleiss, J. A. 1975. A dominant X-linked factor in manic-depressive illness; studies with color blindness. In R. R. Fieve, A. Rosenthal and H. Brill, eds. *Genetic Research in Psychiatry.* Baltimore: John Hopkins University Press.

Perris, C. 1966. A study of bipolar (manic-depressive) and unipolar recurrent depressive psychoses. *Acta Psychiatrica Scandinavia* 42 (suppl.194): 1–188.

Petti, T. A. 1978. Depression in hospitalized child psychiatry patients: approaches to measuring depression. *American Journal of Child Psychiatry* 17:49–59.

Poznansky, E. O.; Krahenbuhl, V.; and Zrull, J. P. 1976. Childhood depression: a longitudinal perspective. *Journal of Child Psychiatry* 15:491–501.

Price, J. S. 1972. Genetic and phylogenetic aspects of mood variation. *International Journal of Mental Health* 1:124–144.

Rosanoff, A. J.; Handy, L. M.; and Plesset, I. R. 1935. The etiology of manic-depressive syndromes with special reference to their occurrence in twins. *American Journal of Psychiatry* 91:725–762.

Rosenthal, D. 1970. *Genetic Theory and Abnormal Behavior.* New York: McGraw-Hill.

Russell, E. W.; Neuringer, C.; and Goldstein, G. 1970. *Assessment of Brain Damage.* New York: Wiley-Interscience.

Slater, E. 1953. Psychotic and neurotic illnesses in twins. Medical Research Council Special Report no. 276. London: Her Majesty's Stationery Office.

Stone, M. H. 1971. Mania—a guide for the perplexed. *Psychotherapy and Social Science Review* 5(10): 14–18.

Weinberg, W. A.; Rutman, J.; Sullivan, L.; Penick, E. C.; and Dietz, S. G. 1975. Depression in children referred to an educational diagnostic center: diagnosis and treatment. *Journal of Pediatrics* 83(6): 1065–1072.

Welner, Z.; Welner, A.; McGrary, B. A.; and Leonard, M. A. 1977. Psychopathology in children of inpatients with depression: a controlled study. *Journal of Nervous and Mental Disease* 164(6): 408–413.

Winokur, G. 1979. Unipolar depression. Is it divisible into autonomous subtypes? *Archives of General Psychiatry* 36:47–52.

Winokur, G.; Cadoret, R.; Baker, M.; and Dorzab, J. 1975. Depressive spectrum disease versus pure depressive disease: some further data. *British Journal of Psychiatry* 127:75–77.

Winokur, G.; Clayton, P. J.; and Reich, T. 1969. *Manic-Depressive Illness.* St. Louis: Mosby.

Youngerman, J., and Canino, I. 1978. Lithium carbonate use in children and adolescents: a survey of the literature. *Archives of General Psychiatry* 35:216–224.

Zerbin-Rudin, E. 1972. Genetic research and the theory of schizophrenia. *International Journal of Mental Health* 1:42–62.

SIDNEY BERMAN

A great deal of attention has been given to the depression which many adolescents experience as they disengage themselves from their parents and embark upon a quest to establish their identities as adults (Blos 1979; French and Berlin 1979; A. Freud 1958; Jacobson 1961). On the other hand, the response of parents to this phenomenon has received scant attention, even though it may well determine how the adolescent resolves the feelings of despair (Anthony 1970; Bell 1961; Newman and San Martino 1976). The purpose of this chapter is to focus on some parental reactions which may be observed in relation to adolescent depression, especially as it applies to a specific segment of the population—the white middle class. Also, since the parents are the central objects of this study, I will forego a critical examination of the contribution of the social matrix to this discussion while recognizing that the current social values and attitudes may shatter the self-esteem of some adolescents and disorganize the judgment of many parents.

Of the many functions of parents, one is to help the child tame the instinctual drives as he progresses from one developmental phase to the next. Another is to prepare the child for the process of separation and ultimately to take his place as an adult in our social system. Within the highly complex transactional process which occurs between parents and child, the gradual integration of these two functions, the mastery of the internal psychological process of the adolescent with the external object-related socializing process of the parents, will determine the way in which the child finally separates from the parents and becomes an adult. This process of separation, as it is experienced by the parents and the adolescent, is significantly important in relation to adolescent depression. In adolescent depression the adolescent is unable to decathect the oedipal and preoedipal aspects of the parental object relationships. As a result, separation becomes intolerable and the adolescent is unable to move toward adult autonomy. Parents, too, demonstrate a difficulty in achieving a psychological separation from the adolescent they infantilize, dominate, or neglect. Regardless of the protean manifestations of adolescent depression, it will cause a striking arrest of psychological and social development and, in the parents, great concern, guilt, confusion, and even anger as they respond to the regressive symptoms and behavior.

The Adolescent Phase of Development

For purposes of this discussion, a brief review of what I would consider to be the normal intrapsychic developmental process for the adolescent and the complementary responses of the parents is in order. We note that adolescents are not inclined to recall significant events in their past life and may convey the impression that their motives and behavior have arisen de novo. However, we know that this is not so, for the past claims an important place in the adolescent's mental life (Spiegel 1972).

Every child, for security reasons and survival purposes in each developmental phase, internalizes certain attributes of his parents through mental processes referred to psychologically as internalization, identification, and superego formation. Unconsciously parents influence the child's mode of thought and behavior and determine the way the he feels about himself and others. Thus this internalization assumes a regulatory function in controlling the child's instinctual drives and social relationships. All of this is well and good during childhood, but when adolescence is reached the adolescent must gradually separate from parents and acquire control over sexual drives. The mastery of these two tasks is essential if the adolescent is to develop relative independence from the parents.

It has been repeatedly stressed that the important factors which force the adolescent to separate from his parents are the physical changes of puberty and the intense increase of the sexual and aggressive drives. When the adolescent experiences intense sexual arousal, there results within the psychic structures a withdrawal of libidinal interest from the parents as love objects to his own body. The ego now responds to the mental representation of the sexual drive by overcoming superego prohibitions of childhood. A realignment of psychic structures begins, and with it there is a gradual disengagement from the parents, mentally and physically. In this process of distancing, although there is an overlapping of psychic functions associated with the psychological separation from the childhood parental object representations, the task in the early subphase of adolescence is the adequate mastery of the sex drive. The task in the middle subphase is the resolution of the oedipal ties to both parents. Finally, in the late-adolescent subphase the task is to achieve psychological separation from the parents and autonomy and sexuality as an adult.

In order for all this to happen, the psychic apparatus, just like the physical body, changes structurally. As the drives increase in intensity, the ego also undergoes new structure formation, both adaptive and defensive to master the drives and alter the superego. In addition to the use of the basic defenses established in childhood to deal with the restrictive aspects of the superego, the ego develops a new mechanism of defense which I have described as the defense of alienation (Berman 1970). This is an intrapsychic process that repudiates those aspects of the superego which in childhood contained the drives and repressed the oedipal conflict. Thus the adolescent ego modifies the superego and the identifications of childhood in order to attain the above mentioned objectives. This mechanism of defense operates throughout adolescence until there is the consolidation of psychic organization in character formation which renders the young adult greatly independent from those forces which determined his behavior in childhood (Blos 1968). These dramatic changes in the adolescent's attitude, behavior, and feelings, including particularly the need to repudiate parental influences, evoke a wide range of complementary parental responses; the parents, too, have to adapt to separation and loss as they experience the gradual decathexis from one they have been very close to for so long.

Parental Response to Adolescent Separation

Very little consideration has been given to the psychic process in parents in relation to the psychic transformation of the adolescent. As the adolescent undergoes a remodeling of psychic structure and attains gradual freedom from the archaic id and superego pressures and a greater freedom from external influences, the psychological task of the parents is to gradually separate from the adolescent as the childhood object of interest.

Although many authors consider parenthood a phase of life for most adults, personally I question the use of that concept of parenthood in the context of psychoanalytic theory. Certainly adulthood is a developmental phase in which there occurs a consolidation of psychic institutions; parenthood, however, is a psychological task within the context of adulthood. Whereas the adolescent is undergoing internal changes, the parents experience parenthood as something outside of themselves to which they have to adapt. The adolescent psychic structures become reorganized whereas the parents respond with a toned-down modification from the childhood object relationship to an adolescent object relationship. This response of the parents, however, depends on multiple factors. These include their mental attributes, both conscious and unconscious; their transferential response to the adolescent based on their own childhood and adolescent experiences; current attitudes toward adolescent society; and their broader family, social, and occupational responsibilities. In this sense parents do not live through a parental phase in terms of psychic structural change—not that the adolescent does not change their way of living. Nor do they usually get what some call a ''second chance'' to relive their own lives through this experience with the adolescent. Such ideas may create false hopes in parents and may interfere with this unique task the adolescent must master in his given point in history. All this does not mean that under favorable circumstances a parent does not improve and refine his character structure, for there is the capacity for self-observation and self-initiated change in relation to the adolescent.

At the same time that the parents are participating with the adolescent in the process of separation they are coping with many other problems of maintaining family stability. This, plus the fact that the separation occurs over the entire phase of adolescence, provides a subtle and gradual emotional detachment from the adolescent. Nevertheless, parents also have to deal with their grief reaction; no longer can they relate to their cuddly, small, dependent child who needs their guidance and protection. The gradual physical and psychological transformation of the boy and girl in adolescence forces the parents to respect the distancing process between themselves and their teenager. As an example, the sexual development and the physical growth of the child evokes the incest barrier and also warns parents that they no longer can control their child by the authority of their size and strength. Additionally, expanding intellectual capacities and intense peer-group relationships become more important factors to the adolescent than the relationship to the parents, making it clear to the parents that they no longer can experience the narcissistic satisfaction which was provided by the child's dependent need for them. The inevitability of these changes in the adolescent compel the parents to assume a more equal relationship regarding mutual dialogue and reasonable expectations.

Although all parents must accept the adolescent's separation from them, the best insurance for maintaining a mutually satisfying relationship is the

370

cultivation of a new relationship with their adolescent as an emerging adult, based on the strength of the adolescent's positive childhood identification, so as to maintain a link of love and respect. When parents realistically and emphatically perceive and respond effectively to the adolescent's phase-specific tasks centered around sexuality and separation, it helps the adolescent to better handle the affective crises associated with mental reorganization and to strive toward the emergence of a new grown-up self.

However, children raised in a home shrouded in a pall of oppressive tyranny, hostility, disparagement, unreasonable parental expectations, death, chronic despair, and pathogenic parental preferences run a high risk of becoming depressed. When such children reach adolescence, the sexual and aggressive drives may overwhelm them so that separation evokes helplessness, futility, and despair. When this occurs, it is not uncommon for one parent to react with intense concern and the other with fierce resentment, or both may feel overwhelmed and confused. It even may aggravate family conflict to the level of a crisis, which places great stress on the bonds of marriage as the parents react with perplexity, confusion, bewilderment, and recrimination.

Depressive Syndromes and Parental Response

Depression in adolescence is a behavioral syndrome, and the natural history of each depression is dictated by its cause. In adolescence, although the core manifestations of depression are self-depreciation, hopelessness, and despair, depression may take many disguised forms, especially when passivity defensively turns to activity that is supported by pathological peer-group relationships. Then it may be expressed as temper outbursts; sadistic, masochistic, and explosive sexual behavior; delinquency; and drug abuse. Only a sensitive diagnostic assessment can clarify if the depression is the core problem or if it is a symptom of other types of disorder. The most common forms of depression during adolescence, up to the age of eighteen years, are the transitory depressive reaction, the psychoneurotic depression, the reactive depression, the masked depression. Endogenous depression, although it may begin to emerge in adolescence, still is not frequently seen.

When there is conflict between the progressive and the regressive forces during adolescence, the symptoms may be those of a mild transitory depression because of the stress of coping with the adolescent process itself. Thus, we may observe cases of a mild depressive reaction in which primary process functioning briefly takes over due to the intense pressure of the sexual drive for satisfaction or to an increase in passivity over activity related to separation anxiety. The history does not reveal significant factors from the past as the cause of the regression or current life experiences which have overwhelmed the progressive forces. This type of regression is in the service of ego development and is commonly observed in adolescence. It quickly runs its course and disappears as the adolescent moves from one subphase of this period to the next. Such temporary fluctuations of development may create great anxiety and concern in the parents who, with help and guidance, are able to bear with the adolescent's discomfort until mental stability is regained.

A common form of neurosis among adolescents is the psychoneurotic depression. Reconstruction invariably demonstrates in one aspect or another the adolescent's high level of ambivalence toward his parents, more so with one than another, dating back to early childhood: the child has experienced a traumatic loss by way of divorce, separation due to death or abandonment, the birth of a sibling, or despair associated with parental incompatibility.

It is not unusual to hear that these adolescents had a lot of trouble adapting to enrollment in nursery school. At that time they may have shown intense sadness or fear about leaving mother, or they may have handled the depressive affect by hyperactive and destructive activity, thereby forcing the teachers and parents to return the child to his home. Invariably this inability to tolerate object loss or loss of love interferes with development during latency. The move from home to elementary school brings no satisfaction or pleasure from playmates or pleasure in growing up. The feeling of loss or abandonment may be so intense that whatever parents or teachers do to intervene only reinforces the repetitious affirmation of this feeling.

A very attractive seventeen-year-old girl of superior intellectual ability suffered from agonizing crying spells, feelings of worthlessness, thoughts of dying, self-pity, insomnia, and deep despair. When she was fifteen months old her brother was born. Although on the surface she accepted this, she reacted with deep pain. When she reached the oedipal phase, she fancied that, because of his aloofness toward her, her father preferred her brother, whereupon she clung to her mother for solace. This symbiotic attachment and feelings of melancholy persisted into high school and ended in a full-blown neurotic depression when she had to prepare to go to college. The sibling rivalry, the unresolved oedipal conflicts, the conflictual parental identifications, and severe hostile superego rendered her helpless to care for herself when she had to face the ultimate separation and individuation of adolescence. Her crying, sadness, self-devaluation, loss of mirth, and disturbing dreams made it necessary to prescribe antidepressant medication, which she took for two weeks. In intensive psychoanalytically oriented psychotherapy she resolved her hostility toward her father and tolerated him as he was. Her resentment toward her parasitic young brother was handled directly with him. She saw her mother as a friend. There was a burst of creative writing, poetry, dancing, and expanding friendships—and a decision to go away to college. Her parents were seen twice in this time. Her father could openly acknowledge that his aloofness was a problem to the family, but felt no need to do anything about it. He acknowledged that his daughter's complaints were valid. The patient accepted this with the same resignation as her mother and no longer felt demeaned by him. The mother restrained herself from infantilizing the patient, who was able to modify her pathological identification with her parents.

When an adolescent suffers from a neurotic depression, one or both parents exhibit certain characteristics which I refer to as applicable to a neurotogenic parent. The adolescent's depressive symptoms and masochistic character formation mobilize intense anxiety and helplessness in these parents. The adolescent's attempt to overthrow a severe superego may cause him to react with hostile behavior, vacillating mood swings, pseudo independence, or despair. In response to this, one parent may withdraw or react with intense anger. The other parent usually attempts some form of restitution by becoming overprotective, reacting with feelings of guilt or seduction, or by becoming frustrated, tearful, angry, or depressed. Such parents are inconsistent, exposing the adolescent alternately to intense involvement and concern or intense outbursts of anger or despair.

Now I would like to consider family issues in relation to reactive depression of adolescence. Although this concept may evoke controversy over its clinical usefulness as a diagnostic entity, I believe it has merit because it defines a special type of depression as to its precipitating cause and its time of onset. A reactive depression is due to a specific traumatic event resulting in a situational loss. The loss of a person, love, job or status, or self-esteem, or failure, or a painful crisis may render the person helpless. Although it may be superimposed on another disorder, the past history is essentially free from evidence of depressive crises.

Parents all too often may precipitate a reactive depression in their adolescent because of marital discord, alcoholism, the death of one parent, divorce, or by applying oppressive control. In any situation like these, the feeling of loss and helplessness may be so great as to cause a severe depression. This demonstrates the fact that every adolescent, even though he is undergoing separation from his parents and his home, needs at the same time external support to affirm that the benevolent caring functions of his parents provide him with a feeling of security. Thus, it assures him a sense of continuity between the past, the present, and the future. When this is lacking, developmental disorganization is to be expected.

Excessive parental control, especially in adolescence, may render the adolescent helpless to deal with the increasingly powerful sexual and aggressive drives. This was the case with an eighteen-year-old daughter of two overly protective and controlling parents. She had gone to college away from home and had become depressed, withdrawn, tearful, and amenorrheal. The separation from her parents and the unconscious need to repress the sexual drive in this vivacious girl precipitated this reactive depression. The parents had created in this patient and her sister severe superego control. However, the parents showed a sensitive understanding of the problem and the patient also responded favorably to brief psychotherapy, which led to a resolution of the symptoms, including the amenorrhea.

Another example of a reactive depression caused by the arbitrary rigid control of obsessional parents was seen in their sixteen-year-old son. He became depressed, agitated, restless, and unable to concentrate. The onset was acute when he felt victimized by his parents who prevented him from playing tennis on a Saturday morning with a girl whose company he enjoyed because her parents were not home. They also delayed his request to take driver education. Throughout childhood he conformed to these restrictive expectations. In adolescence he turned from his parents to his peers for support, and they tried to make him feel better without success.

His mother always smothered him with directives and his father overwhelmed him with logic. He felt he was in "a straitjacket and I flipped. My parents harass me with 'Did you do anything interesting today?' or 'Did you get along better today?' and I don't feel that pitiful." His anger paralyzed him. His greatest worry was how to stop worrying, and he was burdened with a feeling of diffuseness about his own identity.

In psychoanalytically oriented treatment which lasted a year he explored his relationship to his parents, his older sister and a younger brother, his rivalry with his peers, and his expanding peer-group relationships. His depression lifted and he became once again creative, original, and imaginative. Friends enriched his life and he achieved academic success.

His parents were seen twice, and several times there was communication by phone. They stressed academic achievement, proper manners, and social responsibility. Both parents responded to their own adolescent changes with ascetisicm and intellectualization and found little pleasure except in their studies. The patient was held to the same expectations. They were confused and bewildered because whatever they tried in order to help their son failed. The parents eagerly acquiesced to my recommendations and responded more appropriately to the psychological needs of their son, who with tolerance accepted their shortcomings.

When an adolescent is overly depressed parents usually respond with mutual concern. However, the adolescent with a masked depression may create intense anger between parents. This type of adolescent is difficult to live with due to acting-out behavior, such as being disrespectful, flippant, defiant, and delinquent. The adolescent may secretly use marijuana and alcohol, truant, defy curfew, and seek out the companionship of an acting-out group. Obviously, it is difficult for parents to respond with empathy to this type of behavior. Frequently one parent, most often the father, rejects his child while the mother masochistically tries to salvage him. Sometimes other siblings resent the attention the depressed adolescent gets and attack or demean him.

As an illustration of masked depression, a fourteen-year-old adolescent was referred because of rebellious behavior at home and at school. At home he brooded, looked unhappy, felt destroyed by his parents, and was defiantly passive with outbursts of anger. School performance was dismal. He sought the companionship of friends his age who gave him marijuana and other drugs. His mother was depressed and passively withdrew from him. His father, a mathematician with high moral and academic standards, persisted with exhortations and restrictions to try to control him.

The patient came from a large family which appeared to be well adjusted aside from the difficulty experienced with the patient. Until his thirteenth year he was a good student and conformed to his parents' expectations. From then on, with the surge of the increased sexual and aggressive drives overwhelming him, his behavior deteriorated. In the diagnostic study he was confused, defiant, and hostile, especially toward his parents, although he thought his father was fair to him. He was bewildered, wanted closeness and security but felt adrift. Life had no meaning to him, and he had thoughts of suicide. As his parents tried to elicit his cooperation, he became more rebellious and left home. In several days he returned, defeated and in despair. Later he tried to stab himself and his father. Hospitalization was necessary, and there he was seen as a loner, depressed and passive, with an impaired sense of self-esteem.

The parents, devoutly religious, expected uncompromising compliance to which he was too sick to respond. The mother, who came from a broken home and had an unhappy childhood and adolescence, helplessly withdrew from the situation. The father, a stable, kind but stern man, initially responded to his son's illness by attempting to guide him, or by reacting with a feeling of betrayal and anger. The prehospitalization therapy was with the father and son or with the father alone when the son would not come. Treatment was oriented toward the father's need to be logical in order to modify his over-determined punishment and to sustain his empathic concern for his son. He needed to understand the principles associated with decision making. The son, when present, participated in this but was helpless to modify his behavior at home and in school. An antidepressant was prescribed which gave only slight relief. As the crisis was reached, the father, with constant communication with me, effectively arranged for the hospitalization of his son. It is my belief that in this type of depression where alienation is the primary defense of the ego the relationship to the parents is totally repudiated, the intensity of the drives is overwhelming, and the depression carries a guarded prognosis. Prolonged illness may result in character traits of chronic despair, futility, and mediocrity.

Suicide, although it occurs infrequently, is of higher incidence among adolescents. Depressed adolescents often express the wish to die or the fear of dying, and they also reflect this theme in dreams about violence and destruction. Such symptoms always require careful monitoring. No family ever totally recovers from such a tragedy. It invariably remains a dreadful loss and burdens the family with unresolved guilt, remorse, and grief even if it becomes buried as a family secret.

Finally, it is impossible to avoid remarking about the dilemma experienced by parents when they try to decide which adolescent activities they will accept and which they will not tolerate. Pressure on the parents by adolescent society and by changing social values and style of life often cause the parents to react with bewilderment, uncertainty, and at times with helpless compliance. There is no questioning the fact that family mobility, educational trends, economic factors, the entertainment industry, war, and legislation have fragmented the extended and weakened nuclear family. All of these factors tend to increase the burden felt by the parents of depressed adolescents, and these parents need guidance in dealing with such social contaminants. The characteristics of the child's superego formation in adolescence is the crucial factor which determines how the adolescent handles the age-specific tasks of this period of life. If parents are not able to feel secure in the parental role, the resultant defective superego development and fragile identification, although common to all disorders of adolescence, leave adolescents burdened with despair and overwhelmed by the tasks of this period of life.

Conclusions

The focus of this chapter is on the response of parents to a child suffering from depression during adolescence. Whereas the depression is intrapsychic and represents a disorganization of psychic development in the adolescent, the response of the parents is to an external situation, that is, to the depressed adolescent. Their reactions are based on multiple determinants, both past and present, in which structure formation is consolidated.

This parental response is transactional and multidetermined. It depends on the severity of the psychopathology of the adolescent and the character structure of the parents; their transferential reactions based on their childhood and adolescent experiences; their relationship to each other; their ongoing attitudes toward the adolescent society; and their family, social, and occupational responsibilities. The assessment of these qualities in the parents is essential to the treatment of the adolescent.

REFERENCES

Anthony, E. J. 1970. The reaction of parents to adolescents and their behavior. In E. J. Anthony and T. Benedek, eds. *Parenthood*. Boston: Little, Brown.

Bell, A. 1961. The role of parents in adolescence. In A. L. Lorand and H. L. Schneer, eds. *Adolescence: Psychoanalytic Approach to Problems and Therapy*. New York: Hoeber.

Berman, S. 1970. Alienation: an essential process of the psychology of adolescence. *Journal of the American Academy of Child Psychiatry* 9:233–250.

Blos, P. 1968. Character formation in adolescence. *Psychoanalytic Study of the Child* 23:245–263.

Blos, P. 1979. *The Adolescent Passage*. New York: International Universities Press.

French, A., and Berlin, I. 1979. *Depression in Children and Adolescents*. New York: Human Sciences.

Freud, A. 1958. Adolescence. *Psychoanalytic Study of the Child* 13:255–278.

Jacobson, E. 1961. Adolescent moods and the remodeling of psychic structures in adolescence. *Psychoanalytic Study of the Child* 16:164–183.

Newman, M. B., and San Martino, M. R. 1976. Adolescence and the relationship between generations. *Adolescent Psychiatry* 4:60–71.

Spiegel, L. A. 1972. The experience of separation-individuation and its reverberations through the course of life: with special reference to adolescence and adulthood. Paper presented at the meeting of the Association for Child Analysis and the American Psychoanalytic Association, Dallas, May.

ALLAN Z. SCHWARTZBERG

Recent statistics indicate that since 1975 there have been over a million divorces, each one involving an average of 1.22 children. At present, it is estimated that over 10 million children live in fatherless homes because of a rapidly accelerating divorce rate. Approximately one out of six children under eighteen has experienced parental separation and divorce. Currently, only 8.4 percent of children in single-parent families reside with their fathers (Hetherington, Cox, and Cox 1977; U.S. Bureau of the Census 1975). Thus, the most frequently found family situation in the immediate separation and postdivorce period is one in which the children live with the single mother and have intermittent or no contact with the father.

While many studies have looked at the psychological effects of the divorce process upon children, few have considered the reactions of adolescents to divorce. Similarly, there have been few direct behavioral observations of a nonclinical population of adolescents at the time of parental divorce and still fewer controlled studies (Hetherington 1972; McDermott 1968). It is the purpose of this chapter to review some of the significant literature on the psychological effects of divorce on adolescents and to summarize clinical observations of adolescents from single-parent families seen in private psychiatric practice.

Review of Relevant Literature

It is impossible to generalize about the psychological effects of the parental divorce process on adolescents as a whole, and it is difficult to separate clearly the effects of divorce per se from those of the preceding trauma and stress. Anthony (1974) observed that adolescents' reactions depend on age, stage of development, sex, quality of early environment, amount of stress previously experienced, and the ability of the parents to provide security. Bowlby (1952), in an article on the effects of maternal deprivation, noted that reactions also depended on the length and degree of deprivation and the availability of mother substitutes. Additional adolescent reactions depend on the nature and extent of family disharmony prior to the divorce, the parents' and adolescents' personality structures, the parents' relationship during the separation and divorce periods as well as their relationships with the adolescent, and the coping capacity of the adolescent. McDermott (1968) noted the importance of recognizing and differentiating several factors: (1) the direct impact on the child of the strife surrounding the divorce; (2) the immediate reaction of the child to the loss of the parent; (3) the impact of the divorce on the remaining parent and the reverberations of that impact on the child; and (4) the impact at a later date of the loss of the parental model.

Anthony (1974) noted that the first risks for children of divorce are: (1) psychiatric disturbance during childhood, either acute, as in a traumatic neurosis, or chronic maladjustment at home or at school; (2) a rejection of marriage as an unsatisfactory mode of human relationship, or repetition of an unsuccessful marriage ending in divorce; and (3) the development of psychiatric illness in adult life. He described how the nature of marital conflict prior to the divorce influenced subsequent psychological reactions in children and adolescents. A hostile parental relationship resulted in increased irritability and aggressiveness, whereas a neurotic parental relationship—in which children are frequently exploited as scapegoats, manipulators, and allies of the battling parents—led to unconsciously transmitted feelings and excessive guilt. The so-called devitalized marriage, an emotional divorce without overt hostility, created an emotionally blunted reaction in children and adolescents.

In the psychoanalytic literature, many authors have written on the effects of object loss during childhood and adolescence—Deutsch (1937), Laufer (1966), and Neubauer (1960) prominent among them. Most writers tend to focus on the psychological consequences of the loss as it affects the establishment and maintenance of object constancy, the ability to mourn for and to relinquish the lost parent, failure to accomplish developmental tasks, the connection between bereavement and delinquency, and problems in identification and sexual identity. It is surprising to note that relatively few papers consider the specific dynamic interactions of the child or adolescent with the remaining parent and how this relationship may affect future mental health.

Neubauer (1960) described a girl whose father abandoned the family shortly after her birth. He noted that the absence of one parent precluded "oedipal reality'' and concluded that his young patient proceeded in her sexual identification from an initial phallic ambivalence to a state of pseudolatency without having ever mastered the oedipal conflict. He credited the child's relative health to the mother's influence. Neubauer emphasized the increased vulnerability and probability of problems in sexual identification and superego development. He cautioned, however, that the effect of parental loss would be influenced by such variables as the developmental stage of the child at the time of the loss, the child's sex, and, most important, the child's relationship with the remaining parent.

Despert (1962) stated that an "emotional divorce," in which the parents remain together though incompatible, was probably more damaging to children than the legal event of divorce itself.

Westman, Klein, Swift, and Kramer (1970) described divorce as a process rather than an effect. They stated that divorce only alters the form of the family relationship instead of causing the comparatively abrupt loss or bereavement with its associated grief and guilt. Westman et al. noted that approximately one-third of divorces were followed by turbulence that could be pathogenic for children, with conflict situations including: (a) parent-centered postdivorce turbulence related to perpetuation of conflict; (b) child-centered turbulence with manipulation of parents by children in an effort to bring about either continuation of parental conflict or to promote reunion; (c) parent and child turbulence in which one parent and a child are in alliance in manipulating the other parent; and (d) relative-induced turbulence with an exacerbation of conflicts by relatives and in-laws.

Kalter (1977), in a data analysis of 400 children in an outpatient psychiatric population, noted that twice as many children of divorce were seen as other children in the general population.

STRESSES IN THE SINGLE-PARENT FAMILY

Hetherington et al. (1977) have described some of the stresses in the single-parent family. These are: (1) task overload; (2) financial distress; (3) social isolation·and loneliness; and (4) the presence of only one socializing agent. The authors stressed that it was not so much father absence which contributed to psychopathology in children as it was the multiple stresses upon the mother. Task overload includes not only the provision of emotional support, comfort, and financial security but also the need to enhance self-esteem and to provide an effective role model as a single-sex parent. Additional stresses include the need to perform the multiple functions of homemaking, often in addition to holding a job, as well as daily decision making, all without benefit of a spouse. Maintaining discipline is often a problem, frequently marked by inconsistency, overpermissiveness, or overcontrol.

ADOLESCENT DYNAMICS AND THE DIVORCE PROCESS

The tasks of adolescence include coping effectively with aggressive and sexual drives, the development of a stable ego and sexual identity, the development of ego autonomy, appropriate separation-individuation, establishment of a stable moral code, vocational choice, and, eventually, heterosexual object choice. Related issues concern development of peer acceptance with a sense of social belonging and comfort in heterosexual relationships. Blos (1962), Erikson (1959), and Freud (1958) are among the prominent writers to deal with the adolescent's need for appropriate mastery of phase-specific tasks in order to proceed to true adulthood and heterosexual identity formation. Blos (1962) summarized the process as follows: "The adolescent process proceeds from a progressive decathexis of primary love objects to increased narcissism and autoeroticism to heterosexual object finding. It involves a detachment of psychic institutions from the parental influence. This process of detachment is accompanied by a profound sense of loss and isolation equivalent to mourning" (p. 125).

Wallerstein and Kelly (1974) remarked that the interplay between the divorcing adults and between each parent and the adolescent posed a very specific hazard to the normal adolescent process of progressive decathexis of the primary love objects. They observed that, while there was the potential hazard of severely overburdening the adolescent ego, there was also potential for stimulating accelerated growth spurts toward adulthood if the divorce did not occur prematruely, that is, before the normal detachment had begun to take place. These authors described the following reactions to divorce in young adolescents: (1) a temporary interference with entry into adolescence, with regressive-dependent behavior; (2) a prolonged interference with entry into adolescence, with evidence of serious developmental disturbance; and (3) pseudoadolescence, with accelerated sexual and aggressive acting-out behavior.

382

Methodology

This chapter will present some of the effects of the divorce process on adolescents seen in private psychiatric practice. Nearly all of these adolescents were living in suburban, middle-class homes. Information was obtained from one or more consultation interviews or during ongoing psychotherapy. In most instances, one of the parents was also seen in an unstructured interview. In some cases, psychological test data were also available. A total of thirty patients were interviewed, twenty-two girls and eight boys. The length of time from separation to the initial consultation varied from four months to seventeen years, with a mean of 4.7 years. The mean age at initial consultation was 16.2 years. Thus, while psychiatric consultation occurred in mid adolescence, the loss was typically sustained prior to the onset of adolescence.

Results

Diagnostically, at least one-third of the adolescents were moderately to severely depressed; however, depressive symptomatology was present to some degree in nearly all. Depression was characterized by sadness, frequent crying spells, mood swings, easy fatigability, impaired concentration, withdrawal, academic underachievement, and often anorexia and insomnia. Depression frequently alternated with acting-out behavior. Seven patients were borderline and one was schizophrenic. Ten were diagnosed as evolving character disorders, and ten as significantly depressed. Prominent defenses included repression, denial, projection of blame, and acting out. Symptoms included runaway episodes (usually of brief duration), school truancy, stealing, lying, drug abuse, school underachievement, sexual acting-out behavior, and group delinquent behavior. Neurotic conflicts in several adolescents appeared as separation anxiety manifested by brief school refusal.

Six of the adolescents had histories of prior psychotherapy. These teenagers, struggling with already overburdened egos, experienced particular difficulty in coping with the trauma of separation and divorce. Nine were hospitalized at some point following parental separation, often because of suicide attempts by drug overdoses. These cases were associated with onset of parental loss in early adolescence, previous experience with psychotherapy, and preexisting psychopathology. It seemed quite clear that impulse-ridden, acting-out behavior served not only to defend against painful feelings of separation, loss, and abandonment but was also associated with a need to punish the custodial parent. Ten teenagers displayed enough ambivalence about parental divorce to try to find the most satisfactory life-style by alternately living with each parent. Six ended up staying with the father; all but one of these were boys.

In most cases, the initial reaction to the announcement of separation was shock, hurt, disappointment, anger, guilt, and a sense of abandonment, especially when the announcement was sudden and without warning, and when parental relations had previously seemed good. This was not surprising, since 70 percent of the cases studied involved infidelity, primarily by the father. The most intense reactions to the father's infidelity occurred in females who experienced the paternal loss as a kind of sexual rejection, thus complicating final resolution of the oedipal conflict. One fifteen-year-old girl stated: "The separation was a pretty big shock. I used to get pretty mad and angry; I'd yell and scream. Now I get more depressed than anything else." A sixteen-year-old girl whose father had left his wife for another woman after a previously close relationship stated: "I feel like I hate my father, but I love him. I must love him, but he angers me. He just broke up the whole family."

In a small number of instances, the predominant affect was one of denial, detachment, and indifference. A seventeen-year-old, sullen, acting-out young man, when asked his feelings about parental divorce, stated: "If that's what my parents want to do, that's their choice. I don't really know about their situation. I don't care."

A frequent factor prompting psychiatric referral was acute depression brought on by: (1) rejection of a girl by a boyfriend; (2) academic underachievement or failure; (3) social isolation and withdrawal; or (4) a runaway episode. With girls, rejection by boyfriends was quite common and clearly reevoked the original acute sense of rejection triggered by the loss of the father, the original love object. While the girls revealed fantasies of idealized fathers who would be loving, supportive, and protective, the boys were quite ambivalent toward the father's departure. Four of the eight boys interviewed were living with their fathers, and all of them described intensely ambivalent relationships. Five of these boys, diagnosed as borderline, were severely impaired in their psychosexual, social, and emotional development. There were five high school or college dropouts. The remaining boys exhibited considerable acting-out behavior and frequent drug abuse. There was evidence of distinctly impaired identification with the fathers and unresolved oedipal conflicts.

Parental Relationships

The vast majority of adolescents characterized their parents' postseparation and divorce relationships as either very difficult or virtually nonexistent. Only six of the thirty patients characterized their parents' relationships as fairly amicable. Seven adolescents described the relationships with the custodial parent as reasonably satisfactory. Reactions ranged from moderate to intense ambivalence to overt hostility and outright rejection. The girls continued to long wistfully for the departed father, even when he had left for another woman. In a majority of instances, there was a good deal of anger and blame of the mother for somehow "causing" the father to leave. Nearly half of the mothers exhibited a moderate to severe depressive reaction secondary to the separation and divorce. Five mothers became alcoholic. Associated with the depression were regression, loss of self-esteem, bitterness, rage, and a sense of helplessness, hopelessness, and isolation. All symptoms were exacerbated by mobility and a lack of social and family support systems. Since 70 percent of the case series were associated with infidelity on the part of the departing parent (usually the father), there was a profound sense of betrayal and abandonment, along with feelings of intense guilt and failure. Role reversal occurred frequently, the adolescent often feeling a need to assume a parental role, thus additionally frustrating the adolescent's own underlying dependency needs and interfering with phase-specific tasks of adolescence. A common pattern of acting-out behavior among girls included promiscuity and a high incidence of pregnancy and abortion. Another common pattern was a need to date men significantly older in a thinly disguised attempt to recapture the lost father. In general, the healthiest adolescents experienced only temporary regression in coping with developmental tasks. Their good coping ability was related not only to their own basic ego strength but also to a good relationship with the custodial parent (usually mother) who was able to demonstrate genuine caring and good adaptive capacity.

In general, three groups of patients emerged from this study: (1) adolescents with exacerbation of preexisting psychopathology; (2) those with temporary regression; and (3) those who made premature attempts at mastery. In the first group, the separation and divorce process clearly served to exacerbate the problems of their already overburdened egos. Many of these adolescents displayed borderline personality functioning or severe depression. Some were overburdened and required hospitalization.

The second group of patients revealed a pattern of temporary regression. These adolescents had enjoyed a relatively stable family life, had good adaptive capacity, and had a normal ability to cope with the tasks of latency and early adolescence. In these families particularly there had been little, if any, discussion of parental separation prior to the event itself; a conspiracy of silence was common. The resultant shock of parental loss was great, causing a temporary and partial regression; usually, with brief intervention, normal development was resumed. A third group was composed of those adolescents who displayed premature attempts at mastery of drives and separation-individuation. Many spoke about waiting until age eighteen "to split." They displayed precocious and premature sexual acting-out behavior and also had frequent runaway episodes. In girls, the upsurge of sexual drives combined to trigger the reactivation of intense oedipal conflicts and needs to act out the conflicts. In addition to sexual acting out, there was frequent drug abuse and generally poor impulse control. The boys revealed a high incidence of dropout behavior, antisocial behavior, lying, stealing, and drug abuse.

Case Examples

1. EXACERBATION OF PREEXISTING PSYCHOPATHOLOGY

A twenty-year-old girl presented symptoms of dizzy spells, anorexia, frontal headaches, fluctuating mood depression, and easy fatigability. All symptoms had been intensified by her inability to progress at secretarial school, despite prolonged training. As a child she was shy and retiring, a poor student with average intelligence. Her father, strict and self-righteous, had been highly critical during her childhood. In early adolescence, following the loss of a friend, she developed a school phobia and underwent one year of psychotherapy, with improvement. Later, she was sent home from college following a suicidal gesture. Both parents had stressed the need for a religious upbringing; she had attended religious schools all of her life. She was therefore shocked when her father moved out to live with his secretary, whom he had impregnated. The shock led to intense regression and further withdrawal. She remarked, "Mother has stolen my brother (an all-American boy). He gets all the privileges. Dad's got his girlfriend. I've got nothing." At consultation, a diagnosis of borderline personality functioning was made. Despite intensive psychotherapeutic efforts, her limited ego strength and coping capacity were overwhelmed, and she was subsequently hospitalized. Her mother had gone to live with a boyfriend, her father with his girlfriend, and the brother with another family. Total family disintegration had undermined her fragile security and self-esteem. At a three-year follow-up, she remains seriously impaired and clinically at risk.

2. TEMPORARY REGRESSION IN RESPONSE TO SEPARATION

A thirteen-year-old girl was brought in for evaluation and treatment by her mother, who had been successfully treated for depression several months earlier. The household had been quite turbulent and under increasing pressure, culminating in the father's departure for another woman. The teenager felt angry and hurt, yet still wanted her father to return. She described, in a wistful, sad, longing fashion, the idealized father of her childhood, of whom she had many pleasant memories. She stated that, one week after the separation, she confronted her father and told him, "If you really loved us, you wouldn't leave." The father was silent and left the house, making no subsequent contact. She noted frequent crying spells, self-preoccupation, mood fluctuations, and increased difficulty with attention and concentration. Academic performance dropped sharply; she began to experience herself as significantly different from her friends from intact families and felt comfortable only with children from single-parent families. Short-term crisis intervention, in which the therapist was not only supportive but also played the role of a transient ego ideal, allowed her to work through her mourning for the departed father successfully. She has enjoyed a good relationship with her mother, who has shown good adaptive capacity and worked through her own depression. She has come to terms with the fact that her father has not contacted her or the family since the separation. At a one-year follow-up, she is now enjoying school, is doing well academically and socially, and has begun dating.

3. PREMATURE ATTEMPT AT MASTERY

A sixteen-year-old girl was seen in consultation a week after a shoplifting incident. Previously, the family had returned from abroad simultaneously with parental separation. She had been a very bright girl with a high academic performance and a history of emotional stability; now her mother reported that she lied constantly, used drugs, and had recently forged her name to a

$1,000 savings account. In addition to poor academic performance, there were several brief runaway episodes. The mother described the daughter as alternately arrogant and charming. The mother remarked, "She can really snow others but has little depth. She'd like to be a great rock star and has told me that when she's famous she'd like to sing a song saying 'my father never helped me, he ran off with a younger woman.' " The patient presented herself as a cool, sophisticated young lady who acknowledged her desire to be a lead vocalist for a famous rock band. She denied any history of behavioral problems prior to her parents' divorce:

> We were really tight until the divorce, Dad and me, the whole family. I feel now like I hate my father. I hate him but I love him. I must love him, but he angers me. He contacts me once a week. I'm really angry. I feel betrayed. I'd rather learn from my own experience than be punished by being told what to do. I'd like my family to go through the shit they've put me through. It's called revenge. They all tried to run my life, Mom and my sisters. I don't agree with Mother about anything. Yeah, Mom's a nice, warm person, but I just don't agree with her values and bullshit like that. The divorce really didn't hit me for a year, then I felt like shit. I felt the whole thing was stupid. It never should have happened.

In this case, a combination of individual and family therapy interviews, including involvement with the divorced father, succeeded in interrupting acting-out behavior, lessening the intensity of angry outbursts, and improving communication with each parent. Despite repeated threats to leave home prior to high school graduation, the patient allowed herself to go through a delayed mourning process and became more realistic in her appraisal and perception of each parent. Psychotherapy helped her gain insight and greater control over her aggressive and sexual drives. To date, however, she has had no dating experience, feels wary toward boys, and is guarded in interpersonal and peer relationships. She speaks repeatedly of wanting to leave home and threatens to head for California upon high school graduation, never to return.

This case illustrates many of the affective responses associated with separation and divorce: (1) anger, ambivalence, sense of abandonment, loosening of superego and ego controls, acting-out behavior, and a wish for revenge; (2) abrupt deidealization of the father and projection of blame onto the mother because of the latter's being "too polite" to the father following his overt rejection of her for another woman; and (3) delayed response to separation.

Discussion

Anthony (1974) noted that the initial affect experienced by the adolescent following divorce was usually grief accompanied by guilt. Later responses included shame coupled with resentment. He noted that one of the most specific responses to divorce was the "neurosis of abandonment," in which every new relationship was approached apprehensively with the expectation of being rejected or losing love. The neurosis of abandonment has also been characterized by alternations between inner depression and outer aggressiveness, a grieving for the lost family unit combined with feelings of being small, weak, and intensely vulnerable. In this case series, depression alternating with acting-out behavior was prominent in a majority of teenagers. An outstanding feature was the feeling of being abandoned by the father, especially on the part of the girls, combined with an intense longing for an idealized father and projection of blame for the divorce onto the mother. Memories and fantasies of a father who would be supportive, protective, and rescuing were common.

Bach (1946), in a doll-play study of latency children with and without fathers, noted that the "father-separated" children had fantasies of an idealized father, whereas the control children's fantasies more often centered around the father's aggressive tendencies. He corroborated the impressions of Freud and Burlingham (1943), who studied fatherless and orphaned children from post–World War II Europe. They noted a tendency toward fantasy attachment to an idealized father as a characteristic feature of the father-absent group.

Patients most adversely affected were those with preexisting psychopathology whose overburdened egos were overwhelmed by the additional stress of the divorce. The majority of these cases were borderline or severely depressed. Additional stresses resulted in hospitalization or prolonged regression. The best coping responses were made by adolescents who demonstrated prior good ego strength, good relationships with the custodial parent, and minimal parental regression. There was a rough correlation between severity of parental regression with associated loss of self-esteem and severity of adolescent psychopathology. For example, nearly all of the mothers of borderline adolescents were themselves diagnosed as borderline. Loyalty conflicts were common, with intense ambivalence and guilt prominent in the series, as typified by frequent mobility back and forth between parents before final resolution of living arrangements. Many adolescents, during this process, coped with ambivalence by exploitation and manipulation of parents. In six cases the mothers' boyfriends' living in the home triggered feelings of intense anger and rivalry, since these men were perceived as intruders. Not surprisingly, the heightened awareness of parents as sexual objects reactivated oedipal conflicts and triggered further acting-out behavior. This behavior occurred simultaneously with the parents' inconsistent attempts to set limits on their daughters' sexual behavior. Often there was parental regression, with lowering of generational barriers and mother and daughter in direct competition for male attention.

Hetherington et al. (1977), as well as Kestenbaum and Stone (1976), noted that the best coping responses of adolescents depended on the mother's coping and parenting ability. This study is in agreement with those conclusions.

Wallerstein and Kelly (1974), in a survey of twenty-one adolescents seen at random, noted that, despite experiencing the parental divorce process as extraordinarily painful, the majority of the young people studied were able, within a year following the separation, to take up their individual agendas and tasks satisfactorily. They noted that the adolescents who appeared to do best were those who were able to maintain some distance from the parental crisis, a kind of strategic withdrawal, without impairing the capacity for empathy with at least one parent. In this case series, it was surprising to note that symptoms of depression, acting-out behavior, scholastic underachievement, and social withdrawal persisted far longer than has been reported generally in the literature for the normal resolution of crisis, roughly within a two-year period following separation. This may well be associated with a skewed sample representing a somewhat different population than the cases reported by Hetherington and Wallerstein and Kelly. The latter were cases from a nonclinical population not seeking therapy.

Conclusions

Thirty cases of adolescents coping with parental divorce and living in single-parent families have been reviewed. Severe depression was present in at least one-third of the cases, and to some degree in all. Three types of groups were noted—adolescents with (1) exacerbation of preexisting psychopathology and frequent hospitalization; (2) temporary regression with resumption of phase-appropriate tasks of adolescence; and (3) premature attempts at drive mastery and separation-individuation. Symptoms persisted for a far longer time than has generally been reported in the literature for the normal resolution of the crisis of divorce. Acting-out behavior was extensive in both sexes. There was a positive correlation between effective parenting by the custodial parent and good adaptation and coping in the adolescent. Timing of the loss appeared to be of crucial significance, as well as the quality of the custodial parent relationship. Hospitalization was associated with adolescents at high risk who had a history of prior psychotherapy, onset of loss at the preadolescent level, borderline diagnosis, and poor quality of parent-child relationships. There was a positive correlation between effective parenting by the custodial parent and good adaptation by the adolescents, even when the loss occurred in early adolescence prior to normal separation.

While effective psychotherapeutic intervention occurred with many adolescents, it is obvious that effective crisis intervention at the time of separation, when most needed, occurred all too infrequently. Few of the adolescents had the opportunity to work through feelings about the divorce prior to psychiatric consultation. A major effect of the divorce process appeared to be significant delay in resolution of the oedipal conflict as well as impaired identifications with the same-sex parent, particularly with boys. This study is in agreement with Hetherington (1972) that father absence contributes to impaired feminine development, since high evaluation of and reinforcement for feminine behavior for fathers are associated with positive feminine development in girls.

In the last analysis, efforts to help the adolescent cope with the parental divorce process should be preventive. It is important to identify children and adolescents at risk—not only to intervene early in the crisis of divorce but also to prevent the development of severe chronic psychopathology.

Additional data from well-designed research studies with larger populations are needed to further our understanding of the divorce process and its effects on children and adolescents. It is essential that the adolescent be able to integrate his or her losses, to express feelings of anger, loss, sadness, and abandonment, as well as the universal wish for reconciliation. The adolescent who successfully works through the process of mourning at the appropriate time can thus turn the crisis of parental divorce into an opportunity for further growth and development.

REFERENCES

Anthony, E. J. 1974. Children at risk from divorce: a review. In E. J. Anthony and C. Koupernik, eds. *The Child and His Family: Children at Psychiatric Risk*. New York: Wiley.

Bach, J. R. 1946. Father fantasies and father typing in father-separated children. *Child Development* 17:63–80.

Blos, P. 1962. *On Adolescence*. New York: Free Press.

Bowlby, J. 1952. *Maternal Care and Mental Health*. Geneva: World Health Organization.

Despert, J. L. 1962. *Children of Divorce*. Garden City, N.Y.: Doubleday.

Deutsch, H. 1937. *Absence of Grief in Neurosis and Character Types*. New York: International University Press, 1965.

Erikson, E. H. 1959. The problem of ego identity. *Psychological Issues* 1:101–164.

Freud, A. 1958. Adolescence. *Psychoanalytic Study of the Child* 13:255–275.

Freud, A., and Burlingham, D. T. 1943. *War and Children*. Edited by P. R. Lehrman. New York: Medical War Books.

Hetherington, E. M. 1972. The effects of paternal absence on personality development in adolescent daughters. *Developmental Psychology* 7:313–326.

Hetherington, E. M.; Cox, M.; and Cox, R. 1977. *Families in Contemporary America*. Washington, D.C.: George Washington University.

Kalter, N. 1977. Children of divorce in an outpatient psychiatric population. *American Journal of Orthopsychiatry* 47(1): 40–51.

Kestenbaum, C. J., and Stone, M. H. 1976. The effects of fatherless homes upon daughters: clinical impressions regarding paternal deprivation. *Journal of the American Academy of Psychoanalysis* 4(2): 171–190.

Laufer, M. 1966. Object loss and mourning during adolescence. *Psychoanalytic Study of the Child* 21:269–289.

McDermott, J. F. 1968. Parental divorce in early childhood. *American Journal of Psychiatry* 124(10): 1424–1432.

Neubauer, P. B. 1960. The one-parent child and his oedipal development. *Psychoanalytic Study of the Child* 15:287–309.

U.S. Bureau of the Census. 1975. *Current Population Report Series*. P-20. Washington, D.C.: Government Printing Office.

Wallerstein, J., and Kelly, J. 1974. The effects of parental divorce: the adolescent experience. In E. J. Anthony and C. Koupernik, eds. *The Child and His Family: Children at Psychiatric Risk*. New York: Wiley.

Westman, J. C.; Klein, D. W.; Swift, W. J.; and Kramer, D. A. 1970. The role of child psychiatry in divorce. *Archives of General Psychiatry* 23(5): 416–442.

TEENAGE PREGNANCY: AN
ANTHROPOLOGICAL, SOCIOLOGICAL, AND
PSYCHOLOGICAL OVERVIEW

SUSAN M. FISHER AND KATHLEEN RUDD SCHARF

It seems clear, upon sorting out complicated statistics, that what we now have in the United States is an epidemic not of teenage pregnancy but of teenage baby keeping. In 1957, there were ninety live births for every 1,000 teenage girls. In 1974, there were only fifty-eight live births for every 1,000 teenage girls. This drop is less precipitous than the drop in total birthrate, of course, and also less precipitous than the striking drop in babies being put up for adoption. Recent conversations with workers at the Family Planning Center, Fitchburg, Massachusetts, and at the Crittenden-Hastings House of Boston, a long-time placement for girls about to deliver, suggest that most girls referred to maternity homes in the 1950s were middle- and upper-class girls who gave their babies up for adoption, and that the rate of abortion of teenage pregnancies was probably lower than it is today. Now, in the 1970s, both the Fitchburg agency and the Crittenden-Hastings House see primarily lower-middle-class and working-class girls, 95 percent of whom keep their babies. We will not speculate at this juncture on the reasons for this rise in baby keeping or for the increase and lower age of active teenage sexuality. It is clearly the rise in teenage baby keeping that is a major source of the alarm generated throughout the land. (There is also some hysteria in this. Lorraine Klerman of the Heller School of Social Work, Brandeis University, points out in a letter to *Science* that 42 percent of childbearing teenagers in 1974 were married eighteen- and nineteen-year-olds.)

Some basic sociological points must be made. Though there are, obviously, vast individual differences in the psychological meaning of a pregnancy for each girl regardless of her social class, there are class differences in patterns of adolescent pregnancy outcome. For example, counselors at the Fitchburg family-planning agency report that most of their childbearing adolescent clients come from working-class families in the relatively depressed industrial towns of Fitchburg and Gardner. Many of these young mothers' own mothers were teenage parents; the main change seems to be about a two-year drop in the age at first birth. Women in such communities have long married young, often in response to pregnancy (Rubin 1976).

The notion of early childbearing as an interruption of career plans has little appropriateness in many communities like Fitchburg; most women expect intermittent low-level factory employment, initiated and interrupted in response to family needs. In such towns, the childbearing rate rises with the unemployment rate. For such girls, the high school diploma seems irrelevant to realistic life expectations. Similarly, when South Boston High School was closed or boycotted during the 1974 busing crisis, the pregnancy rate among nominal South Boston High School students soared.

It is important to note that working-class sixteen-year-olds with babies are not dramatically worse off than their contemporaries without babies. For some of these girls, heretic as it seems, beyond the filling of inner emptiness and the resolution of intergenerational symbiotic conflicts, pregnancy represents a thrust toward mastery and individuation. The Fitchburg observers find that pregnancies are seen by some of their adolescent clients as means to leaving the parental household.

As anthropologist Carol Stack argues in her study *All Our Kin* (1974), having babies also allows the formation of kin ties among the displaced black families she studied in a Midwestern city. A stable community network, often extending beyond the confines of the city itself, can be constructed through the exchange of child care and financial resources; even nonmarital parenthood creates such kin links. There are whole sections of American society where adolescent childbearing, with or without marriage, has long been common and will continue to be so. At the same time, abortion has become a relatively accepted solution to the pregnancies of middle- and upper-class American girls; a statistical rise in the abortion rate among such girls would be hard to prove since such abortions were usually done illegally before 1973, but long-time observers believe that they are seeing a rise in adolescent abortions.

Despite class differences in pregnancy outcomes, individual pathology may be the same for middle-class and working-class girls. The different maternity rates may only reflect the greater push for abortion by middle-class families and a greater number of alternative channels to displace the emptiness and psychological disturbance that can characterize all these girls, regardless of social class. The dynamics of the parent-child relationship can be the same, but sociocultural opportunities may make delay of instinctual gratification via pregnancy and motherhood more tolerable for the middle-class girl. The ability of middle-class girls to move readily into lessons, activities, college plans, and an open-ended orientation toward the future does not necessarily reflect genuine sublimations but may merely express alternative ways other than pregnancy to escape inner and outer conflicts.

One conclusion we have reached is that some girls are going to get pregnant no matter how extensive the intervention and prevention—not only for complex social and traditional subcultural reasons, but because of the peculiarly tenacious quality of the symbiosis within the maternal line. The pregnancy may reflect several overlapping psychodynamic issues: an attempt to replace a lost object, an attempt to cure the mother's depression, an attempt to avoid separation, or an attempt to overcome early deprivation through identification with the new baby. The baby may be a hostage to the mother/grandmother for the daughter's own liberation, with a subsequent development arrest at a phallic level.

These points were illustrated in supervising a twenty-four-hour intensive outreach program at Tufts–New England Medical Center. For some highly delinquent and depressed girls there was great success in defusing explosive aggressive behavior and in improving self-esteem and the quality of socialization. But where there are severe early deficits in nurturance and in the stabilization of an adequate self-concept leading to the need to have a baby early—be it as a gift to mother, a buying off of mother's hostility or despair, a continuation of a tie to mother—this dimension of character is most unresponsive to intervention. This is not as pessimistic as it might seem, however, because, regardless of the unconscious roots of the need for a child, the outcome of the pregnancy and the quality of maternal care given the new baby are deeply influenced by other changes that have already taken place in the teenager and her availability to guidance from her social worker.

Beyond these severely deprived teenagers, there are other girls, less deeply disturbed, who are amenable to briefer intervention and for whom pregnancy reflects an attempt to resolve an intense triadic conflict. Although there are always pregenital issues for such girls—just as for the previously described profoundly damaged ones there are always oedipal issues—the preponderance of oedipal conflicts makes this group of teenage mothers a happier prospect for psychotherapists and community workers.

The cohort of age nine to fifteen adolescent mothers presents a special phenomenon quite different in its impact on both mother and child from the fifteen to nineteen cohort. These little-girl mothers constitute a very small group with a proportionately high abortion rate and other special characteristics. The baby for the girl ten to fourteen is often a toy or cuddly creature representing, at best, a transitional object, at worst, nothing at all, a thing to be left in a corner.

The issues for the girl aged nine or ten to fourteen usually revolve around very early problems with mother; there has frequently been no fathering at all and, as among delinquent girls, there is a great longing for fathering. The difficulty is not only that the little-girl mothers' psychopathology may be greater; they simply have not experienced as much of life as older girls. Whatever intrapsychic meaning any experience has for an older girl—failure, achievement, separation—even meanings that seem to controvert any real value, they are still real-life experiences that can be the basis for later re-working and integration. The pubescent girl, if she delivers, becomes the mother shattered by the experience of childbearing. Her body image is not coherent enough to tolerate such massive change. Her physiology is simply not ready to handle another being growing within her and emerging from her. And, just as trauma is defined as that which shatters or deforms the enclosing vessel, so for these little girls there can be irreparable ego damage.

In general, then, we characterize three groups with obvious overlap: a group of psychologically deprived, perhaps profoundly damaged girls for whom a baby fills a deep narcissistic need related to faulty self-concept and primitive object ties to the mother; a group of better-integrated girls attempting an oedipal resolution through pregnancy; and another group for whom pregnancy represents an attempt at maturation, a rite de passage, kin ties, economic skill utilizations, or a tradition of their social group.

Perhaps we can understand better the diverse meanings of pregnancy for these different groups if we reflect for a moment on the general fate of adolescents in the United States when menarche occurs so much earlier and teenage life starts earlier and lasts longer. Latency in the United States is markedly shorter than it used to be. Teenage life, with its appropriately sexualized concerns, begins in many urban centers at age ten or eleven. A generation ago, these years would show conventionally ascribed latency tasks in full flower—the development of hobbies, same-sexed peer relationships around activities, solitary pursuits of great significance in developing resources for later aloneness and self-discipline, and the strengthening of autonomous ego structures.

Another change in teenage life, however, has functioned as a corrective to the deprivations for ego development that such a shortened latency could produce. There has been a shift in the character of object relationships among teenagers such that there is more nonsexualized interacting among boys and girls as friends and persons, a quality of relating reminiscent of latency. Sharing in groups coexists with the relationships that are (happily) based on sexual interest—and there are friendships reflecting genuine interest in each other based on qualities of personality that are not organized by heightened hormonal change. This provides a second chance for the peer group experiences of latency and is an enriching addition to teen culture.

Unfortunately, those girls, locked out of the gifts of latency by the culturally aborted premature adolescence, who then become pregnant and are prematurely and of necessity adult in their focus, do not have this second chance to develop the ego resources they need so much. Their psychological development is limited thereby. What is arrested in these girls is the completion of the tasks of adolescence which, for some, may already have been difficult because of earlier deprivations and conflicts. By tasks, we mean the following irreducible human developmental issues—not class bound: (1) nonsexualized socialization with a variety of peers, male and female; (2) the opportunity to regress in adolescence and thereby reexperience closeness and nurturance to gather strength for intimate relations at a more mature level; (3) reworking the superego by opening up identifications and testing boundaries—all in a more realistic manner, so that harsher, more magical superego structures are ameliorated; (4) developing skills and hobbies that further enhance autonomous ego functions to provide strength for disciplined tasks and the capacity for aloneness; (5) making a career choice—the preparations for nonlibidinal pleasures of adulthood; and (6) autonomous physical self-care.

To the extent that it is possible to effectively intervene to interrupt the impulse to bear a child in the psychologically vulnerable girl, the effort must be made ahead of time to promote self-worth and self-esteem in some setting that will gratify basic emotional needs. Relevant as birth-control information is, many observers suggest that perhaps only 10 percent of girls who become pregnant do so because they do not understand contraception. It is also clear to us that the setting required to help prevent pregnancy in the vulnerable girl has the same characteristics as the setting required to help the young pregnant woman. Such a setting must (1) provide a peer group of similar girls of the same age; (2) provide models of nurturance who nurture young mothers while showing them how to nurture their own babies; (3) provide models of admonition, rule givers who gently discipline young childbearing clients where indicated and become models of limit setting for the young; (4) provide structures to maintain and teach age-appropriate skills; (5) provide educational and career facilities for the further development of the childbearing girl; (6) provide adequate physical care for the pregnant girl and her baby; (7) recognize the role of the father, and acknowledge and involve him whenever possible; and (8) continue services and client contact beyond the separation-individuation phase of the child.

This last point is of great importance, although it is frequently difficult for nonprofessionals to perceive. Mother and child must be involved in continuous contact with the program-setting and modeling persons because it is at this time that these mothers have the most difficulty. It is at this juncture that most abuse and foster placements, as well as new pregnancies, occur, for this is the developmental phase that these mothers have never struggled beyond to achieve genuine autonomy for themselves. It is also at this point that the mother's overidentification with her child can make the toddler's first attempts at independent self-assertion most upsetting, provoking the ill-equipped mother to abuse or neglect. It must be noted that this aspect of the successful program setting seems to be the most controversial; it is at this point that social institutions and the community at large express the greatest hostility to young unmarried mothers. The most vulnerable moment for the mother and child is also the moment at which they are most subject to the punitive thrust of the community. Therefore, the need for this kind of institutional support is all the more profound.

Two programs illustrate these recommendations; one is in the northeastern United States and the other is in the South.

The northern program was started in 1969 as a continuing education program for pregnant girls. It was designed to remove girls who were continuing pregnancies from the public schools on the theory that they would "contaminate" other students by their very presence in public high schools; there was also some concern for their physical safety. Although pregnant girls have, since 1971, been legally able to attend regular public schools in the entire country, the northern program still serves thirty-five full-time students each school year. After primarily educational beginnings, it has gradually added a range of services which aim at assuring the physical and social well-being of pregnant teenagers. The education program, funded in part by the city public school system, employs five full-time teachers and provides a full range of academic subjects. There is a federally funded hot-meal program. Through a pastiche of local, state, and federal sources, the program now provides a full-time nurse for prenatal examinations and education. Crucially, three counselors, including one bilingual in English and Spanish, conduct a steadily expanding effort to develop the girls' self-image and ability to plan realistically for the future.

Counselors make home visits immediately postpartum and refer clients to other agencies in the urban area for needed services. Recently the program was able to add child care for babies aged one month to two years and nine months, allowing mothers to continue their high school education on the premises. A job training and placement program is presently being developed;

this will also include fathers of program infants. All services are located in a YWCA, which also maintains a preschool nursery which continues the care of client children when they are too old for infant care. Counselors report that their students encounter psychological and practical difficulties as their babies start to walk and talk, and that the extension of child care, employment, and counseling services from the prenatal to the nursery school period is crucial to the avoidance of further early pregnancies, welfare dependency, psychological problems, and even child abuse.

The program has already posted a very good record: In an area of very high repeat pregnancy rates among teenage mothers, administrators report only a 5 percent program dropout rate and an astonishing 5 percent repeat pregnancy rate.

A second program, in a southern state, was originally developed by a local school system. It had additional funding from several federal sources and received services from a local medical school. Originally developed as a separate academic school for pregnant girls, the school social service program requested a prenatal care program because of concern with pregnancy complications. The school had a part-time nurse and social worker who connected the absent or late prenatal care pattern of these adolescent mothers with financial and legislative problems. The medical school became interested in training medical students and residents in these high-risk pregnancies. Recruitment of two other part-time nurses then occurred, both mature women with several children of their own and a great deal of experience in community programs for school-age girls. They rapidly were cast in the role of mothering these adolescent girls.

Through innovative leadership, all the junior high school and high school programs were stretched to expand their functions so as to provide opportunities of understanding and social models. The English class read *Romeo and Juliet* instead of *Julius Caesar*. In the hot-lunch program, the cook became a teacher of nutrition. Child development, parenthood roles, and adolescent issues were addressed within the prescribed high school curriculum. In time, a peer community of girls developed with lots of sitting around, giggling, working together, and interacting with this variety of nurses, cooks, and teachers. The girls formed a club with pink and blue colors and a slogan, Babies Are Our Most Important Business.

Once babies were born, a special ancillary program was developed and funded to run child care through the second year of life. Observers found that the girls who had previously given babies up for adoption grieved for them while in this program, acknowledging a loss they themselves said they had not previously experienced. However, girls who left the program to have an abortion tended to repeat the pattern of further pregnancy and abortion. The girls who went through the program, however, and had their babies in this setting were less likely to repeat their pregnancies for at least a two-year period. The lesson learned was that quality child care takes time and can have more gratifications than repeated childbearing. The extended child care component of the program had the greatest resistance from the local established schools and social institutions; it was the last to be added and funded, the first to be dropped, and it provoked the sharpest punitive response to the girls from the larger community.

The programs described share a number of attributes addressed to developmental problems of adolescence and childbearing. It often appears that the problems associated with adolescent childbearing are in large part the same problems experienced by new mothers of all ages, exacerbated not only by maternal immaturity but by the withdrawal of social support in response to deviant behavior. Older, married first mothers are more able to elicit or purchase social and physical support services of the kind described in the program examples. Young childbearing is not abnormal in human terms; important social issues are obscured by the assumption that the problems of young unmarried mothers are the inevitable outcome of their own pathological behavior. Although the later age at menarche which characterizes most nonindustrial societies creates a biologically determined tendency to delay childbirth until the late teens and early twenties, ethnographic data suggest the importance of certain kinds of social and physiological support which can be recreated in our own society. Our society has the unfortunate convergence of a diminishing age at menarche and an increasing age at socially defined maturity. It is clear that many of the social problems of teenage mothers in Western societies are really an exaggerated, even caricatured, version of the problems of adult American mothers: isolation, the nonhormonal components of postpartum depressions, and lack of support and training for role change.

The anthropological literature describes many non-Western, nonindustrial societies with networks of social support and education for the incipient mother. The qualities of mothering are taught through communal task sharing that provides modeling and the opportunity for admonition as well as the opportunity to rework possible defects in the pregnant girl's approach to her forthcoming role. The capacity to share work in nonindustrial societies appears to be related to the ability to tolerate a pregnancy and become a good mother.

Films of the !Kung (Bushmen) of Southern Africa made by John Marshall (1975) reveal three generations of women—some pregnant, some nursing,

400

some grandmothers—holding children of mothers scarcely younger than themselves, laughing and playing while working at female tasks. There is a remarkable and moving quality of cooperation and enjoyment between these generations and an atmosphere in which the learning of skills and roles is lived out in the communal ties.

Those familiar with the classic ethnographic photographs and films of Margaret Mead and Gregory Bateson (1954) in Bali are struck by images of young children carrying and caring for children hardly younger than themselves; care for younger siblings and friends is a normal part of Balinese childhood, and adult supervision is provided in a continuous way such that girls approach their first pregnancies with considerable assurance of competence and the certainty that their childbearing years will be supported by a wide network of co-childraisers.

English anthropologist Audrey Richards (1961) notes the formalization of such expectations of lifelong childbearing support among the Bemba of Rhodesia. For the Bemba, age grades, ritually recognized peer groups constructed at the point of menarche among girls, entail ties of emotional and material support stronger even than kin ties. This kind of peer support will buffer new mothers who can share the needs of their developmental level with each other throughout life. The Bemba also display a series of institutionalized means of easing the transition from childhood to adult responsibilities; marriages are contracted before menarche, and the marital partners pass through a graduated process of brideservice, cohabitation, puberty rites, and parenthood. This is a culture that acknowledges incipient sexuality (puberty rites involve songs with heavy sexual references), tolerates such awareness, and yet separates sexuality from childbearing. In contrast, an obvious difficulty of American life is the ideal of bringing mature sexuality, marriage, economic adulthood, and childbearing together at once.

In his study of Southeast Asian birth customs, Hart (1965) describes culturally constituted mechanisms of physical nurturance, physiological admonition, and emotional support which also permit dependence on adult females outside of potentially difficult intergenerational kin relationships. Hart relates the pregnancy experience of Bisayan Filipinos: as soon as a young woman becomes pregnant she contracts with a midwife who begins a program of massage intended to maintain correct fetal positioning and prevent a breech birth. This massaging is accompanied by the inculcation of culturally approved rules for the pregnant woman, which include dietary and behavioral injunctions, as do American obstetrical visits. The mother/midwife relationship, however, is at once more egalitarian and more intense than most mother/

obstetrician relations; the midwife can provide a very maternal kind of nurturance and admonition while avoiding any of the separation anxieties between biological mothers and daughters.

Cultural bypass of a potentially troublesome intergenerational dynamic is not by any means universal. Hagaman (1977) reports that young mothers among the Lobir of Ghana usually stay in their natal households until after the birth of the first child. In this matrilineal society, female relatives other than the biological mother take care of the new mother as well, whether or not the biological mother is still present.

The two successful programs for pregnant teenagers described seem to replicate what anthropology has observed about those cultures which have to deal with pubertal mothers, that is, an institutional or cultural pattern involving a combination of modeling, rule giving, and nurturance. In the unconscious transplantation of the "primitive" models of teaching for motherhood, two problems for Western girls are solved simultaneously, problems that seem to be paradoxical. One satisfies the need for mothering by using a mother substitute who can effectively meet the basic needs of any pregnant woman as well as the special needs of the deficiently mothered girl, but one does it in a form that is tolerable to the adolescent girl who is so ambivalent about acknowledging such needs. A more mature woman, who has finished adolescence, can turn to her own mother for help because she has more or less solved her adolescent issues with her mother. Having a child early in adolescence before the separation process is completed complicates the normal regressive identification with the positive mothering experience.

Part of normal adolescent development is the quest for an ego ideal. The different role models in both these programs present a range of such available models in the external environment. The same figures that can nurture and educate these often inadequate psyches and be internalized as ego ideal figures for the adolescent part of the self can also be used to ameliorate early developmental failures, but this is done in a form that is tolerable to the girls in an age-appropriate setting.

Conclusions

Winnicott (1956) has discussed excellently the normal dedifferentiation of ego boundaries during pregnancy and after delivery. This state of openness and regression with the temporary fluidity of defensive structure that is normal in pregnancy can provide a very fruitful reworking and "second chance" for infant mothers in a proper setting. Perhaps these programs work best in separate facilities—their own school, with their own club slogans—outside the shared, nonpregnant culture, because they create a "holding environment" in which the mother-to-be is properly nurtured, perhaps for the first time in her life, and is, therefore, better able to hand down this newly discovered experience to her own offspring.

REFERENCES

Hagaman, B. 1977. Beer and matriliny: the power of women in West African Society. Doctoral dissertation, Northeastern University, Boston.

Hart, D. 1965. From pregnancy through birth in a Bisayan Filipino village. In D. Hart, P. Rajadhon, and R. Coughlin, eds. *Southeast Asian Birth Customs*. New Haven, Conn.: Human Relations Area Files.

Marshall, J. 1975. *The Wasp's Nest*. Cambridge, Mass.: DER Productions.

Mead, M., and Bateson, G. 1954. *Bathing Babies in Three Cultures*. New York: New York University Films.

Richards, A. 1961. *Chisungu*. New York: Humanities Press.

Rubin, L. 1976. *Worlds of Pain*. New York: Basic.

Stack, C. 1974. *All Our Kin*. New York: Harper & Row.

Winnicott, D. W. 1956. Primary maternal preoccupation. In *Collected Papers*. London: Tavistock.

CARLOS SALGUERO, EDILMA YEARWOOD, ELIZABETH PHILLIPS, AND
NANCY SCHLESINGER

Pregnancy and parenthood in the adolescent needs careful scrutiny because of the serious implications they bring to the young mother and her child. Each year we read of the dramatic increases in statistics on childbearing and abortion patterns. In 1976, for example, birth among fifteen- to nineteen-year-old women numbered 558,744 or 17.6 percent of all births. Births to females under age fifteen numbered 11,928. The number of abortions for females age fourteen and under were 13,291 compared to 11,639 in 1974. For fifteen- to nineteen-year-old women there were 300,956 abortions, up from 237,294 in 1974 (Center for Disease Control 1978).

The sociological and medical implications that these pregnancies and abortions bring to the adolescent population have been extensively reviewed (Furstenberg 1976; Grant and Heald 1970; Stepto, Keith, and Keith 1975; Zelnick and Kantner 1978). Psychiatric studies have been conducted to understand the intrapsychic motivations that lead the adolescent to become pregnant (Babikian and Goldman 1971; Baizerman 1977; Barglow, Bornstein, Exum, Wright, and Visotsky 1968; Cobliner 1974; Shaffer, Petigrew, Wolkind, and Zajicek 1978). Just as important are the psychological events triggered by the pregnancy which have profound effects not only in the psychosexual development of the adolescent but also in her mothering attitudes toward her offspring. Of special concern should be how the emotional well-being of each pregnant adolescent and her child are affected by this event. For the adolescent, who is in the midst of profound life changes before having successfully negotiated the crisis of adolescence and who is in the process of developing a sense of self, the impact of motherhood and a baby, who will soon attempt to assert his own autonomy and individuality, may prove overwhelming.

This chapter is an initial report of our experiences in a comprehensive teenage pregnancy program for infants and their adolescent mothers who live in an inner-city neighborhood and who were considered by the program to be at risk for failure to thrive and for child abuse and neglect.[1]

The Teenage Pregnancy and Parenting Program (TAPPP) was developed to provide continuous psychological and social support to sexually active adolescents, pregnant adolescents, and young mothers and their children and to coordinate the services offered to them by the Hill Health Center.

The Center is a community controlled health facility that provides comprehensive health services. This is accomplished by three interdisciplinary teams made up of (1) physicians (pediatricians, internists, and obstetricians); (2) nurses (public health, pediatric, midwives, and family practitioners); and (3) community health workers, nutritionists, dentists, and mental health specialists (child psychatrists, social workers, special education teachers, and psychologists). A pharmacy and a laboratory provide support services. The number of persons presently enrolled at the Center is 12,500. Hospital services are provided by Yale–New Haven Hospital, six blocks away from the Center. The local middle and high schools are within walking distance.

The population of the community is 21,000 according to the 1970 U.S. Census. Forty percent are black; 30 percent Hispanic, and 20 percent white. Thirty-nine percent of this population is comprised of children and adolescents, ages thirteen to eighteen. Over one-third of the population are on state or city welfare. The median income for a family varies from $3,500 to $7,000 a year. The unemployment rate is 12 percent and in the Hispanic population this figure is significantly higher.

The TAPPP program is able to offer a full range of services to its clientele. In addition, a teenage health, parenting, and family life consortium, drawing from the expertise of its component agencies, is developing educational strategies to prevent adolescent pregnancy. It also assists the pregnant adolescent to remain in school and, when appropriate, to continue after the baby's birth. Young mothers who do return participate in special parenting activities as part of their high school curriculum.

Several concerns led the Center's mental health services department to develop the teenage pregnancy and parenting program: (1) Data obtained for the year 1976 revealed that a high number of adolescents at the local high school were pregnant. Of the 113 children referred for clinical evaluation and treatment, forty-two (37 percent) were born to adolescent mothers. In the same year, of the fifty-five cases diagnosed as child abuse and neglect, 34.5 percent were born to adolescent mothers. (2) Surveys revealed that adolescent girls did not use readily available prenatal and other allied services until the last trimester of pregnancy. Except for individual cases known to us or referred by obstetricians, very little was known of the adolescents' social, educational, and psychological situation prior to or after having the baby. Often, our only follow-up occurred when the adolescent became pregnant a second time. (3) The most important reason was our serious concern that the psychological trauma of pregnancy would damage the adolescents' emotional well-being and increase the risk potential for the infants' emotional and physical development—especially for failure to thrive and for child abuse and neglect. Our staff was painfully aware of the many circumstances which led many of the adolescents to become pregnant and the poor social conditions existing in the catchment area which made them vulnerable to early pregnancies. Yet, the most important question we asked ourselves was, Which adolescents are ready for parenthood? and Which factors separate the ones who are prepared from the ones who are not? If adolescents are trying to define their own identities, is it possible for a teenage mother to be ready to recognize her child as separate from herself and to have developed the inner psychological mechanisms to be attentive to her infant's needs and establish a meaningful and long-lasting relationship? Thus, protecting the often fragile mother-infant bond has become one of the most important goals of our program.

The program, initiated in 1976, is a service delivery model and is open to any adolescent who comes to the Center. The data collected in our studies have been obtained through regular clinical interviews with the adolescents seeking health care at the Center. One hundred fourteen teenagers participated in the program from November 1977 to November 1978, the first year the grant was funded. Of the 114 pregnancy test results, forty-six (40 percent) had a negative test result, and sixty-eight (60 percent) had a positive test result. Eighteen teenagers with negative pregnancy tests returned for a second test of which nine were positive and nine were negative. Two adolescents returned a third time, one had a positive and another a negative test. Seventy-eight of the teenagers, therefore, became pregnant during the year. Of these, fifteen proceeded to terminate their pregnancy while the overwhelming majority chose to carry to term. Only one of the fifteen teenagers choosing abortion was Hispanic.

Typically, an adolescent becomes involved with TAPPP when she requests a pregnancy test. She is then assigned a primary worker (PW), who is usually a social worker. The PW shares the results of the pregnancy test with the adolescent, makes an assessment of those factors leading to the request, and provides her with contraceptive counseling. There is clinical follow-up for those teenagers with negative pregnancy tests and those choosing termination of pregnancy. Teenagers choosing to carry to term are followed closely by the PW to ensure that they keep all prenatal appointments and receive nutritional counseling and dental care. Efforts are made for the adolescent to remain in school. When the adolescent reaches her seventh month of pregnancy, she is invited to participate in parenting classes and discussion groups to prepare her for labor and delivery and for her return home with her baby. At the same time, a clinical determination of how much at risk her child will be for failure to thrive, for neglect, and for abuse is made. This is based on a series of factors that are reviewed after the birth of the baby and every three months during the child's first year of life; thereafter every six months for infants considered at minimal risk; and every three months for those at high risk and moderate risk until the child is four years old when he can receive the benefits of other special state and federal programs if needed.

The need to make an assessment of how much an infant is at risk for abuse, neglect, and failure to thrive was derived from our observations that some adolescents were quite happy and accepting of their pregnancies. These adolescents continued to do well after delivery and provided excellent mothering care. We considered their infants as being at minimal risk. By contrast, another group of adolescent mothers did not appear to relate at all to their pregnancies. After delivery, this detachment either continued or their home situation worsened. Often their babies ended up in the hospital with medical problems and/or failure to thrive (high risk). Still another group related to their pregnancies in an ambivalent fashion; at times they felt overwhelmed but responded well to environmental support, especially when it was lacking in their home or the home situation was chaotic (moderate risk).

A working definition of the different at-risk levels was developed to assess and determine the clinical course of action to be taken by the primary worker for each child and his mother. All children born to adolescent mothers were considered to be at minimal risk since they are potentially more vulnerable to suffer from attachment difficulties, medical problems, and suboptimal growth and development than children born to adult mothers. In addition, if appropriate psychological and social supports are lacking, they are at higher risk for failure to thrive, child abuse, and neglect. It was decided that the one to be placed at risk was the infant since it is totally dependent on maternal care.

The following are the at-risk definitions developed.

Minimal-risk child. A child considered under this category suffers only from minor or no medical problems at all. Physical and emotional development is within normal limits for age. Mother is in tune with needs and keeps all appointments for herself and her child. She also makes appropriate plans for both and is coping well with the stresses of young motherhood. She receives or avails herself of emotional and social supports when needed.

Moderate-risk child. This is a child who suffers from a reversible medical condition and/or developmental interference or delay. Another criterion for moderate risk is a child whose mother cannot cope successfully with the demanding tasks of motherhood due to ongoing personal, family, or social problems. These problems interfere with the mother's ability to care optimally for her child and are manifested by not keeping appointments for herself and her child and often feeling overwhelmed by her child's demands. The young mother does express positive feelings toward her child.

High-risk child. A child who is suffering from a serious medical condition is at high risk for failure to thrive, for child abuse, and neglect when mother is definitely not coping with her mothering responsibilities. This may be due to serious problems of a personal, family, or social nature which have led to a negative perception of herself and her child, observed by a very poor quality of interaction with her infant, expression of negative feelings, total failure to keep appointments, and poor child care. A child can also be at high risk when his mother is facing acute problems which interfere with her ability to relate to her baby. By giving an at-risk designation to each case, it is felt that therapeutic strategies to help the young mothers can be better directed. A number of prepregnancy and prenatal factors are taken into account during the review which, when considered together, help the team decide into what risk category the infant and his mother should be placed.

Of great importance has been the isolation and study of those predictive factors that are believed to correlate directly with the different at-risk categories, since they further validated our clinical predictions. Lynch and Roberts (1977) have determined predictive factors for possible child abuse and neglect. These authors compared fifty children referred because of actual or threatened abuse with fifty controls born at the same maternity hospital. Five factors were significantly more common in the abused group than among their controls: (*a*) mothers under twenty at birth of first child; (*b*) evidence of maternal disturbance; (*c*) referral of family to hospital social worker; (*d*) baby's admission to special-care unit; and (*e*) recorded concern over the mother's ability to care for her child.

Servici (1979) reviewed a number of maternal variables of the first thirty-four teenage mothers followed by TAPPP in 1977 and correlated them with various measures of infant outcome at six months and one year. It was felt that, by better understanding these variables, the prenatal assignation of risk could attain greater validity, especially if certain maternal characteristics were

408

found to have more weight than others in the prediction of infant risk. Servici found that, of all the prenatal factors, two reached statistical significance in correlating with infant outcome: (*a*) the number of social problems in the mother's clinical chart and (*b*) the degree of the social worker's (SW) concern. He found that the more social problems noted in the mother's chart, the more problems noted in the child's chart. The comments written in the chart by the SW (degree of SW concern) were examined and scored as pointing to minimal, moderate, or maximal concern that the child would be at risk for subsequent neglect or abuse. This index of SW concern correlated most closely with the total number of social problems in the chart for the mother ($r = .49$; $P < .005$) and with the total number of maternal psychiatric problems recorded before and during pregnancy. The number of problems in the child's chart also increased with greater SW concern during pregnancy. The trend was similar both for the number of infant problems at six months and twelve months. Degree of SW concern correlated highly with the presence of pediatrician concern once the child was born. With a χ^2 value of 19.91 ($P < .005$) at six months and 10.45 ($P < .01$) at twelve months. Feeding difficulties were more common in the children of mothers about whom a high degree of SW concern was expressed during pregnancy.

Although the sample reviewed in this study was relatively small, it illustrated that certain predictive factors were consistently present which correlated with infant outcome. The most important of these factors was the index of SW concern. It also provided us with good justification to continue assessing the degree to which infants are at risk. As we have continued our at-risk assessment in our population of young mothers, we have found certain characteristics and trends for the minimal-, moderate-, and high-risk groups.

The determination of how much at risk an infant is often proves to be a difficult task. A young mother may be doing well when underlying problems surface or unsuspected circumstances arise that may place her child at high risk. Being at minimal risk certainly does not mean that adolescents can cope with all the demands and frustrations of motherhood. They should be considered as not fully mature, but as children who are better equipped than other adolescents to deal with the added pressures and demands of pregnancy. These adolescents still need active support and help from their families, other people, and agencies.

For example, Estela was sixteen years old when she became pregnant by her twenty-two-year-old boyfriend. She initially wanted an abortion, but then decided to keep her baby. She had good prenatal care. Labor and delivery of a 6 pound 9 ounce baby girl were normal. When her case was reviewed three months after Maria was born, Estela had married her boyfriend. The couple was living in their own apartment. Estela expressed and exhibited positive feelings toward her baby and kept all medical appointments. Baby Maria was placed at minimal risk. Estela was described as an assertive, mature teenager who, at times, was noncompliant with counseling and guidance because she wanted to try things her own way and because she perceived suggestions as being critical of her own mothering abilities. When Maria was six months of age, problems developed over a short period of time. Estela was upset by her husband's spending too much time with his friends and not being available at home. At the same time she tried to return to school but dropped out because Maria was making too many demands and was crying too much, especially at times of separation. Estela felt quite angry and resentful at Maria for crying and preventing her from going to school; at the same time, she felt guilty for having these feelings which were so contrary to her mothering image. She became anxious and depressed. She was seen in crisis intervention by her PW who by then had established a positive therapeutic relationship with her. Maria was placed at high risk.

The following factors are assessed at each review session to determine the degree of risk.

1. *Age.* It is felt by the clinical staff that most adolescents fifteen years old and under relate in a very immature, often childlike, fashion to their pregnancies. The younger they are, the less they exhibit maternal feelings. Very young adolescents center their attention on how the pregnancies affects them and their bodies: "It hurts when they draw blood," or "Will I be able to ride a bike?" are typical comments made by this age group. The infant's grandmother takes over the mothering role in many cases, while, in others, the infant has multiple caretakers. Greater difficulties arise in the fifteen- and sixteen-year-old group who are in the process of wanting to assert their own autonomy. They often rebel against their mothers, leave home, and live with other relatives. They may become "emancipated" minors and move to their own apartments. They lack, however, the necessary skills and strengths to fend alone with their babies and most soon feel overwhelmed by the many daily demands and responsibilities they encounter. Many adolescents in this group welcome the support given by programs such as ours. Older adolescents are more psychologically prepared to look after themselves and their babies. In their case, factors other than age play an important role in determining how they will relate to their babies.

2. *Adolescent's medical and prenatal history.* It is felt that an adolescent has good prenatal care if she has more than eight medical visits and three nutritional visits during her pregnancy, has fair care if she has between five and eight medical visits, and poor care if she has less than five visits or started her care in the third trimester.

3. *Infant health history.* Neonatal history, labor, delivery, and newborn information are reviewed. This includes type of delivery, use of anesthesia, birth weight, Apgar score, emotional condition of the young mother during labor and delivery, and hospital stay. Later, health-care history, growth, and development are constantly monitored.

4. *Maternal-infant relationship (MIR).* Our staff follows Bibring's (1959) observations on the psychological aspects of pregnancy. Bibring observed that an expectant mother after experiencing "quickening" begins to relate to her baby as another person, and develops appropriate preparatory anxiety about how she will mother her baby after birth. In our program, a great deal of attention is paid to the way a pregnant adolescent relates to her pregnancy—for example, making spontaneous comments about her baby, having or not having fantasies, dreams. A positive MIR score is noted when the expectant mother makes a direct positive comment about her pregnancy and her future baby. A "not known" MIR is noted when it is not possible to determine if the adolescent has any positive or negative feelings toward the baby. A negative MIR score is noted when it is felt clinically that the adolescent is not relating to the pregnancy or the baby at all. Soon after birth, the mother's attitude is reassessed in view of any neonatal or delivery complications, any changes in the mother or her family in regard to the baby, and the developing maternal-infant interactions.

5. *Family situation.* The relationship the adolescent has with her family, especially her mother who provides her with a positive or negative role model, is carefully examined. Interactions with other family members are also assessed, including the baby's father when he can be reached. While some of our adolescents have a history of being abused by their mothers, the most important variable in our family assessment is the presence or absence of a person who has provided the adolescent with maternal behavior and emotional continuity from which the young mother can draw in forming an attachment to her own baby.

6. *Marital and living situation.* The presence or absence of a boyfriend and his degree of involvement and support are considered. Only a few adolescents in our sample are legally married. Most adolescents do not have the idea of marriage in mind when they become pregnant, although some do expect financial help from and some do live with their boyfriends. Marriage itself cannot be considered a sign of maturity or stability, since, in most cases, for those who do marry, it is the girl's family who pressures her to do so. One of our cases, fourteen-year-old Carol, got married at thirteen, before she delivered her baby, and is getting a divorce at fourteen. She now has two babies. In the Hispanic population, younger pregnant teenagers traditionally move to their boyfriend's family home while sixteen- and seven-

411

teen-year-olds often move to their own apartment. Their boyfriends are usually in their twenties. Black pregnant teenagers tend to remain with their families and only a few move to their own apartments (Salguero, Suarez, Yearwood, and Schlesinger 1979).

7. *School attendance.* Many of the adolescents were experiencing school problems, and the trauma of pregnancy only precipitated their decision to drop out. This is especially true in the Hispanic population who, with few exceptions, have all dropped out and have not returned to school.

Many other contributing factors are considered at the clinical conferences, such as income, religion, and medical and psychiatric problems of the adolescent before, during, and after pregnancy. In addition, the continuous follow-up provides the PW with an understanding of the teenager's personality, strengths, and difficulties.

A very helpful tool in our program has been the review of the pregnant adolescent and the mother-infant dyad every three months. Many events take place in their lives during this period, and they help us to determine the type and the manner of intervention that seems most appropriate. For example, an infant considered at minimal risk at one review can be placed at moderate risk if an intercurrent illness occurs, or at high risk if there is a crisis at the next review. In ten of the fifty-nine cases reviewed, the infants were changed from one risk category to another.

In reviewing these factors at scheduled times, the main focus in assessing risk is how they affect the quality of the MIR. Poor mother-infant reciprocity, as described by Brazelton (1975), prevents the infant from learning successful mastery of his environment and may lead to severe failure to thrive in the first year of life and to definite signs of neglect and abuse later on. When the mother cannot experience affirming interactions, she is less apt to care for her infant appropriately. Thus, when the young mother is in need of support, the assessments during the infant's first year of life are important in determining how best to provide it.

Results

The cases reviewed in this chapter are fifty-one mother-infant pairs that were followed by TAPPP from December 1977 until April 1979. We have included in one of the three at-risk categories cases that have moved from one category to another and cases which have only one at-risk review (four cases) (see table 1).

TABLE 1

DISTRIBUTIONS OF INFANTS AND MOTHERS ACCORDING TO DEGREE OF RISK

Characteristics	Minimal Risk (N = 25)		Moderate Risk (N = 12)		High Risk (N = 14)	
Median age at delivery	17.7 years		16.4 years		16.3 years	
Prenatal care:						
Very good	18		3		3	
Fair	4		3		3	
Poor	3		6		8	
Mothers with 2 children	3		1		4	
Mothers with 3 children	0		0		1	
Maternal-infant relationship:	7-Month Prenatal	After Delivery	7-Month Prenatal	After Delivery	7-Month Prenatal	After Delivery
Positive	20	25	5	12	2	3
Not known	5	0	3	0	1	0
Negative	0	0	4	0	11	11
P W comments about mothers	Stable, happy, mature		Immature, passive, naive		Impulsive, noncaring	
Living arrangement:						
With family	16		7		9	
With boyfriend	6		3		3	
On their own	3		2		2	
Emotional support:	Family	Boyfriend	Family	Boyfriend	Family	Boyfriend
Positive	16	10	3	4	0	0
Nonsupportive	5	6	5	5	12	7
Not known	4	2	4	3	2	7
School:						
Return after delivery	13		2		3	
Did not return	12		10		10	
Not known	0		0		1	
Infant's health and growth	50th percentile height & weight; higher at one year; had all health checkups; 1 hospitalized (diarrhea)		40–50th percentile height & weight; missed some pediatric appointments; 2 hospitalized (diarrhea)		Under 40th percentile height & weight; missed scheduled appointments; 2 hospitalized (failure to thrive and diarrhea)	
Adolescent's psychological profile	Good ego-strengths; stable object relationships		Depressive elements; regression		Poor object relationships	

413

CHARACTERISTICS OF MOTHERS AND OF INFANTS
CONSIDERED AT MINIMAL RISK

Twenty-five of the fifty-one mother-infant pairs studied were mothers of infants at minimal risk. Their median age was 17.7 years at delivery. The youngest became pregnant at sixteen. Eleven became pregnant at seventeen. The prenatal care for this group was on the whole very good: eighteen had very good prenatal care, four had fair prenatal care, and three had poor prenatal care. In spite of receiving good prenatal care, four had cesarean sections due to cephalo-pelvic disproportion; a reminder that adolescents have a higher number of delivery complications than the adult population. For three mothers, this was their second baby. The MIR was characterized by an appropriate warm attitude toward their pregnancies and their babies by the majority of this group of mothers. At the seventh month of pregnancy follow-up it was felt by the PW and other staff that twenty mothers related positively to their infants. They expressed feeling happy about being pregnant and were looking forward to motherhood. A ''not known'' MIR was noted for the remaining five. Of these, one expectant adolescent stated that the reason for becoming pregnant was because ''I like children.'' The others appeared more concerned about how they were feeling at that precise moment in their pregnancies and associated little to their future babies. After delivery, the twenty-five mothers felt positive during the third-month and sixth-month postdelivery review. Only one mother had difficulties with bonding during delivery.

With few exceptions all the mothers were described as stable, happy, mature, motivated, and independent. At times, this independence had the flavor of adolescent rebellion. The adolescent wanted to feed the baby or raise him ''her way'' and, once she proved her point, she would follow the nutritionist's or pediatric nurse's advice.

As noted in table 1, sixteen of the twenty-five mothers lived with their own families and relatives, six lived with their boyfriends, and three lived on their own. The majority had a good relationship with their mothers (sixteen cases) and tended to follow their advice. For five, it was nonsupportive and for four it was not possible to determine. Typical of this group of mothers was their ability to mobilize their inner resources to elicit emotional support from their families, friends, and authority figures. Except for seven Hispanic mothers who did not return to school, thirteen mothers returned to continue their education. The remainder either chose to stay home or encountered difficulties that prevented them from returning to school.

All infants enjoyed excellent health and were brought to all health checkups and immunizations. Although their height and weight percentile dropped from the median of 55 and 65 to 35 and 40 during their six-month measurement, these percentiles have tended to even out at 45 and 50 at the end of the first year. Only one of the infants was hospitalized—for diarrhea.

In summary, it has been our impression that the young mothers in the minimal-risk group had very good ego strengths and stable object relationships. In spite of the many reasons for getting pregnant, they appeared to have accepted and felt quite comfortable with their experience. Yet, it did not stop them from pursuing their own interests or goals after having their babies, such as returning to school or working. Their ability to relate well to their babies and their positive self-esteem acted as a stimulus for growth in their infants while, at the same time, the mothers were well cared for and nurtured by their families or other significant persons.

CHARACTERISTICS OF MOTHERS AND OF INFANTS CONSIDERED AT MODERATE RISK

Twelve of the fifty-one mothers (24.5 percent) were considered to be at moderate risk. Their median age at delivery was 16.4 years. The youngest one became pregnant at thirteen. The remaining ages were scattered between fourteen and eighteen. Half (six) had poor prenatal care owing to their delay in applying. Two had therapeutic abortions before becoming pregnant a second time; and two wanted abortions, waited too long, and had to go to term. For one it was her second child. It was clear that these adolescents were ambivalent about their pregnancies. As a result, at their seventh month of pregnancy, five had a positive MIR but were placed at moderate risk because after delivery, detrimental family and environmental factors prevented them from providing their infants with optimal care, for example, bringing them to their health checkups. In three, it was not possible to determine how they felt about their baby. However, after delivery they related more positively to their infants. Four had a negative MIR during their seventh month of pregnancy. This changed after delivery to a more positive relationship but was still clouded with fears, anxieties, and ambivalent feelings toward the baby.

In nine cases, the presence of elements of pre- and postpartum depression was striking. During their seventh month of pregnancy review, seven girls appeared depressed and overwhelmed by the pregnancy itself, by the prospective new responsibilities they had to face, and by the demands that the babies would make on them. Other PW's comments made about this group were that they were immature, innocent, naive, and passive. Of the fourteen adolescent mothers, seven lived with their families, three lived with a mate, and two lived alone. Only three felt supported by their families, but for the majority, no emotional support existed and practical help was lacking. Their boyfriends, on the whole, were nonsupportive, and only four out of the twelve expressed positive feelings toward their boyfriends. Only two of the twelve returned to school.

These infants had a high number of missed regular pediatric visits. Two of the infants were hospitalized for diarrhea and vomiting in the first six months. One was born with a pulmonary-valve obstruction and another with an undiagnosed heart murmur. A third suffered from a congenital bilateral hip rotation. Half were behind in their immunizations at six months of age. At one year of age the infants remained in the 40–50 percentile in height and weight.

The psychological profile in this group of mothers is that of a fifteen-year-old teenager who becomes pregnant in order to deal with conflicts. Her wish is that the baby will bring her the care or nurture she so much wishes for herself. However, as delivery approaches in the third trimester, she realizes that the baby will make more demands than she expected. After delivery, many of the mothers go through alternate periods of depression and well-being. Plans to return to school usually do not crystallize. This group was receptive to therapeutic and emotional support. When problems arose, they sought help and assistance from those with whom they were acquainted and trusted.

CHARACTERISTICS OF INFANTS AT HIGH RISK AND THEIR MOTHERS

Fourteen of the fifty-one infants (or 27.5 percent) were considered to be at high risk. The mothers median age was 16.3 years old at delivery. Four of the mothers had a second child, one had a third child. The youngest became pregnant at thirteen years of age. Eight had poor prenatal care, while only three had good prenatal care. One adolescent wanted a therapeutic abortion but was too late.

Eleven mothers were characterized by a total inability to relate to their babies during pregnancy or after delivery. For example, a main reason for pregnancy in a fifteen-year-old was to get back at her mother. In four others, it was to please their boyfriends. These girls were generally described as immature and impulsive. Becoming pregnant was part of the very disorganized sociopsychological background they came from. Two related well to their pregnancies but faced serious problems at home. None of the fourteen adolescents came from supportive families. Seven lived with their families and/or other family members who had a serious history of alcoholism. Often there was overcrowding with other younger siblings in the home. Two young mothers lived with a sister. Two lived alone in an apartment and three with a boyfriend; seven did not feel supported by their boyfriends. Of the fourteen mothers, only three returned to school. Most of these mothers' infants missed their appointments and health checkups. Two infants were hospitalized at three and four months of age, one with failure to thrive and one for diarrhea and dehydration. Five other infants went steadily down from the forty-fifth percentile in height and weight at birth to the tenth and fifteenth percentile, respectively, at six months. As Servici (1979) reported in her study, this group of mothers had poor knowledge about nutrition and the introduction of foods to their infants.

In contrast to the moderate-risk group, many of the high-risk mothers were not described as depressed. They appeared to be more concerned and involved in their own lives and problems and did not appear to be receptive to therapeutic help. They were relatively unconcerned about the well-being of their infants and were quite comfortable in allowing their mothers to become the primary caretakers. The program's ability to make meaningful contact and to establish a therapeutic working relationship with these young mothers usually met with rejection. They did not want anything to do with agencies, professional people, or their babies. In spite of these limitations, TAPPP did everything to encourage mother and child to come to the Center. In cases where there were definite signs of parental neglect, signs of developmental delay, or a serious unexplained drop in the baby's height and weight percentiles, the protective services agency was notified. This agency was involved with seven of the fourteen mothers before the baby was born and with a total of ten after the birth. In other cases, mothers of infants placed at high risk wanted to relate and care for their babies, but serious problems, usually with the family, made it difficult if not impossible for them to do so. For example, fifteen-year-old Yolanda could not return to her home after delivering her baby because of the negative relationship she had with her mother.

417

Because a place could not be found for both, the baby was placed in one foster home while Yolanda was placed in another by the protective services agency. The baby was, therefore, considered at high risk, since Yolanda was unable to care for or attach to the baby.

Discussion

The purpose of this chapter is to give a preliminary report on a particular segment of the teenage-mother population that lives in a slum area where both psychological and sociological factors contribute to the high incidence and prevalence of teenage pregnancy. Due to the relatively small sample, our findings cannot be generalized, and most of the infants have not yet been followed into their second year. However, this preliminary study (Servici 1979)—by using infant-at-risk criteria based on a number of clinical factors— clearly indicates that all adolescent mothers cannot be lumped together or assessed adequately through cross-sectional observations or short-term studies. Adolescent mothers face similar problems but vary in their attitude toward themselves and their babies according to intrapsychic, developmental, and environmental factors, age, and the availability and acceptance of emotional and practical support from helping persons or agencies.

We developed our at-risk categories from the observed patterns of behaviors and personality characteristics exhibited by the young mothers and the strengths of the family support system. These categories are descriptive and not diagnostic. The staff were sensitive to the need for flexibility in using at-risk categories. At times there were clinical disagreements among the reviewers, but it was possible to delineate three clusters at the certain time checkpoints.

The changes observed in young mothers also was evident when there were two children, and a mother would relate quite differently to each child. In one case, the first child had always been placed at moderate risk due to his mother's ambivalence toward him. He had been the product of an unwanted pregnancy when the mother was fifteen years old. The second child, when she was seventeen, was wanted, and she felt happy about having him. She began to relate better to her first child, but never with the positive feelings she showed for the second.

Adolescent mothers whose children consistently remained at minimal risk had, on the whole, very good ego strengths which helped them to mobilize their inner strengths to cope with the crisis of pregnancy and to elicit the support of other people and agencies. These same strengths permitted them to look after their babies in as realistic a fashion as an adolescent can. Their object relationships were characterized as stable and mature. At times they wanted and were eager to try their own brand of mothering, but had realistic expectations of their babies and were in tune with their needs. Their own mothers were supportive and acted as good role models. This healthy mother-teenager relationship was a very significant predictor in the adolescent's own positive identity as a mother.

Adolescent mothers whose infants remained at moderate risk appeared depressed and unhappy. They used pregnancy as a means of dealing with their conflicts and low self-esteem by creating the fantasy of the "all giving and happy infant." In this group, were adolescents who wanted to have "something of their own." Depression, therefore, was a clinical symptom late in their pregnancy and during their baby's first year of life. Many were receptive to therapeutic intervention and slowly appeared to mature and to like and accept their babies. Yet they paid a high price. They were unable to keep or make new friends and appeared isolated and withdrawn. The demands of the new babies brought these girls' adolescence to an end and many seemed at risk for another pregnancy.

Mothers of infants consistently placed at high risk presented serious characterological and borderline characteristics. They appeared either to feel negative and unconcerned about their babies or to see them as a burden. Becoming pregnant was a form of acting out. Their babies were at very high risk for failure to thrive during the first year and for abuse and neglect during their second year. Their family backgrounds were chaotic, and there were no role models for these mothers to emulate. Their own mothers were in some cases having more children of their own and had very little time or love to give these adolescent daughters. The multiple traumas these young mothers experienced took away some of the necessary ego strengths needed to relate meaningfully to others or to feel attached to their infants.

From a programmatic point of view, the decision to place infants at minimal, moderate, and high risk has permitted the program to intervene with different levels of therapeutic intensity. The decision is not a therapeutic artifact but the result of observations the staff felt were valid and significant. Inherent in our sample is that all of the adolescents who have participated in our program have been followed continuously by our staff. Therefore, much of what has happened to them and their infants has been influenced by the nature of our interventions. From November 1977 to April 1979 only one of the cases developed failure to thrive as compared with six in 1976 before TAPPP was inplemented. So far, no child has been physically abused as compared with six in 1976. Yet, as we have noted, many of these infants will continue to be at risk physically and emotionally.

Conclusions

Extensive data have been gathered in our program about the social, educational, and medical problems a teenage mother encounters. The mental health needs of this special population as well as their infants' protection must be addressed. To date, there are only a few comprehensive programs that provide the protection of the emotional well-being of adolescents and their children as the main goals. The TAPPP program uses established mental health principles to implement an intervention program where each adolescent is monitored in health, social, educational, and mental health aspects. Assessments are made at regular intervals as to how much at risk her infant is for failure to thrive, abuse, and neglect. At the same time, TAPPP has developed therapeutic programs to help infants and young mothers. Our preliminary findings introduce the concept that pregnant adolescents and young mothers differ in their abilities to cope with their pregnancies and their relationships to their babies.

The importance of developing programs such as ours is obvious. Our concern should not only be that there is an epidemic of teenage pregnancies in the United States, but how to alleviate the trauma of pregnancy on the mothers and on their infants' mental health.

NOTE

1. The Teenage Pregnancy and Parenting Program (TAPPP) was developed by the Hill Health Center's Mental Health Services Department, New Haven, Connecticut. The Teenage Health, Parenting, and Family Life Consortium consists of TAPPP, the Yale University Child Study Center, and the New Haven Board of Education.

REFERENCES

Babikian, H., and Goldman, A. 1971. A study in teenage pregnancy. *American Journal of Psychiatry* 128(6): 755–760.

Baizerman, M. 1977. Can the first pregnancy of a young adolescent be prevented? A question which must be answered. *Journal of Youth and Adolescence* 6(4): 343–351.

Barglow, P.; Bornstein, M.; Exum, B.; Wright, M. K.; and Visotsky, H. 1968. Some psychiatric aspects of illegitimate pregnancy in early adolescence. *American Journal of Orthopsychiatry* 38(4): 672–687.

Bibring, G. 1959. Some considerations of the psychological processes of pregnancy. *Psychoanalytic Study of the Child* 14:113–121.

Brazelton, T. B. 1975. Maternal-infant reciprocity. In M. H. Klaus, P. Leger, and M. A. Trause, eds. *Maternal Attachment and Mothering Disorders*. Piscataway, N.J.: Johnson & Johnson.

Center for Disease Control, Atlanta, Ga. 1978. *Morbidity and Mortality Weekly Report* (November 17).

Cobliner, G. 1974. Pregnancy and the single adolescent: the role of cognitive functions. *Journal of Youth and Adolescence* 3(1): 17–29.

Furstenberg, F. 1976. *Unplanned Parenthood*. New York: Free Press.

Grant, J. A., and Heald, F. 1970. Complications of adolescent pregnancy: survey of the literature on fetal outcome in adolescence. *Clinical Pediatrics* 11:567–570.

Lynch, M. A., and Roberts, J. 1977. Predicting child abuse: signs of bonding failure in the maternity hospital. *British Medical Journal* 1:624–627.

Salguero, C.; Suarez, J.; Yearwood, E.; and Schlesinger, N. 1979. *Report: Teenage Pregnancy and Parenting Program*. New Haven, Conn.: Hill Health Center.

Servici, I. 1979. Adolescent pregnancy at the Hill Health Center: factors predicting infant development in the first year of life. Ph.D. diss., Yale University School of Medicine.

Shaffer, D.; Petigrew, A.; Wolkind, S.; and Zajicek, E. 1978. Psychiatric aspects of teenage pregnancy in school girls: a review. *Psychological Medicine* 8:119–130.

Stepto, R. C.; Keith, L.; and Keith, D. 1975. Obstetrical and medical problems of teenage pregnancy. In J. Zacker and W. Brandstadt, eds. *The Teenage Pregnant Girl*. Springfield, Ill.: Charles C. Thomas.

Zelnick, M., and Kantner, J. F. 1978. First pregnancies to women aged 15–19: 1976 and 1971. *Family Planning Perspectives* 10:135–142.

33   ADOLESCENT HOMOSEXUAL PATTERNS: PSYCHODYNAMICS AND THERAPY

LILLIAN H. ROBINSON

The realtive scarcity of studies dealing with adolescent homosexuality may be attributed to the acceptance of an allowable homosexuality in adolescence which, under favorable circumstances, is gradually replaced by heterosexual development (Adatto 1967; Fraiberg 1961; Group for the Advance of Psychiatry [G.A.P.] 1968). Although some have objected to this concept (Secarides 1978), those who accept a normal homosexual stage consider homosexuality in early adolescence comparable to sleep disturbances or enuresis in very young children who are expected to have these developmental problems and to outgrow them.

The purpose of this chapter is to examine the relationship of dynamic factors to prognosis and to consider the issue of psychotherapy for adolescents who are conflicted about sexual object choice and sexual identity—the conflicts which are the core of the intense identity struggle at this stage of maturation (Blos 1953).

Psychodynamic Factors in Homosexuality

Personality development is complex and every outcome is multidetermined. Disturbances in childhood relationships with parents are known to alter the development of object relationships in psychosexual development.

In infancy, strong attachments develop to caretakers. These ties persist through the toddler phase when the child struggles with efforts to become autonomous but still tries to cooperate and conform enough so that important relationships are not jeopardized. During the oedipal phase children develop erotic attachments to the parents, and upon giving them up shift some of their interest to friendships with peers of the same sex.

When sexual feelings are stirred up they are often directed toward these peers. The latency-age boy commonly has homosexual fantasies and engages with peers in such activities as comparing the size of the genitals, mutual masturbation, and seeing who can urinate farther. The choice for the object of his affection is narcissistic—someone like himself, or someone he admires and would like to emulate. This is the so-called normal homosexual stage which usually lasts into early to mid adolescence and has positive value because it contributes to the development of the ego ideal (Blos 1962).

Homosexually oriented activities are also quite common among latency-age girls. Adatto (1967) states: ''Spending the night with each other or exchanging sexual talk leads to considerable excitement. . . . Homosexual activity (during this period) is a step toward sexual mastery (both for boys and girls) . . . involving another person who is in some way safe for the time being.'' During adolescence, the choice must be made whether to move on to heterosexuality, and there is often much conflict during this period though most youngsters seem to handle it very well (Offer and Offer 1971).

The preference for a homosexual object choice in latency and early adolescence has been explained as a defense against castration anxiety (Pearson 1958). The boy avoids girls because the girl's lack of a penis is frightening to him. Similarly, the girl's preference for girls can be a means of denying feelings about boys' anatomical advantages. She may become a tomboy to prove that she is not to be outdone by boys. A crush on a best friend gratifies the repressed wish for a close relationship with her mother whom she rejects and criticizes. During this phase, if homosexual attachments are intense and exclusive more overt homosexual activity is likely to occur, and there is less motivation to make the advance to heterosexuality.

Fraiberg (1961) outlined some guidelines for distinguishing between adolescents whose homosexual tendencies will subside in normal development and those who will continue to be homosexual. These include the adolescent who acknowledges and exhibits homosexuality, who has had a gratifying homosexual experience, or who has fallen in love with a homosexual partner, particularly an adult partner. Such a youngster is more likely to be satisfied to continue as a homosexual and is less motivated to progress, despite anxiety, to the opposite sex than the ''uncommitted'' adolescent who experiments with homosexual activity.

In considering psychodynamic factors, one must examine both gender identification and object choice. Individuals who choose a homosexual love object may not have gender identity problems, but individuals with gender identity confusion are prone to a homosexual adaptation, and these cases can often be identified in early childhood (Whitam 1977). Except for the youngsters with extreme gender identity confusion, it is questionable whether there are any valid criteria for prognostically separating adolescent homosexual experimentation from future homosexuality (Gadpaille 1969).

Factors which predispose to homosexuality can be divided into four catagories: (1) problems in child-parent relationships, (2) early traumatic sexual experiences, (3) inferior feelings about the sex role, and (4) nonsexual determinants.

PROBLEMS IN CHILD-PARENT RELATIONSHIPS

An overly close relationship or a poor relationship with either parent can predispose to continuing homosexual orientation (Bene 1965; Ferenczi 1909; A. Freud 1958; S. Freud 1905, 1922; G.A.P. 1968; Kaye, Berl, Clare, Eleston, Gershwin, Gershwin, Kagan, Tardo, and Wilbur 1967; Looney 1973; Lorand 1930; Swanson, Loomis, Lukesh, Gronin, and Smith 1972; Tessman and Kaufman 1967).

For the boy or girl to be able to relinquish the romance with the parent of the opposite sex, the *parent* has to be willing to give up the erotically charged relationship. If, instead, the parent is disappointed in the marital relationship and enjoys the romantic attentions of the child too much, the child may be unable to get free. Thus, an overly close, troublesome bond develops between mother and son or father and daughter. If, in addition, the parent of the same sex is punitive and frightening, absent, cold and distant, or hostile to the child, identification with this parent may not occur.

The absence of the father or the presence of a weak or very frightening father can cause a boy to become overly attached to his mother. He may want to be like her and may very early develop a feminine identification. Stoller (1974) believes the early symbiosis, which babies have with their mothers, encourages feminine identification and can interfere with a boy baby's developing masculinity, especially if the mother is conflicted and unable to encourage separation and support his growing sense of mastery. Feeling like a woman usually leads a boy to continue to seek love and sex with males rather than females during adolescence. However, even if he does not identify with her, a boy who is overly close to mother may become homosexual if his wishes to remain faithful to her cause him to give up other women permanently. On the other hand, absence of the mother and an overly close relationship between a boy and his father can lead to powerful love feelings

424

for father and a male object choice for sexual activity even though the identification is masculine.

Intense castration anxiety is thought to be an important factor playing into continuing homosexual object choice for a boy. With a very frightening father, he may give up not only his mother but all women, and then submit himself to the father by taking him symbolically as his love object, thus avoiding father's wrath and at the same time getting someone to love. The high value set upon the penis and fear of its loss can also lead to intolerance of its absence in a sexual partner.

When the anal zone continues to have great erotic significance, homosexual object choice is more likely. A man who wishes to be a woman, like his mother, can express this wish by using his anus as a vagina.

Several authors have emphasized an oral basis for homosexuality (Arlow 1952; Eidelberg 1956). Their studies have shown that many homosexual men resented and resisted being weaned as babies and had subsequently shifted their interest from the breast to the penis, which they enjoyed sucking.

Problems in child-parent relationships in females which contribute to homosexual object choice include a strong attachment to the father with the incest taboo deterring heterosexuality because every boyfriend symbolizes father; early fixation on the mother at oral, anal, or negative oedipal levels; difficulty in the mother-child relationship due to hostility or coldness of the mother; reaction to mother's envy of her daughter, leading to withdrawal from men to avoid mother's hostility; distaste for mother's role as dominated or abused by father, leading to difficulty in identifying with mother; paternal rejection of the oedipal or pubertal girl, causing her to give up all hope of ever being accepted by any man.

Some authors have stressed the importance of identification with the parent of the opposite sex for the persistence of a homosexual way of life (Pearson 1958). Nagera (1975), however, points out that an essentially "feminine" girl may be homosexual if her move toward father has been severely interfered with by the father's massive rejection and disapproval of the girl's oedipal strivings toward him. Fixation to the mother at oral or anal levels may also lead to continuing homosexuality in girls with a predominantly feminine identification.

EARLY TRAUMATIC SEXUAL EXPERIENCES

Anxiety about heterosexual activities or interests can result from early sexual overstimulation, strong parental disapproval of early heterosexual interests and activities, and childhood seduction. It has been shown that sexual overstimulation in early childhood can interfere with heterosexual development (Greenacre 1952). A young child who witnesses intercourse by seeing or hearing it may have a very distorted, confused concept of heterosexuality. Often, in our culture, a child who witnesses intercourse misperceives sex as violent and dangerous. The child may fear that the woman will be injured or there may be deep-seated fears that the penis will dissolve or break off inside the body of a woman.

Another early experience which can favor homosexual object choice is early parental disapproval of even harmless heterosexual manifestations in children's behaviors. If parents overreact and forbid heterosexual interest and exploration in such a way that the child concludes that this interest is wrong and objectionable, a strong inhibition may develop which can interfere with subsequent heterosexual development.

Seduction by a close relative or family friend occurs significantly more frequently in the childhood of homosexuals than is found in the backgrounds of heterosexual individuals. Seduction of girls by fathers and stepfathers has received more attention in the literature than seduction by brothers, though the latter probably occurs more frequently. Sexual play among siblings is likely to be emotionally damaging when it is painful, thereby intensifying preexisting fears of mutilation, and when guilt about sexual feelings is reinforced by being discovered and blamed.

INFERIOR FEELINGS ABOUT SEX ROLE

Dissatisfaction with an inferior position may cause a girl to resist feminine identification. Many researchers believe that cultural factors are more important than anatomy as a cause for girls to envy boys (Romm 1965). Parents' preference for boys can also play into a girl's inferior feelings and her efforts to be a boy, just as parents' preference for girls can cause a boy to strive to be feminine.

NONSEXUAL DETERMINANTS OF HOMOSEXUALITY

Wishes for strength and power are often motivators of homosexual object choice by males (Bibring 1940; Nunberg 1938; Ovesey 1965). A man who feels weak, impotent, and castrated may seek homosexual activity with a man he admires and whose strength he wishes to incorporate. A type of "pseudohomosexuality" has been described by Defries (1976) in women college students who are struggling with identity conflicts and who have temporarily merged ideological issues about the feminist movement with sexual identity issues. Although they function as homosexuals, they are basically heterosexual.

Therapy: To Treat or Not to Treat?

Gay-liberation groups maintain that homosexuality is a normal, even superior, alternate life-style. Although their efforts to eliminate discrimination against homosexuals are commendable, it seems unfortunate that they sometimes take the position that homosexuality in innate and inescapable, when, in fact, many conflicted homosexuals can be helped to understand and overcome their fears of heterosexuality. On the other hand, Szasz (1965) has pointed out that treatment aimed at heterosexual adaptation should not be forced on unwilling homosexuals. As with other conditions, motivation has to belong to the individual for any meaningful change to occur. The therapist's role is not to sell patients on heterosexual object choice but rather to help them face fears and become aware of opposite wishes in order that they can weigh one against the other and decide which to gratify.

There is no uniform agreement on the necessity or the advisability of treating adolescents for homosexual problems. Horney (1934), in discussing homosexuality in girls, stated that favorable life circumstances may effect a "cure" in many cases. Erikson (1956) also drew our attention to the delicate balance that may throw decisions of identity in one direction or another during adolescence. Winnicott (1965) emphasized the beneficial effect of the passage of time which allows for maturational processes.

Marmor (1965) states that "psychiatric intervention is prophylactically indicated for children or adolescents who seem to be failing to make appropriate gender identifications . . . [because] as long as . . . society . . . regards homosexuality as an undesirable deviation, the ultimate adaptations of . . . children to their inner and outer worlds will be potentially better if they can be prevented from developing homoerotic patterns."

Fraiberg (1961) pointed out the good fortune of youngsters who are in psychotherapy at the time of engaging in a homosexual act: "They have the advantage of our therapeutic attitude in addition to anything else that we bring them in the way of insight." She agreed with Blos (1953) that often it is necessary to postpone analysis of homosexual tendencies until the adolescent has achieved his "sex-appropriate orientation" in view of the fact that while a young adolescent is testing sexual identity in the unstable period of early adolescence, analysis of homosexuality may intensify the conflict and add to doubts about sexual identity. Fraiberg stated that it is necessary to make an exception where the adolescent reveals that homosexual tendencies are not working toward establishment of the appropriate gender identification and where a homosexual tendency has achieved a powerful reinforcement. She suggested that there is a good possibility of changing the orientation while anxiety and guilt about homosexual tendencies are still present.

Many homosexuals seek treatment because of depression. They sometimes maintain that their only problems relate to ostracism which they encounter. Although occasionally they ask for help because they are uncomfortable with their homosexual urges, they frequently are not aware of any conflict. Complaining that they have been coerced into treatment by a family member or a friend, they attempt to externalize the inner conflict, preferring to struggle with a parental figure or therapist rather than deal with the struggle within.

When heterosexual interests are slow in appearing, normal adolescents often worry that perhaps they are homosexual (Coons 1971). In such cases, the parents do not fit the predisposing stereotypes. These youngsters continue to enjoy the friendship of members of the same sex and when they reach college realize that their peers are preoccupied with heterosexuality. They then become anxious and assume that they must be homosexual, despite the fact that they do not feel a compelling sexual attraction to friends of their own sex. These cases respond very favorably and quickly to intervention. In therapy, the "pseudohomosexual" young women described by Defries (1976) gradually determine their sexual preference on personal grounds rather than accepting homosexuality as a matter of policy.

It is usually assumed that when homosexuality is overdetermined by multiple dynamic factors, treatment is more difficult. This may be a dangerous assumption since the thereapist's expectations tend to influence outcome.

CASE EXAMPLE

Jean was the youngest of three children. She felt inferior to her four-year-older brother and two-year-older sister and thought that her mother had always been disappointed in her. Jean's parents quarreled frequently about the father's drinking and his objections to his daughters' music and dancing lessons. Even as a preschooler, Jean felt she should have been able to mediate the quarrels.

When Jean became frightened at night, or when she was ill, she slept with her parents. However, she frequently felt that both parents ignored her. She recalled that her father was always engrossed in reading or his work, and her mother had seemed preoccupied and sometimes forgot to pick her up at school and dancing class. She admired and looked up to her brother and sister with whom she tried to tag along and join in their activities.

Because Jean was intellectually precocious she entered first grade at age five and skipped fourth grade. She often felt uncomfortable with her older, more mature classmates.

At age ten, Jean repeatedly engaged in sexual play with her brother and three of his friends. The boys kissed and hugged her and attempted intercourse. When her sister discovered them, Jean thought all of the blame was placed on her. She often wished she were a boy. It seemed to her that boys had more privileges and were not held responsible for their behavior. She became a tomboy and devoted herself to climbing trees and playing football until early adolescence, when she became shy in the company of boys. She had several crushes on girls, but was not sexually involved with any of them. She could not recall any masturbation and said the subject was repulsive to her.

At college, she was crushed when the sorority to which her mother and sister belonged rejected her. She concluded that she was not pretty or feminine enough to be accepted by girls as a girl. A few weeks later, after a few beers, she reluctantly engaged in some petting with a date. When she began to feel sexually excited, she became nauseated, acutely anxious, and returned to her dorm. Her roommate's expression of sympathy and concern produced overwhelming feelings. She professed love for the girl and attempted to hug and kiss her.

The following day she was summoned to the dean's office, where she was met by her concerned parents. She was humiliated, frightened, and angry at the dean's implication that she was a homosexual. She transferred to another college where she dated a lot, drank heavily, and made frequent painful attempts to have intercourse.

Jean developed a strong attachment to a female physical education instructor who gave her special attention, praised her athletic talents, and invited her to her home for some additional coaching in tennis. After the tennis lesson and a candlelit dinner with wine and soft music, they engaged in mutual cunnilingus, Jean's first pleasurable sexual experience. Following this, she often dropped in on her teacher without an invitation. She was envious of her relationship with other friends and was quite reluctant to leave her to attend graduate school. When her friend encouraged her to go, she feared this meant that she was not loved or valued. In graduate school, she became sexually involved with another teacher.

It was due to this friend's insistence that she sought therapy at age nineteen. She was rather depressed, lacked self-confidence, and felt chronically disappointed in her friend, who behaved seductively but granted sexual favors rarely and then became punitive and rejecting.

Initially, during her sessions, Jean rarely made eye contact, and she avoided all feelings about the therapist. Later she told of fears that the therapist disliked her and dreaded her therapy hours. She nervously watched the clock to make certain she was receiving her full time.

Her dreams revealed fears of violent, aggressive encounters with men and wishes for an accepting, loving relationship with her mother. She became aware that her concept of an ideal man, to whom she could feel attracted, was a man like her brother—"big, athletic, gentle, intelligent, and interesting." However, when she involved herself with such a person, she always experienced overpowering fears of being mutilated. Afterward, she felt dirty and degraded as if she had been caught again by her sister in an incestuous relationship, and she would promptly retreat to a homosexual involvement.

During the year of therapy, she developed some awareness of her resentment of her mother, the therapist, and her friends for not accepting her and meeting her needs unconditionally. She became more in touch with wishes and fears about heterosexuality. As graduation approached, she reported having more dates, even though she still had mixed feelings about being close to men. She expressed a wish to find an unattached football player to love. The therapist suggested that she would probably find more eligible men when she became more comfortable with her sexual feelings.

Completion of her graduate degree necessitated interrupting her therapy to accept a position in another state. During her last therapy hour, Jean talked of her wishes and fears about having a baby, something she had always wanted to discuss with her mother, who had evaded her questions and placed in her room a book about sex and reproduction. She quickly added that she did not want to hear her therapist's thoughts about the matter. She responded to the suggestion that she was afraid of being controlled and forced to have a baby, by talking, for the first time, of how forceful and controlling her mother had seemed. On one occasion, when she had tried to be close to her father, her mother became upset and threatened to leave home. She was accepting of an interpretation that her fear of being hurt by sex and childbirth, as well as her fear of losing mother, made homosexuality seem a good

430

compromise solution for her dilemma. She said she would like to overcome these fears, marry a powerful man, and have his baby. On parting, she spoke sadly of her reluctance to give up her therapy and said she had become more comfortable with loving feelings and dependency wishes toward the therapist.

DISCUSSION

Jean's behavior was overdetermined. She had experienced a lasting and very gratifying homosexual relationship with an older woman whom she loved and initially had little awareness of any desire to give up homosexuality. Her fears of heterosexuality went back to frightening primal scene memories as well as to memories of painful sex experimentation with her brother and his friends. Guilt and humiliation over heterosexual impulses were strong, and derived from her mother's reluctance to discuss sexual matters and her sister's denunciation upon discovering her in incestuous heterosexual activity.

Identification with her brother and father was strong. Her feminine identification had been discouraged and negatively reinforced, as for example, by her father's objections to her dancing lessons, by being "abandoned" when her mother forgot to pick her up, and later through being rejected by the sorority.

During college, when she felt a failure because of her fear to relate sexually to boys, she was branded a homosexual by the friend to whom she turned for reassurance and acceptance. At her second college, she was so determined to overcome her fears that she attempted to rush into sexual intercourse without the background of a caring relationship. This was always painful and thus reinforced the anxiety which was associated with heterosexual activity. All efforts to relate to men ceased after she became involved in a sexual relationship with her teacher and fell in love with her.

The multiple roots of Jean's behavior include almost every life experience which has been found to predispose to continuing homosexuality, including castration anxiety associated with sexual activity; incomplete resolution of the oedipal conflict with the incest taboo deterring heterosexuality; early fixation on the mother; difficulty in the mother-child relationship; reaction to mother's envy, leading to withdrawal from men to avoid mother's hostility; dissatisfaction with the feminine role because of envy of boys and fears that she could never measure up to mother or sister; an incestuous relationship. Jean had unresolved feelings associated with the painful attempts to have intercourse with her brother and his friends. Her later frantic attempts to have

431

sex with any boy who took her out constituted an effort to reenact and master the earlier traumatic experiences. She enjoyed male company and preferred masculine men, as do most homosexual women (Wilbur 1965).

Despite the fact that seeking therapy had not been her own idea, Jean never missed a session and was always punctual. This is not surprising in view of the fact that conscious motivation is not a prerequisite for successful therapy; however, there must be conflict about some behavior for any lasting change to occur. Chafetz (1961), Myerson (1957), and others have reported significant improvement with very difficult, involuntary alcoholic patients who initially had no motivation for treatment and no conscious wish to change.

During the year of therapy Jean became hopeful that she could overcome her fear of relating to men. She also became aware of mixed feelings about "mothers" from whom she wanted unconditional love and acceptance to make up for the deprivation she had suffered because of her own mother's seeming indifference and preoccupation. As termination approached, she was sufficiently motivated to continue in therapy that she considered giving up the position which necessitated her moving away, even though she would have had to repay her scholarship had she refused a position in her home state.

Having experienced an intimate, trusting relationship with the therapist without sexual seduction or rejection, Jean may be less hungry for relationships with women and more able in the future to identify with her mother and the therapist. Although her homosexual relationships had been pleasurable and less anxiety provoking than many of her heterosexual relationships, she was disenchanted with their ambivalent and superficial nature. Awareness of this dissatisfaction, greater self-confidence, and some diminution of her fears may enable her to continue efforts to relate warmly to men.

Conclusions

Some authors, including Freud (1920), have expressed doubts about the homosexual's ability to change, whereas many others, including Bacon (1956), Bieber (1967), Blos (1953), Deutsch (1948), Fraiberg (1961), Horney (1934), Ovesey (1965), Romm (1965), and Socarides (1978), have reported success with analytic therapy, particularly in adolescence and young adulthood. Pessimism about therapy of homosexuals of any age is often ascribed to a presumed irreversibility of homosexual object choice, particularly for individuals with preoedipal predisposing factors, once the choice is made and the individual has become sexually active and adjusted to the choice. This attitude seems to ignore developmental factors and human adaptability. Whether or not we like the term "normal homosexual stage," by preference, little boys love little boys, little girls love little girls, and if nothing interferes, their tastes change as they grow older. When this development is blocked, it is sometimes possible to intervene and remove the block.

The pessimism may be related, in part, to therapists' negative feelings about patients who make them uncomfortable (Robinson and Podnos 1966). If the concept of a normal homosexual stage is a valid one, all of us have, in the past, experienced some conflict about love object choice, therefore we may have a sense of superiority and feel disdain for those who have failed to make the switch to heterosexuality. Therapists must be aware of counter-transference feelings which could cause them to discharge a homosexual patient as "unmotivated" or "hopeless," when the patient is eager to have help in understanding and mastering feelings of anxiety and depression which often will be found to be related to conflict about homosexual behavior.

Because it is easier to change a pattern when it is conflictual and not well established, late adolescence is an opportune time for a youngster, predisposed to homosexual object choice, to have help from a therapist. Youngsters with gender identity problems should receive this help much earlier, preferably as soon as it is recognized. Many adolescents with homosexual conflict benefit from therapy, regardless of whether they seek it voluntarily or are coerced into it by friends or family members. While therapy may not always lead to heterosexual object choice, it provides a safe arena for struggling with opposing wishes and often enables youngsters to gain self-understanding and a higher level of maturity.

REFERENCES

Adatto, C. 1967. Inner life of the adolescent. In G. Usdin, ed. *Adolescence*. Philadelphia: Lippincott.

Arlow, J. A. 1952. Psychodynamics and treatment of perversions (Panel report). *Bulletin of the American Psychoanalytic Association* 8:315–327.

Bacon, C. L. 1956. A developmental theory of female homosexuality. In S. Lorand and M. Balint, eds. *Perversions: Psychodynamics and Therapy*. New York: Random House.

Bene, E. 1965. On the genesis of female homosexuality. *British Journal of Psychiatry* 111:815–821.

Bibring, G. L. 1940. On an oral component in masculine inversion. *Internationale Zeitschrift für Psychoanalyse* 25:124–130.

Bieber, T. 1967. On treating male homosexuals. *Archives of General Psychiatry* 16:60–63.

Blos, P. 1953. The treatment of adolescents. In M. Heiman, ed. *Psychoanalysis and Social Work*. New York: International Universities Press.

Blos, P. 1962. *On Adolescence*. New York: Free Press.

Chafetz, M. E. 1961. Alcoholism problems and programs in Czechoslavakia, Poland, and the Soviet Union. *New England Journal of Medicine* 265:68–74.

Coons, F. W. 1971. The developmental task of the college student. *Adolescent Psychiatry* 1:245–274.

Defries, Z. 1976. Pseudohomosexuality in feminist students. *American Journal of Psychiatry* 133:400–404.

Deutsch, H. 1948. On female homosexuality. In R. Fliess, ed. *Psychoanalytic Reader*. New York: International Universities Press.

Eidelberg, L. 1956. Analysis of a case of a male homosexual. In S. Lorand and M. Balint, eds. *Perversions: Psychodynamics and Therapy*. New York: Random House.

Erikson, E. 1956. The problem of ego identity. *Journal of the American Psychoanalytic Association* 4:56–121.

Ferenczi, S. 1909. More about homosexuality. In *Problems and Methods of Psychoanalysis*. Vol. 3. New York: Basic.

Fraiberg, S. 1961. Homosexual conflicts in adolescence. In S. Lorand and H. I. Schneer, eds. *Psychoanalytic Approach to Problems and Therapy*. New York: Harper.

Freud, A. 1958. Adolescence. *Psychoanalytic Study of the Child* 13:255–278.

Freud, S. 1905. Three essays on the theory of sexuality. *Standard Edition* 7:3–243. London: Hogarth, 1953.

Freud, S. 1920. Psychogenesis of a case of homosexuality in a woman. *Standard Edition* 18:147–172. London: Hogarth, 1955.

Freud, S. 1922. Some neurotic mechanisms in jealousy, paranoia and homosexuality. *Standard Edition* 18:223–232. London: Hogarth, 1955.

Gadpaille, W. J. 1969. Homosexual activity and homosexuality in adolescence. *Science and Psychoanalysis* 15:60–70.

Greenacre, P. 1952. Perversions: general considerations regarding their genetic and dynamic background. *Psychoanalytic Study of the Child* 23:47–63.

Group for the Advancement of Psychiatry. 1968 *Normal Adolescence*. New York: Scribner's.

Horney, K. 1934. Personality changes in female adolescents. In *Feminine Psychology*. New York: Norton, 1967.

Kaye, H. E.; Berl, S.; Clare, J.; Eleston, M. R.; Gershwin, B. S.; Gershwin, P.; Kagan, L. S.; Tardo, C.; and Wilbur, C. B. 1967. Homosexuality in women. *Archives of General Psychiatry* 17:626–634.

Looney, J. 1973. Family dynamics in homosexual women. *Archives of Sexual Behavior* 2:329–341.

Lorand, S. 1930. Fetishism in status nascendi. *International Journal of Psycho-Analysis* 11:410–427.

Marmor, J. 1965. *Sexual Inversion*. New York: Basic.

Myerson, D. J. 1957. A three year study of a group of skid row alchoholics. In H. Himwich, ed. *Alcoholism, Basic Aspects and Treatment*. Washington, D.C.: American Association of Advance Science.

Nagera, H. 1975. *Female Sexuality and the Oedipus Complex*. New York: Aronson.

Nunberg, H. 1938. Homosexuality, magic and aggression. *International Journal of Psycho-Analysis* 19:1–16.

Offer, D., and Offer, J. 1971. Four issues in the developmental psychology of adolescents. In J. G. Howells, ed. *Modern Perspectives in Adolescent Psychiatry*. New York: Brunner/Mazel.

Ovesey, L. 1965. Pseudohomosexuality and homosexuality in men: psychodynamics as a guide to treatment. In J. Marmor, ed. *Sexual Inversion: The Multiple Roots of Homosexuality*. New York: Basic.

Pearson, G. H. J. 1958. *Adolescence and the Conflict of Generations*. New York: Norton.

Robinson, L. H., and Podnos, B. 1966. Resistance of psychiatrists in treatment of alcoholism. *Journal of Nervous and Mental Diseases* 143:220–225.

Romm, M. E. 1965. Sexuality and homosexuality in women. In J. Marmor, ed. *Sexual Inversion: The Multiple Roots of Homosexuality*. New York: Basic.

Socarides, C. W. 1978. *Homosexuality*. New York: Aronson.

Stoller, R. J. 1974. Symbiosis anxiety and the development of masculinity. *Archives of General Psychiatry* 30: 164–172.

Swanson, D. W.; Loomis, S. D.; Lukesh, R.; Gronin, R.; and Smith, J. A. 1972. Clinical features of female homosexual patients: comparison with heterosexual pateints. *Journal of Nervous and Mental Diseases* 155:199–210.

Szasz, T. S. 1965. Legal and moral aspects of homosexuality. In J. Marmor, ed. *Sexual Inversion: The Multiple Roots of Homosexuality*. New York: Basic.

Tessman, L. H., and Kaufman, I. 1969. Variations of a theme of incest. In

O. Pollack and A. S. Friedman, eds. *Family Dynamics and Female Sexual Delinquency*. Palo Alto, Calif.: Science and Behavior Books.

Wilbur, C. 1965. Clinical aspects of female homosexuality. In J. Marmor, ed. *Sexual Inversion: The Multiple Roots of Homosexuality*. New York: Basic.

Winnicott, D. W. 1965. Adolescence: struggling through the doldrums. In *The Family and Individual Development*. London: Tavistock.

Whitman, F. L. 1977. Childhood indicators of male homosexuality. *Archives of Sexual Behavior* 6(2): 89–96.

ARTHUR D. SOROSKY AND MARLIS B. STICHER

The French dermatologist, Hallopeau (1889), introduced the term trichotil-lomania to refer to alopecia caused by patients suffering from an irresistible urge to pull out bodily hair. The name is derived from the Greek: *tricho* ("hair"), *tillo* ("to pull something from oneself"), and *mania* ("psychosis"). A number of articles describing this entity have appeared in dermatologic and psychiatric journals, and case reports have included children, adolescents, and adults. While various diagnostic entities and a variety of psychodynamic explanations have been entertained, the purpose of this chapter is to focus on trichotillomania as it manifests itself during the adolescent years.

Symbolic Meaning of Hair

One of the earliest references to hair occurred in the biblical story of Samson. His Phillistine wife, Delilah, discovered that his strength lay in his long locks. She secretly cut off his hair and turned him over to his enemies. During his years in prison his hair grew back, his strength gradually returned, and with renewed power he pulled down the Phillistine temple with his bare hands. The story illustrates the virility attributed to hair, along with the castrating effects experienced by having it cut off. The undoing of the castration is represented in the resumption of strength regained after the hair grew back.

The unconscious significance of hair was first described by Berg (1936), who used dream material to demonstrate displacement from the pubic area to the head. Anxious reactions to the cutting of scalp hair are viewed as a form of castration anxiety with concerns about hair becoming thin, falling out, or developing grayness as manifestations of that anxiety. Sperling (1954) saw hair as having male-female attributes. Because hair is located on the body of both sexes, and grows back spontaneously when removed, it lends itself particularly well for use as a bisexual symbol. In women, at a conscious level long hair represents femininity, whereas at an unconscious level it may be a symbol of maleness.

Psychodynamics of Hair-Pulling

The symbolic meaning of hair is important in attempting to understand why some persons choose habitually to pull out their hair. In reviewing the literature on trichotillomania it becomes obvious that we are not dealing with a distinct clinical entity, but rather a symptom which may be associated with a variety of psychiatric disorders: retardation, behavior disorder, psychoneurosis, borderline disorders, and schizophrenia. Furthermore, the hair-pulling problem has been described in both sexes, although predominantly female, and at all ages. In some cases, even though there are areas of missing hair, actual diagnosis can be made only after a careful clinical examination, because the patient has denied pulling out the hair because of shame and embarrassment. The typical clinical picture encountered is that of ill-defined plaques of nonscarring alopecia of the scalp (Muller and Winkelmann 1972) with incomplete hair loss, including short broken strands alongside long and normal appearing hairs (Oguchi and Miura 1977). When necessary, the diagnosis can be confirmed histopathologically by punch biopsy of the scalp.

In Buxbaum's (1960) psychoanalytic study of hair-pulling, she viewed the symptom as a fetish and multidetermined by a variety of unconscious conflicts. According to her formulation, hair-pulling may represent any of the following: (*a*) transitional phenomena secondary to separation anxiety; (*b*) autoaggression (anger turned inward) secondary to ambivalence felt toward the parents; (*c*) autoerotic activity designed to counter feelings of loneliness, insecurity, and anxiety; (*d*) displacement of castration fears secondary to a wish to pull the parent's hair (especially the ''castrated'' mother for the girl); (*e*) an amalgamation of painful and pleasurable sensations (the early symptoms of masochism); (*f*) signs of despair and mourning; and (*g*) a means of reassuring the person of his/her existence through the bodily sensations experienced.

Greenberg and Sarner (1965) approached the problem as resulting from multiple fixation points at all levels of psychosexual development. At the oral level, the pulling, saving, or eating of hair symbolizes an incorporation and

438

identification with the mother, as well as a reassurance against her loss. At the anal level, the hair plucking expresses rage and frustration directed toward the object and the internalized superego, with the symptom becoming a depressive-equivalent. At the genital stage, hair-pulling in the female demonstrates to her mother that the girl is willing to deny her femininity and give up the oedipal struggle. For both sexes, hairlessness is seen as symbolizing a return to innocent childishness in which the patient has renounced all claims to genital sexuality.

The pregenital aspects of this habit disorder have been emphasized by many authors who have observed disturbances in the mother-child relationship with early emotional deprivation leading to a hostile symbiosis and problems in separation (Greenberg and Sarner 1965; Mannino and Delgado 1969; Oguchi and Miura 1977; Rechenberger 1976; Stadelli 1963). The hair-pulling can be viewed, in this context, as an autoerotic turning to the self because of the nondependable mother (Delgado and Mannino 1969). Another explanation is that an unconscious attempt at reunion with the abusive mother, through an identification with her, can be brought about symbolically by the hair-pulling (Monroe and Abse 1963).

A few authors have demonstrated that the mothers of hair-pullers are controlling and aggressive, whereas the fathers tend to be passive and uninvolved (Delgado and Mannino 1969; Greenberg and Sarner 1965). In one study, the ordinal position was implicated as a factor, with a higher incidence of oldest children, suggesting that a greater intensity of parent-child interaction may be a contributing factor (Takaishi, Fujii, and Ohmi 1959). Furthermore, the affected child can be seen as compensating for feelings of intimidation and helplessness through a preoccupation with control over hair (Delgado and Mannino 1969). These anal control issues are exemplified by the fact that hair-pulling is not infrequently associated with an obsessive-compulsive neurosis (Greenberg and Sarner 1965; Philippopoulos 1961).

The hysterical aspects of the illness were discussed by Winnik and Gabbay (1965), who viewed the hair-pulling act as a defense against castration anxiety by switching from a passive to an active role. Furthermore, the hair-pulling experience results in the achievement of libidinous, orgasm-like satisfaction. Monroe and Abse (1963) saw the hair-pulling as a renunciation of femininity, and a depreciation of the girl's sexual value, as her solution to the oedipal conflict. Basically, the girl was seen as dissatisfied with her feminine status, resulting in penis envy. Also, there was a repetition of the fantasied castration, and reassurance through watching the hair regenerate itself. Delgado and Mannino (1969) demonstrated that some of the female hair pullers had been overstimulated sexually by exposure to their parents' genitals at the same time that their aggressive feelings toward the parents had been inhibited from expression. In some cases the child had experienced repeated beatings which had become eroticized, resulting in a perpetuation of masochistic sexual pleasure through the self-punishing, self-stimulating hair-pulling (Monroe and Abse 1963).

Hair-pulling has also been considered to be a depressive-equivalent, with the symptom occurring after the loss of a significant love object (Greenberg and Sarner 1965). An exacerbation of the symptom has been associated with anxiety-producing events (birthdays, examinations, family reunions, etc.) (Delgado and Mannino 1969) or following traumatic experiences (Muller and Winkelmann 1972). It has been reported in families where the child has been subjected to physical abuse, including the use of hair-cutting as a means of punishment (Monroe and Abse 1963). It has also been seen following certain illnesses, such as flu syndrome, and after experiencing specific trauma to the scalp (Delgado and Mannino 1969; Greenberg and Sarner 1965). Furthermore, it has been found in connection with a variety of other neurotic and behavior problems, including hypochondriasis, eating disorders, school problems, and peer difficulties (Greenberg and Sarner 1965). It has also been found in association with similar body-related habit disorders: nail biting, nose picking, picking at the clothes, compulsive masturbation, and rapid eating (Delgado and Mannino 1969).

An organic explanation has been offered for the problem by Bartsch (1956) and Huber (1959), who viewed the hair-pulling as resulting from seizure-like motor discharges from the brain. Furthermore, Mehregan (1970) and Muller and Winkelmann (1972) have deemphasized the psychiatric or neurologic aspects and have portrayed the problem as a predominantly dermatologic illness.

Age of Onset

A number of authors have stressed that the illness can be expected to have a more benign course if it has its onset in childhood and preadolescence, and that the problem is more serious when it begins during adolescence (Greenberg and Sarner 1965; Oguchi and Miura 1977; Sanderson and Hall-Smith 1970). In contrast, a review of cases by Muller and Winkelmann (1972) did not confirm the opinion that trichotillomania in the adolescent is a more serious condition. These observations are particularly significant in that one study demonstrated the incidence of hair-pulling to be greatest during the adolescent years (Greenberg and Sarner 1965). When the illness has its onset in adulthood it appears that there is a greater likelihood of it being associated with a psychotic illness (Oguchi and Miura 1977).

Treatment Approaches

There are few reports of treatment outcome in the literature. Buxbaum (1960) reported the success of psychoanalysis in treating two girls, ages three and six, and Philippopoulos (1961) reported a successful analysis of a sixteen-year-old girl seen over a two-year period. Monroe and Abse (1963) described moderate success in treating a twenty-two-year-old borderline girl, and Zaidens (1951) had fairly good results in treating those patients who pulled hair from their eyebrows, eyelashes, and pubic hairs, in contrast to poorer results obtained with patients who pulled hair from their scalp. In contrast, Bartsch (1956) viewed psychotherapy as being predominantly unsuccessful. Successful treatment results have been reported by behavior therapists utilizing "feedback" methods (Bayer 1972; de L. Horne 1977), "competing responses" (Azrin and Nunn 1973), and "thought stopping" techniques (Taylor 1963).

Case Reports

Case A: Barbara was seen initially at the age of seventeen, at which time she had been pulling out her hair for four or five years and had been covering the bald spots on her scalp with a wig. She was depressed, had little self-confidence, was overweight, and had the uncomfortable feeling that people were always making fun of her. She felt very inadequate in her peer relationships and had a fear of meeting new people. She was doing average work in school and had no behavior problems or conflicts with her teachers.

Her family life was filled with tension. She and her mother fought continuously, and it occasionally escalated to a physical level. Once her mother phoned the police after being threatened by the patient. At the onset of treatment Barbara's parents had been separated for two years and divorced for one year. She took out all of her frustrations on her mother, often blaming her for the divorce. She also resented her mother's attention to her two younger sisters, with whom she had always felt much rivalry. Furthermore, Barbara felt very rejected by her father because he also showed more attention to her sisters and was constantly belittling her about her sloppy appearance.

Barbara was extremely guilt ridden and felt responsible for everything that had gone wrong in her family, including the divorce. When she was not blaming her mother, she would insist that she was the cause of the divorce because of her provocative behavior. Conversely, she also felt guilty about the fact that her birth had allegedly prevented her parents from divorcing years earlier. She had suicidal fantasies and had made a number of suicidal gestures in the preceding years. She had begged her parents to send her to a therapist, but they had minimized her problems and failed to respond to her pleas for help.

Barbara's birth was without complication. She was breast fed for six weeks, at which time her mother terminated abruptly, complaining that she did not enjoy it and was finding it a nuisance. Barbara was colicky and a very poor eater. She cried irritably almost nightly until she was nine months old. Her physical development proceeded normally, including toilet training around the age of two. However, there was excessive stranger and separation anxiety unless she was left with close relatives. Because of these problems she did not attend nursery school. She adapted to entrance into elementary school without too much difficulty, however, and never complained about going to school throughout her elementary school years.

Barbara was three years old when her next oldest sister was born and four when the youngest arrived. She was very competitive toward both of them, whom she viewed as more attractive, intelligent, and personable. Her menarche began at eleven. On the surface she seemed to handle the experience well, but it coincided roughly in time with the onset of the hair-pulling problem. She began petting with a number of boys around the age of twelve and had intercourse for the first time at fourteen. Subsequently, she was somewhat promiscuous. She also felt sexually attracted to other girls and feared that she might have homosexual tendencies.

Barbara was seen once a week in both individual and group psychotherapy for eight months, at which time the individual sessions were decreased to every other week. After another six months the individual therapy sessions were terminated, and her group sessions stopped around three months later. The total period of treatment spanned over a period of one and a half years. The therapeutic approach was eclectic, utilizing analytically oriented techniques along with humanistic and behavioristic methods.

In the initial sessions, Barbara expressed ambivalent feelings toward her father. She felt love for him but could not handle the frustration resulting from his continual rejection of her. She found herself competing with her sisters for her father's attention, as well as with his step-daughter from a current remarriage. Her step-sister was her age, and her father was always comparing Barbara to her unfavorably.

Barbara was open about her sexual feelings, fantasies, and activities. She masturbated regularly and found it to be a pleasurable experience. In contrast, she had never found sexual intercourse to be enjoyable and admitted that she did it more for approval and the pleasure of her boyfriends. She recalled a dream in which she asked a girl to go steady with her, but the girl's father became angry and refused to let the two go out because he did not want his daughter dating another girl. Barbara had also read some literature on lesbianism and was afraid that her dream and attraction to girls might be an indication that she was on the way to becoming a homosexual.

She described a deep conflict in expressing angry feelings. For example, if her friends did anything to annoy her, she immediately suppressed the feeling and attempted to block out the memory. Furthermore, she complained of recurrent feelings of rejection and disapproval from others and was continually placing herself in positions of being taken advantage of. She was also quite impulsive, sloppy, and disorganized.

As the therapy sessions progressed, she recalled a number of traumatic and seductive experiences that had occurred with her father. As a child, he would beat her uncontrollably, once hitting her head against the wall. She began to recognize that she often provoked these beatings as a means of getting his attention. Her father repeatedly told her that he would have preferred her to have been a boy. She had obliged him by wearing her hair short and engaging in tomboyish activities. Barbara gradually became more aware of the guilt she felt about the seductive quality of the relationship existing with her father.

Barbara felt guilty about her overall lack of motivation and achievement in most areas of her life. She felt good about her commitment to therapy and her growing psychological awareness. She produced a number of dreams for analysis and delighted in coming up with her own dynamic interpretations. In one dream, she was sleeping inside a water bed surrounded by fish. She was able to associate this to a repressed memory of witnessing her mother kissing her boss in the ocean when she was eleven years old, at a time when her parents were still married. In another dream, she was driving in an old car when she was picked up by two ugly and repulsive policemen who arrested her for drug possession. Her associations led to experiences she had had with her father in earlier childhood. The two used to take long drives together to a very poor and dilapidated section of town, where he apparently engaged in shady business dealings. It also helped her to recall a discovery she had

443

made of her father's pornographic collection of pictures, books, and movies in his desk drawer when she was only ten years old. This discovery was very upsetting to her and she recalled wondering at the time why he needed such stimulation when he was married to her mother. She also recalled that she and her father had taken showers together for a number of years, and that she had found the experience to be sexually stimulating. She was quite aware from early childhood that there was a lack of love and affection displayed between her two parents and had been concerned for some time that they might eventually divorce.

Other dreams included one in which she was ill and her mother told her she might be dying. She protested vehemently because she felt she was too young to die. Her therapist made a visit to her house to examine her and held her hand while he took her pulse. He discovered that her sickness resulted from eating a poisoned chicken. It was too late to save her, however, and she died. She continued to beg to be brought back to life but the therapist said that nothing more could be done. She associated to a general feeling of helplessness and an inability to rely or depend upon the adults in her life. Furthermore, the poisoned chicken was seen as relating to her guilty oedipal feelings and the fact that she was damaged beyond repair. She also viewed the chicken as representing her inability to control her hair-pulling problem, that is, "being chicken." It also reminded her of family stories of her grandparents plucking chickens on the farm. The relationship of plucking chickens and hair-pulling was very interesting to her.

In another dream, she had cut off her dog's ear and was holding it out the window as she rode alongside her mother in a car. When they came to a red light she became sick to her stomach and the dog's ear fell out of the car. Exploration revealed a long history of sexual stimulation and experimentation. When she was six or seven years old, she began to engage in sex play with a neighborhood boy, which continued into her adolescence, although it never terminated in intercourse. Around the age of nine or ten, she observed a man masturbating on a park bench. She herself began to masturbate regularly in childhood and experienced much guilt, until she read in a book that it was acceptable behavior. Also, when she was thirteen or fourteen, she engaged in mutual breast fondling with a girlfriend. This experience was particularly stimulating and guilt provoking. Thus, the dog's ear in the dream symbolized penis envy and castration fears.

The dream analysis and progress in psychotherapy made it quite apparent that she was reluctant to let go of her hair-pulling symptom because of the secondary gain accrued through the attention and concern tendered by her family, friends, therapist, and fellow group members. However, she gradually began to feel less anxious, depressed, and guilt ridden. She was more open with her friends and less embarrassed about her hair-pulling problem. The wig she had worn for a number of years was now becoming a source of shame to her rather than an object she held onto for security and dependency gratification. The habitual aspect of the hair-pulling problem was now becoming more significant than the underlying dynamics. To enable her to become more successful with symptom resolution, hypnotic interviews were included during her therapy sessions, providing her with posthypnotic suggestions aimed at breaking the hair-pulling pattern.

The patient gained a great deal of support from her fellow group members, who encouraged her to expose her bald spot to them. She was very frightened at first and it took her a number of weeks to prepare herself for this event. Finally, she selected the two group members she felt closest to and took them into the office bathroom, where she closed the door and pulled off her wig. When the three youngsters returned to the group meeting and shared their experience, there was a great deal of excitement and celebration. It was not long afterward that she gradually began to expose her scalp to her friends, family members, and eventually her classmates. Her hair grew back in, yet she held onto her wig for a number of months as insurance lest she suffer a relapse. When she felt she no longer needed it, she presented the wig to her therapist as a gift.

At the time of termination, her hair-pulling problem had ceased and her general emotional state was markedly improved. Her sexual experiences became narrowed to one boyfriend, and she described deep feelings of love and affection for him. She experienced a sense of accomplishment in her growth in therapy and also took pride in her physical appearance. She graduated high school and after a few years of college and various jobs, she decided to marry, at the age of twenty, the boy she had been dating for the past three years.

Case B: Sandra was seen for the first time at the age of fifteen and had been pulling out her hair for three years, keeping her head covered at all times with a wig. Her behavior at home, and in school, was characteristically irresponsible, negativistic, and defiant. She found it difficult to relate to her father, whom she viewed as controlling and uncommunicative. Her mother was a frustrated and unfulfilled housewife, and Sandra was extremely hostile and resentful toward her because of the weak, passive role she played in the family. Sandra felt jealous of her younger sister's close relationship with her father and the special attention afforded her younger hyperkinetic brother.

Sandra was also doing poorly in school, where she was underachieving and having behavior problems. She presented problems to her parents because of her lack of self-discipline and overall sloppiness. For example, she kept misplacing and losing her orthodontic retainers. Furthermore, she neglected to wash the wig that covered her bald spot, and her parents found it to be a repulsive sight. She was extremely sensitive to criticism and responded with a surly, negativistic retort. She was also still enuretic, a problem which dated back to the age of four when her sister was born. She seemed untroubled by the bed-wetting, and her mother felt angry because she saw it as her daughter's means of punishing her. The patient was also concerned about being overweight and was constantly trying to keep herself on a diet.

Sandra's parents viewed her as being two different people, when she was with her family and when she was with her friends. At home they viewed her as tense, uncommunicative, withdrawn, and spending most of her spare time isolated in her bedroom. In contrast, when she was with her friends, she appeared to be somewhat more outgoing and full of fun. Her parents were also concerned that Sandra might have been affected by a "family secret." They had had a Mongoloid child a year or so after Sandra's birth who was immediately placed in a permanent foster home. No one had discussed this child, but Sandra had inadvertently come across the child's birth certificate in a bureau drawer and had inquired about it. The parents had become very uncomfortable and concocted a story that another child had been born but died prematurely. The parents were not sure if Sandra had ever accepted this story or not.

The patient's pregnancy was unplanned, and the mother suffered from nausea and vomiting for the first four months of the gestation period. The delivery was uneventful, but the mother was extremely depressed in the postpartum period. Sandra was bottle fed for two and a half years and had become very attached to her bottle, showing considerable resistance at the time of weaning. Her development proceeded normally, and she was toilet trained around the age of two, although she began to wet again at four after her sister was born. There is no history of excessive stranger or separation anxiety. Her initial adjustment to nursery and elementary school went well, but she began to suffer from school phobia at eight, after moving to a new neighborhood requiring a school transfer. Her grades remained at least at average level until junior high school, at which time they began to decline markedly.

There was little communication in the family. Her mother kept to herself and her father's only meaningful interaction was with Sandra's sister, who was four years her junior. She was an exceptional tennis player, and her lessons and tournaments occupied much of the father's free time. This created considerable envy and jealousy from the mother, patient, and Sandra's younger hyperkinetic brother. The brother was five years younger than the patient and was constantly getting into trouble and receiving negative attention from everyone. Needless to say, Sandra felt squeezed out, neglected, unloved, misunderstood, and quite resentful.

Sandra was very mistrustful and apprehensive when she started in therapy. She gradually relaxed and formed a therapeutic alliance. During her second session, she described a dream in which she was sitting on a park bench when a man came up to her. He presented her with flower seeds and then threw them into a pond of water. They both watched the seeds turn into flowers, and then Sandra began to pick the flowers out of the water. At this point she became aware that there was also a baby nearby. This particular dream opened up many discussions about sexual fantasies, petting experiences, and a general tendency to drift off into a fantasy world rather than dealing with a real world which was viewed as frightening and lacking in nurturance.

Some of the initial sessions were held with the entire family present in order to get a better grasp of the family dynamics. The mother saw the worst of herself, as well as her mother-in-law, in the patient, which made it very difficult for her to relate to her. She was extremely frustrated in her marriage and in her own unfulfilled life, displacing much of her anger onto the children. The younger brother was eventually referred to another therapist and placed on stimulant medication, which helped to alleviate some of his problems and the tension level in the family. Marital therapy was recommended but refused by both of the parents. Sandra was then seen in weekly individual psychotherapy sessions and in combined individual and adolescent group therapy after two or three months had elapsed. After a year, she was seen exclusively in group therapy with only occasional individual therapy sessions. Treatment was terminated after a total time of three and a half years had elapsed.

During the treatment, she began to open up considerably and expressed feelings which she had never shared previously. She spoke about the bed-wetting problem and related it to a period in her earlier childhood when her father would routinely check her pants in the morning to see if she had wet herself. Whenever he discovered she had wet he would beat her. She had become very frightened by these beatings and would enlist her mother's alliance in protecting her from her father. There was obviously a sense of excitement that she received from this reaction on her father's part and a fusion of pain and pleasure vis-à-vis the enuresis and spankings. She traced this pattern into adolescent dating activities in which she often placed herself in dangerous masochistic positions with boys, although she always stopped herself short of having sexual intercourse. She denied masturbating at any time in her life, and felt somewhat repulsed by the idea.

447

After a number of months, she had a dream in which a boy grabbed her arm and injected it with a syringe filled with heroin. This was very upsetting to her and caused an intensification of her hair-pulling. It reminded her that smoking marijuana in the past had often led to an increase in her hair-pulling problem. These drug experiences brought out a fear of losing control of both her sexual and aggressive impulses, which were symbolically defended against by the hair-pulling.

At one point in the treatment she began to inquire about the "hidden sibling." Her parents found it impossible to discuss this with her and asked the therapist if he would do it. After the discussion, she seemed rather relieved and remarked that she had always felt there was something that had been withheld from her. A year later, her therapist accompanied her to the foster home where she met her brother for the first time. It was a very exciting experience for her, and although she never visited him again, she sent him cards and small gifts on holidays. She described this experience as providing her with a more complete sense of understanding her family dynamics and, in turn, with a truer sense of her own personal identity.

In her group-therapy activities, she experienced considerable rivalry with the more assertive, attention-drawing members. She eventually worked these feelings through, and it helped her to deal more effectively with similar feelings she encountered with her siblings. At first she was extremely embarrassed about her bald spot and the need to wear a wig. Finally, she was able to share her hair-pulling problem with the other group members and took pride in reporting to them about her progress in controlling the impulse to pull out her hair. It was an exciting day for her when she was able to take off the wig during a group-therapy session and display the bald spot with the short, stubby hairs growing back in.

At the time she terminated therapy, she was feeling better about herself and had conquered the hair-pulling problem. She was very proud of her long, beautiful hair and delighted in running her hands through it, almost continuously. A follow-up of Sandra at the age of twenty-three revealed that she had never experienced a recurrence of the hair-pulling. She was still emotionally immature, however, and had transferred her dependency from her family to a boyfriend with whom she was living. She worked part time as a waitress, yet relied on her father for financial support. She described occasional bouts of depression, but had required no further psychotherapy.

In addition to her own changes, marked changes had occurred in the family structure as well. Her brother had outgrown his hyperkinesis and had settled into a less hectic, although somewhat borderline, life-style. The younger sister had gone through a period of depression in her high school years and had been seen by the same therapist in both individual and group therapy. Her conflicts resolved around the close oedipal attachment to her father, a weight problem, and a fear of sexual involvement with boys. Finally, the mother began to assert herself and found a career direction and a truer sense of identity. Her newfound independence, fostered by psychotherapy, brought her to a point of improved self-esteem but increasing dissatisfaction with her marriage. Her husband finally gave in to her demands and entered into marital therapy with her. They have made mutual compromises, but their marital prognosis is guarded.

Discussion

These two cases have many features in common. Both are nonpsychotic, passive-dependent girls with hysterical features. Both experienced seductive, and at the same time rejecting, behavior from their fathers. Both of them were uncomfortable in their feminine identity and had difficulty modeling after their ineffectual and rejecting mothers. Furthermore, both reacted to their hair-pulling problem with shame and embarrassment, keeping their head covered at all times with a wig, which had taken on the significance of a transitional object, as described by Winnicott (1953). The successful outcome in treatment resulted in the giving up of the wig and a transfer of cathexis to adult-like heterosexual objects.

The start of hair-pulling in both cases had its onset in puberty. In order to understand why the symptom developed at this time, it is important to keep in mind the pressures, both conscious and unconscious, confronting such youngsters. At a more conscious level there is a need to make quick adjustments to a rapidly changing physical appearance, as well as learning to deal with the physiological stresses created by hormonal imbalance. The unconscious psychological conflicts have been comprehensively outlined by Blos (1962). He viewed the period of early adolescence as a time of revival of the Oedipus complex at the same time that the youngster is attempting to disengage from the primary love objects. Heterosexual object choice is gradually made possible through the abandonment of previously held narcissistic and bisexual positions. In the case of the young adolescent girl there is a tendency to defend actively against a regressive pull to the preoedipal mother by a forceful and decisive turn toward heterosexuality. The girl's fear of this regressive pull may also cause her to react in an extremely negativistic manner toward her mother. The frustration, insecurity, and anxiety resulting from

449

these unconscious conflicts may be countered somewhat in masturbation fantasies, although in some youngsters there remains a marked resistance and inhibition of masturbatory impulses.

Both of our cases have features in their background and developmental history which makes it obvious why entrance into adolescence was such a struggle. They both experienced fixations at all levels of psychosexual development. When they reached puberty there was a strong regressive pull to each of these fixation points. At the oral level both experienced deprivation, which was more pronounced in Sandra, whose mother had suffered a post-partum depression. In both, the frustrated oral dependency needs led to the development of passive-dependent personality structures. In Barbara these oral features were expressed further in overeating, whereas in both there was a perpetuation of separation concerns and depressive tendencies. Both the strands of hair which were pulled out, one by one, and the wig which was used to cover the resulting bald spots, represented transitional objects which helped them to defend against feelings of separation and loneliness. Furthermore, the resulting hairlessness and baldness could be seen as a symbolic means of returning to a period of childish innocence and total dependence.

The girls remained, to some degree, at a narcissistic level of development in which they continued to rely upon themselves for pleasurable sensations. The hair-pulling provided them with a tingling feeling of the scalp, similar to that which must be felt when an infant's head is stroked. Autoerotic activities are common in small children, especially at a time of fatigue, illness, or insecurity. For our two subjects, the entrance into adolescence was such a trauma that they resorted to infantile autoerotic practices to pacify themselves.

At the anal level, both were still dealing with unresolved control issues at the time they were entering chronological adolescence. As oldest children in their families, both were subjected to intensified parental pressures and controls. The act of hair-pulling provided some sense of control, similar to the accomplishment of learning to control the bowels and bladder. In the case of Sandra, there was a continuation of bladder-control problems throughout adolescence. In both, there was an opportunity to displace aggressive affect from the ambivalent love objects to the individual strands of hair. Or, looking at it another way, the hair-pulling experience provided them with an opportunity to identify with the aggressor. These autoaggressive activities were also associated with an exhibitionistic sense of pride and achievement. It was as if the girls were saying, "Look what I can do!" while at the same time they were guiltily covering their achievement with a "dirty old wig." In Barbara these anal features were further manifested in her unkempt, sloppy appearance.

At the genital level, both girls found themselves in the uncomfortable position of having to deal with a seductive father while lacking a stable, mature mother with whom to identify. Barbara's father was overtly seductive, with his exhibitionistic nudity and display of pornography. Sandra's father was less overt in his seductive behavior, but his overconcern with her enuresis was stimulating because of close proximity of the urethra to the vagina and the pleasurable sensations associated with urination. Both fathers attempted to control their own sexual responses to their daughters by rejection and corporal punishment. This behavioral inconsistency only served to confuse the girls and to trigger a process of unconscious fusion of pleasure and pain. In this vein, both girls described the sensation derived from plucking out the hairs from their scalp as both "feeling good" and "irritating." Thus, the hair-pulling can be viewed as a masochistic repetition compulsion of the early experiences with their fathers.

The hair-pulling can also be seen to relate to unresolved penis envy. The individual strands of hair are phallic symbols, and the plucking experience served to perpetuate the fantasy that the castrated penis can grow back. The resulting bald spots were symbolic of the castration and served as a punishment for the fantasied oedipal wishes. These fantasies were kept hidden from conscious awareness by the ever-present wig, which served as a disguise to the outside world and the punitive superego.

The lack of oedipal resoltuion led to sexual immaturity in both girls, manifested in Barbara by bisexual conflicts and in Sandra by masturbatory inhibition. Barbara fought against her homosexual impulses by engaging in promiscuous heterosexual behavior. This nondiscriminatory sexual behavior was also a way for her safety to act out her sexual desires for her father. For Barbara the hair-pulling can also be viewed as a means of renouncing her femininity so that she could please her father, who had always made it clear that he would have preferred her to be a boy.

For both girls the reawakening of unresolved oedipal strivings was intensified by the heightened physiological changes occurring during early adolescence. In addition to these unresolved pregenital and oedipal issues, adolescence also brought into play other insecurities associated with school and peer pressures, as well as the need to begin making commitments for the future. With all of these internal and external pressures bombarding these two girls, it is easy to see how the hair-pulling habit served as an obsessive preoccupation and a compulsive ritual which isolated frightening affects from entering into conscious awareness. The hair-pulling, resulting bald spots, and wearing of the wig provided the secondary gain of attracting considerable attention, albeit negative, from the rejecting parents, as well as caring and concern from the therapist and fellow group-therapy members.

451

The treatment consisted of an uncovering of the repressed incestual and aggressive strivings, especially in the individual therapy sessions. The adolescent group-therapy experience enabled the patients to push toward adolescence and to counter the regressive pull to the pregenital fixation points. The other group members served as role models, and the sharing with them of the hair-pulling secret symbolically represented a revealing of unconscious penis envy and castration fears. Once they were freed of these conflicts, the patients were able to move on to healthier heterosexual object attachments.

The basic character structure of both girls probably will continue to be predominantly passive-dependent with hysterical features, but they are less likely to utilize the unhealthy defenses of repression and denial as an outcome of their therapy. Hence, they should be able to function as adult heterosexual women, even though they both appear to have transferred their unfulfilled dependency needs to their boyfriends or husbands. The hair-pulling no longer serves as a transitional experience or as a means of working through unconscious conflicts resulting from disturbances in psychosexual development.

Conclusions

Hair-pulling is a multidetermined habit disorder which can have its origins at any of the pregenital fixation points or develop as an outgrowth of unresolved oedipal issues. It can be found in association with almost any psychiatric diagnostic entity, although the two cases described in this paper are nonpsychotic adolescent girls with passive-dependent personalities and hysterical features. The notion that the onset of hair-pulling in adolescence is a poor prognostic sign needs to be reexamined in light of the successful treatment outcome in these two cases. The use of peer-group psychotherapy as an adjunctive means of undoing the regressive pull to pregenital levels of psychosexual development should be given strong consideration as an effective means of treating this problem. Finally, the term trichotillomania should probably be discarded from the psychiatric nomenclature, as it is extremely misleading, implying that a psychotic illness is responsible for the disorder.

REFERENCES

Azrin, N. H., and Nunn, R. G. 1973. Habit reversal: a method of eliminating nervous habits. *Behavior Research and Therapy* 11:619–628.

Bartsch, E. 1956. Contribution towards the aetiology of trichotillomania in infancy. *Psychiatrie, Neurologie und Medizinische Psychologie* 8:173–182.

Bayer, C. A. 1972. Self-monitoring and mild aversion treatment of trichotillomania. *Journal of Behavior Therapy and Experimental Psychiatry* 3:139–141.

Berg, C. 1936. The unconscious significance of hair. *International Journal of Psycho-Analysis* 17:73–88.

Blos, P. 1962. *On Adolescence.* New York: Free Press.

Buxbaum, E. 1960. Hair pulling and fetishism. *Psychoanalytic Study of the Child* 15:243–260.

Delgado, R. A., and Mannino, F. B. 1969. Some observations on trichotillomania in children. *Journal of the American Academy of Child Psychiatry* 8:229–246.

Greenberg, H. R., and Sarner, C. A. 1965. Trichotillomania. *Archives of General Psychiatry* 12:482–489.

Hallopeau, X. 1889. Alopecia par grottage (trichomania ou trichotillomania). *Annals of Dermatology and Syphilology* 10:440.

Horne, D. J. de L. 1977. Behavior therapy for trichotillomania. *Behavior Research and Therapy* 15:192–195.

Huber, E. G. 1959. Trichotillomania as a free wheeling mechanism. *Zeitschrift fuer Psychotherapie und Medizinische Psychologie* 9:77–81.

Mannino, F. B., and Delgado, R. A. 1969. Trichotillomania in children: a review. *American Journal of Psychiatry* 126:505–511.

Mehregan, A. H. 1970. Trichotillomania: a clinicopathologic study. *Archives of Dermatology* 102:129–133.

Monroe, J. T., Jr., and Abse, D. W. 1963. The psychopathology of trichotillomania and trichophagy. *Psychiatry* 26:95–103.

Muller, S. A., and Winkelmann, R. K. 1972. Trichotillomania. *Archives of Dermatology* 105:535–539.

Oguchi, T., and Miura, S. 1977. Trichotillomania: its psychopathological aspect. *Comprehensive Psychiatry* 18:177–182.

Philippopoulos, G. S. 1961. A case of trichotillomania (hair pulling). *Acta Psychotherpeutica* (Basel) 9:304–312.

Rechenberger, H. G. 1976. Dynamic psychiatric interpretation of a disease model of trichotillomania. *Zeitschrift fuer Psychosomatishe Medizin und Psychoanalyse* 22:126–131.

Sanderson, K. V., and Hall-Smith, P. 1970. Tonsore trichotillomania. *British Journal of Dermatology* 82:345–350.

Sperling, M. 1954. The use of the hair as a bisexual symbol. *Psychoanalytic Review* 41:363–365.

Stadelli, H. 1963. The choice of the symptom of trichotillomania. *Praxis der Kinderpsychologie und Kinderpsychiatrie* 12:122–127.

Takaishi, N.; Fujii, H.; Ohmi, S.; et al. 1959. Psychiatric study of trichotillomania. *Skin* (Tokyo) 122:126.

Taylor, J. G. 1963. A behavioral interpretation of obsessive compulsive neurosis. *Behavioral Research and Therapy* 1:237–244.

Winnicott, D. W. 1953. Transitional objects and transitional phenomena: a study of the first not-me possession. *International Journal of Psycho-Analysis* 34:89–97.

Winnik, H. Z., and Gabbay, F. 1965. On trichotillomania: a study in minor autoaggressions. *Israel Annals of Psychiatry and Related Disciplines* 3:131–147.

Zaidens, S. 1951. Self-inflicted dermatoses and their psychodynamics. *Journal of Nervous and Mental Diseases* 113:400–402.

PART IV

THERAPEUTIC APPROACHES IN ADOLESCENT PSYCHIATRY

EDITORS' INTRODUCTION

The world of the adolescent is not the world of the adult. Many of the stresses faced by adolescents, such as poor family and peer relationships, school difficulties, sexual conflicts, and the struggle for identity and independence, are quite different in nature and content from the stresses of adult life. Thus, adolescent development theory and treatment modalities must reflect these differences.

This part explores in depth a number of different therapeutic approaches to the special world of the adolescent and his family. The approaches range from intensive psychoanalytic treatment of the neurotic adolescent to specific intervention with seriously disturbed adolescents requiring hospitalization and combined individual and family therapy. Effective therapeutic intervention must be specific and tailored to highly individualized needs. Only an approach embracing developmental, genetic, psychosocial, socioeconomic, and biological factors will allow this perspective. Knowledge of family systems must share equally with awareness of psychoanalytic theory. Similarly, grasp of the interaction between society and adolescent process is essential.

Moses Laufer examines reconstruction in psychoanalytic treatment: the rebuilding with a patient of what happened during development, how he experienced his past life, and what part was played by fantasy and by distortion. In adolescents, however, Laufer believes the nature of the psychopathology is different and, therefore, the direction and function of reconstruction must reflect adolescent process. Reconstruction of the preadolescent past makes little sense to the adolescent while he is experiencing failure in his immediate life. Unless interpretations and reconstructions are first placed within the context of the adolescent's current struggles, the central purpose of analysis in adolescence is lost.

Derek Miller writes about the treatment of seriously disturbed adolescents and the importance of specific interventions to prevent the development of chronic intractable states. The production of serious disturbance is viewed from developmental, genetic, psychosocial, socioeconomic, psychotraumatic, and biologic perspectives. Careful balance of these various factors in treatment planning with specific transference dilemmas to be avoided are seen as necessary to prevent development of neglect disorders or chronic ilness states.

Judith A. Ashway discusses the changing needs of female adolescents living in a society where they are freer to choose occupations, natures, and roles than ever before. She notes, however, that change of any kind holds both promise and burdens. Female adolescents receive conflicting messages in the areas of family relationships, peer relations, sexuality, and self-esteem that have to be approached in a holistic fashion during treatment. Ashway believes that psychotherapists should have knowledge about adolescent growth and development; patience and a sense of humor; flexibility and availability; respect for the adolescent's struggle for autonomy and identity formation; competency to deal with the emotional and physical aspects of sexuality, pregnancy, and abortion; and she raises the issue of using female psychotherapists to provide a same-sex role model. The goal is to assist women to emerge as more secure, self-respecting, productive adults.

John G. Looney, Mark J. Blotcky, Doyle I. Carson, and John T. Gossett examine the impact of psychotherapy and hospitalization on emotionally disturbed adolescents. They are concerned about the quality of care provided and believe that a model program should utilize the concept of a well-functioning family system. Using a five-level system of family function (optimal, competent but pained, dominant-submissive, conflicted, chaotic) they illustrate how they assess the impact of their program on adolescent patients and attempt to achieve maximal effectiveness in their treatment approaches.

Loren H. Crabtree, Jr., and Douglas F. Levinson studied the social processes of an adolescent therapeutic community as a general system. They found that there are definable stages of organizational development, elaboration, and eventual deterioration. Large groups undergo, in addition, discrete cycles of tension that are challenges to management. Crabtree and Levinson discuss the diagnostic and leadership abilities necessary to reverse these entropic developments and provide creative program alternatives.

Reed Brockbank examines group process in adolescence and discusses those developmental factors served by the peer group. He found that displacement of unresolved parental dependency, elaboration of homosexual and heterosexual object ties, and reworking of group and individual identity are the significant factors that the group provides on the way to adulthood's intimacy and commitment. In group therapy these characteristics are emphasized, complicated by action and regression. Brockbank warns of the vicissitudes in adolescents while participating in group therapy and the therapeutic value to be gained from dealing with narcissistic impulses in a group setting.

MOSES LAUFER

In psychoanalytic treatment we take it for granted that reconstruction is fundamental both to our theory and to our day-to-day work with patients. Early in his psychoanalytic writings, Freud compared our analytic tasks with our patients with those of the archaeologist—looking for signs of the past, drawing conclusions or completing a map from the foundation which is unearthed, putting together a picture of the overall edifice from a large number of pieces which may not fit exactly. He reminded us of the authority of the past, showing us that psychological life must be viewed as a continuum, with each previous developmental phase influencing and directing future phases. Psychopathology means for us a history of conflict, compromise formations, compulsions to repeat, and the unreal power of the affective and historical past on the present, especially if it remains alien to the ego. By the ''past'' we mean the infantile or childhood past, whether that is preoedipal, oedipal, or preadolescent; and with our adult patients our eyes are always on this past—examining, looking for more evidence, rebuilding together with the patient what happened, how he experienced his past life, and what part was played by fantasy and by distortion. In the course of what I wish to say about reconstruction in adolescent analysis, I will try to show that what we have borrowed from our experience with adult patients only partially fits the adolescent. This is because adult pathology and adolescent pathology are very different from one another.

The role of reconstruction in analytic work has not been discussed very much since Freud's 1937 ''Constructions in Analysis.'' Greenacre's 1975 paper is the exception. I will use these two studies as my main sources of reference and comparisons with what I will say about reconstruction in adolescent analysis. Freud used the terms ''construction'' and ''reconstruction'' interchangeably, meaning primarily that "one lays before the subject of the analysis a piece of his early history that he has forgotten. . . ." Interpretation, on the other hand, is "something one does to some single element of the material, such as an association or a parapraxis" (1937, p. 261). Greenacre not only discusses the work of the analysis but also differentiates between the reconstructions of the analyst and those of the patient, reminding us that the undoing of pathology is based on insight and that insight is tied to reconstruction, but that reconstructions require a constant remodeling as new facts or new evidence emerges, especially through the transference.

As regards the treatment of the adolescent, there are many different points of view about the pros and cons of analysis, about technique, and about the part played by the period of adolescence in one's mental life (Klumpner 1975). Some writers think that analysis should not be undertaken during adolescence, believing that the treatment process goes contrary to the needs of the adolescent and to the inherent developmental push. Some writers see the acute difficulties in treatment as predictable and feel that a range of parameters may be introduced both as a safeguard to the treatment and as a way of meeting the need of the adolescent. There is also the view that, if we rely on reconstructing the past in the undoing of pathology, we must expect difficulties (often insurmountable ones) with the adolescent patient. Yet another view is that the adolescent insists on denying the past, whereas we work with the assumption that the past is central to one's life and to an understanding of what may have gone wrong developmentally; that interpretations which are related to the past, and which are followed over a period of time by reconstructions, are often experienced by the adolescent as a confirmation that he remains regressively tied to those objects which he feels he must give up if he is to develop toward psychological adulthood. Such understandings are, I believe, theoretical formulations that at the same time contain the stuff which may either drive the adolescent away from analysis (and from coming into touch with the history and the meaning of his illness) or may participate in resistances that are used to avoid the pain of the present reality.

It is understandable, in terms of the history of psychoanalysis, that we have made use of our experience with the adult patient and have tried to apply it to the analysis of the adolescent. But I think that the nature of adolescent pathology, and the acute anxiety which surrounds this pathology, is such that the role of the past and its recollection is different for the ill adolescent than for the ill adult, and, therefore, the direction of analysis is different. This then implies that reconstruction in adolescent analysis has a function which seems to be different from that in adult analysis.

How much of what Freud and Greenacre have discussed about reconstruction is applicable to the analysis of the adolescent? Why do we so often come up against impossible resistances when we try to reconstruct the past of the adolescent? Or, even if we do interpret and then reconstruct the past, we are met with the fact that nothing really alters the life of our adolescent patients, or, worse still, we find that the usual approaches to reconstruction may even encourage the adolescent to run away from analysis.

My views about reconstruction in adolescent analysis come from my experiences at the Centre for Research into Adolescent Breakdown, where I have had the opportunity to follow the analyses of a number of seriously disturbed adolescents. The patients I have in mind have come with presenting problems of anorexia, attempted suicide, homosexuality, or psychotic-type functioning. In each instance, I came to the conclusion that the pathology of the adolescent could not be understood or altered except through individual analysis, since contact with parents, schools, or police was to no avail.

The young people who come to me for help may present a whole range of disturbances, but in my selection of adolescents who are suitable for analysis, I look for signs in their behavior or functioning which convey to me that a developmental breakdown has taken place. The assumption I make about developmental breakdown is that, for some adolescents, physical sexual maturity precipitates what seems to be a sudden overwhelming of the ego, with the result that the sexual body image throughout adolescence is rejected or denied expression (Laufer 1978). Such an experience must endanger the function of adolescence which may, in summary, be described as the establishment of a final sexual organization (Freud 1905).

In the adolescents studied, their experiencing at puberty emerging sexual impulses adds new meaning to earlier oedipal or preoedipal fantasies. Unconsciously they are overwhelmed by their incestuous wishes, with the accompanying fear that they may live out these wishes. The defenses which they have used up to puberty now suddenly prove to be inadequate. If they are not psychotic (and my patients are not), they try to defend against these wishes by rejecting their sexuality or by distorting the unconscious wishes. This experience at puberty is, for these adolescents, equivalent to a trauma. They feel overwhelmed and frightened; and at the same time, the anxiety which is attached to this experience is of such intensity that they are constantly fearful that this loss of control might happen to them again.

Privately, or perhaps secretly, these adolescents continue to feel abnormal. Their fantasies or secret sexual actions are proof to them that something is seriously wrong with them. Analysis for these adolescents is both frightening and an enormous relief (because it offers hope to them that something can be done to change their lives).

462

Reconstruction in the analyses of these adolescents is a critical experience. Even though the adolescent does not know why he often feels dissatisfied with the direction or the progress of his treatment, he is aware that his present life is in disarray, his present anxieties, fears, and relationships continue to make him feel abnormal, and his fantasies convince him that he is crazy. He cries, "Why don't you help me understand what is going on now?" In terms of the nature of his present pathology, the adolescent is right, and his discomfort is something that we must take note of in the analysis.

The analysis of the adolescent patient must enable him to reexperience and relive the breakdown which took place at puberty, but this time it is reexperienced and relived within the transference. The function of reconstruction, then, is to first put the patient in touch with this traumatic experience and the accompanying affects, and then, through the transference, help him to see why this breakdown had to take place at puberty and why it took the form it did. Unless this is done, the power of the trauma at puberty continues to operate and prevents the adolescent from undoing the immediate past and integrating the experience of the breakdown. The transference relationship allows the piecing together of the adolescent's core fantasies, that is, fantasies which are central to the life of the adolescent and which are active now in his sexual life (Laufer 1976). There is no purpose in piecing together fantasies and experiences of the oedipal or preoedipal past while the adolescent is experiencing sexual fantasies now which make no sense to him, and while the more recent breakdown which took place at puberty is still experienced as a traumatic event.

In the analysis of adolescents there is danger that we may reconstruct the wrong thing at the wrong time. Here we may be ignoring what the adolescent is telling us or, perhaps, unable to tell us but wanting us to know about in order to help him understand. We may make the mistake of assuming that earlier or deeper is better and more therapeutic. Concentration on the wrong things and reconstructions of the wrong past may be why so many adolescents run away from analysis.

It is of help to me in my work with adolescent patients to think of them as having two pasts—the more immediate past, which contains the traumatic experience at puberty; and the preadolescent past, which has woven into it the preoedipal history, the oedipal resolutions, and the experience of latency. Both pasts need understanding and reconstruction, but, unless the immediate past makes sense to the adolescent patient, the reconstruction of childhood is an intellectual experience and of little help affectively.

I do not want to give the impression that we must stay away from trying to understand the preadolescent past until we have reconstructed and helped the adolescent to work through the breakdown at puberty. We must keep in the forefront of our thinking what it was that brought the adolescent to analysis. Very often, the adolescent and his environment (parents, school, and various professional people who have contact with the patient) will try to get us to forget why the adolescent came for treatment. I have experienced this most often with adolescent patients who have attempted suicide, where everyone (including the patient) wants to believe that the event was something which is now past and is best forgotten. I take a different view and let the adolescent know that I cannot forget or pretend. Often, the adolescent conveys that he knows unconsciously that the recent events are more painful and more frightening than the long-past ones. But if we allow the patient to resist understanding his recent past and what it means to his whole life, we deny him the possibility of integrating the trauma of the breakdown at puberty and helping him to believe that he can take an active part in creating a continuity to his life (rather than feel passive in relation to his past and future).

By the time the adolescent comes to analysis, there is already some integration into the ego of his distorted sexual body image. The extent of this integration varies a great deal with patients and will depend on the quality of the gratification from his core fantasies (central masturbation fantasy), on the severity of the regression which has taken place, and on the extent to which the adolescent's function of reality testing is intact. But, in every instance, the integration of the distorted sexual body image will express itself in present object relationships. What we may see is anything from a total absence of sexual relationships to those which contain obvious elements of perverse development.

The adolescent will not say "there is something wrong with my sexual body" but may instead complain of loneliness and isolation, and that relationships never have the meaning he seeks. The anxiety about his own distorted sexual body image and his failure to alter this is expressed through his feelings about these relationships. Whatever else may feel wrong to the adolescent, he is unconsciously aware that he is failing as a sexual being. His superego never lets him forget this, even though he may have available a wide range of ways to help him deny his failure.

In analysis, then, reconstruction of the preoedipal or oedipal past makes little sense to the adolescent while he is experiencing failure in his immediate life. His anxiety is tied to the experiences of puberty and adolescence. His self-worthlessness and unconscious feeling of being out of control need to make sense to him in the transference before reconstruction of childhood takes on meaning. Dependence on the analyst, a wish for mothering, a wish to replace the oedipal parent, and early fantasies of having destroyed the parent or a sibling may all be historically correct, but initially interpretations which lead to such reconstructions create a feeling in the adolescent that treatment has no meaning. Unless interpretations and reconstructions are first placed within the context of the adolescent's present sexual life, the central purpose of analysis in adolescence is lost.

The importance of first resolving the pubertal trauma which is distorting age-appropriate adolescent experiences is illustrated by the following clinical example:

An eighteen-year-old, in the first interview, described his loneliness and depression at length. He was having difficulty in his studies and was uncertain about which road to take, being gifted in philosophy and art. It took a number of interviews to establish that analysis should be the treatment of choice, as at first his story did not fit together. I recommended we meet a few times to try to define what it was he thought I could help him with.

He related that all of his relationships were homosexual, and he felt that he was now deciding to live a homosexual life. Although nobody knew of this, he had had a large number of ongoing relationships with men, each one being a sexual one at some point. He described the sexuality as including anal intercourse, fellatio, being overpowered and overpowering, and occasionally joining an orgy which meant a range of sexual experiences in one night with a number of young men.

He knew from the start that I did not accept his view that homosexuality was as normal as any other form of sexuality. Coming to analysis meant giving up his various plans and moving to a university in London. He was clearly a highly gifted young man, but his functioning contained elements of psychotic-type organization, and he worried me.

His early communications in the analysis revolved around the closeness to his mother, who, he reported, had experienced a number of episodes of madness during his childhood. His father, although highly successful in his work, was considered a failure at home. His memories of his early life were of an isolated child, revered by his parents. He was considered brilliant but frightened of other children at school, who usually ignored him. He remembered spending many free hours painting landscapes for his mother, who would sit by him in ecstasy. He had his first sexual relationship with another boy when he was aged six. This relationship continued throughout his preadolescence and consisted of mutual masturbation, fellatio, and hugging. At other times he reported masturbating to pictures of male athletes.

In the transference, I soon became the failed father who could not do anything right. I also was the person who was to take away his homosexuality. He wanted to feel close to me, but he felt I was distant. He went into considerable detail about his art and his staying up to read books on philos-

465

ophy, and every so often he would tell me of the man with whom he had spent the previous night. He began to taunt me with a long list of beautiful men who loved him.

My interpretations at this point were directed mainly at his disappointment and his feeling that these men still left him feeling alone and empty. His frustration with these men helped him feel that I was a failure. I called attention to his fear of coming to treatment, but I did not try to interpret this because I did not know what it might mean. I could have guessed at its meaning—fear of closeness, fear of giving in, wish for my closeness so that he could then destroy me. Instead, I repeatedly referred to the discrepancy between his belief that the world would be perfect if he had a beautiful sexual partner and his private feeling that nothing was worthwhile and that he must never allow himself to feel sad.

He reported a dream of a man lying on a diving board in a swimming pool—the man and the diving board being under the water. The man looked contented but dead. This led to his telling me of the hours he was spending in his room lying on the floor, feeling unable to get up. At his work, before coming to London, he had had a sexual relationship with another male employee, after which this person did not even bother to greet him on the street. My patient then went to his room, contemplated suicide, and subsequently spent about seven hours lying on the floor feeling that something in him had died. He became so frightened by this, thinking that he would jump out the window (as he claims his mother threatened to do when he was aged six), that he ran out of his room and wandered the streets for most of the night. His fear of continuing the analysis had to do with his immediate fear that I would force him to remember what had happened that day. He accused me of taking away the men who made him happy, saying that he had never again thought of that episode until I forced him to have a dream and to remember this terrible experience. The excitement in the sessions, of my getting into him and making him one with me, was included in my interpretations, but I did not lose sight of the fact that, for the present, this was much less important than the anxiety and the meaning of the experience of feeling so desperate when he lay on the floor for hours. Nothing was any good, and his own physical beauty meant nothing if I reminded him of this inability to hold onto someone who could love him.

The reconstruction of the breakdown at puberty now had begun—but we were far from a full answer. He recalled his astonishment at being able to ejaculate and the accompanying feeling that his mother would be horrified if she knew. He tried for nearly two years after puberty to continue to speak in a high-pitched voice. He remembered secretly lying on the floor during this period, crying and wishing for his mother to tell him that she would go on loving him for his art. The longing for his father had never been conscious. I did not interpret this other than to call attention to the fact that he found it impossible to accept that his father was very taken up with his own work. I also mentioned that my patient must continue to feel that his father was responsible for his mother's mental state.

He talked of his past, but his memories were restricted. He was clearly frightened about coming into touch with a childhood which he felt he has lost. But my focus at this point throughout the sessions was on the immediate past and on the affective experiences which were still alive and frightening. Transference interpretations were directed primarily at the different ways he now experienced me in relation to his male sexual partners. I noted his longing for me as a sexual partner and his wish both to be loved by me and to destroy my potency. I did not interpret his hatred of his mother and his accusations toward her, which occurred in dreams. Instead, my concentration was on his fear of women and his discomfort in being treated as a potent man.

I am excluding here details of the piecing together of his core fantasy, except to say that these details came via the repetition of sexual experiences with men, the efforts to force me to attack and hit him, and the satisfaction he described himself as getting from men after anal penetration and being hugged. At this point, the patient was in touch with the extent of the anxiety he experienced if not touched after penetration. He felt prepared to give in to men in any way, even though this giving in often left him feeling that he was crazy during this period—a union with the object, but with the underlying fear of being thrown away.

Conclusions

In adolescence, the patient is more vulnerable to giving in to hopelessness and to feeling that nothing can ever change. If we accept the view that a main function of adolescence developmentally is the establishment of a final sexual organization (an irreversible sexual identity by the end of adolescence), reversibility of pathology during this period is critical. Reconstruction, then, of breakdown following puberty is essential if we are to influence this outcome. The understanding of the reasons why this breakdown had to take place following puberty is essential for insight and to free the adolescent to be responsible actively for the direction of his future social and sexual life.

REFERENCES

Freud, S. 1905. Three essays on the theory of sexuality. *Standard Edition* 7:123–243. London: Hogarth, 1953.

Freud, S. 1906. My views on the part played by sexuality in the aetiology of the neuroses. *Standard Edition* 7:271–279. London: Hogarth, 1953.

Freud, S. 1937. Constructions in analysis. *Standard Edition* 23:255–269. London: Hogarth, 1964.

Greenacre, P. 1975. On reconstruction. *Journal of the American Psychoanalytic Association* 4(23): 693–712.

Klumpner, G. H. 1975. On the psychoanalysis of adolescents. *Adolescent Psychiatry* 4:393–400.

Laufer, M. 1976. The central masturbation fantasy, the final sexual organization, and adolescence. *Psychoanalytic Study of the Child* 31:297–316.

Laufer, M. 1978. The nature of adolescent pathology and the psychoanalytic process. *Psychoanalytic Study of the Child* 33:307–322.

DEREK MILLER

Epidemiological studies reveal that a good many disturbances of adolescence automatically correct themselves. At any one time some 15 percent of high school–aged adolescents show symptoms of psychological disturbance; about 3 percent are seriously disturbed (Feinstein and Miller 1979). The larger percentage includes those who appear to recover either by the chance appearance of psychological support or through supportive therapy.

In the treatment of seriously disturbed adolescents, however, a multiplicity of determinants of illness are relevant. The important issue is the decision as to where the weight of maximum therapeutic intervention should occur. A failure here can create a state of intractable illness which becomes unresponsive to treatment. Seriously disturbed adolescents require specific interventions (Knesper and Miller 1976) and cannot be left for the possibility of self-righting mechanisms to occur.

The Production of Serious Disturbance

Many disturbed adolescents have become pubertal but have never become psychologically adolescent. These boys and girls reach their teenage years, become physiologically mature, and show the psychological responses to this process, but do not have the emotional capacity to develop a truly autonomous sense of self (Miller 1978b). Often such individuals have had seriously disturbed childhoods and may suffer from a variety of neuroendocrine disorders or severe nurturing deficits. The characterological distortion that occurs before puberty makes the possibility of secondary separation-individuation resolution, a sine qua non of adolescence, effectively impossible (Mahler 1972). When postpubertal and physiologically adult, it is clear that such individuals are, psychologically, almost exactly the same individuals as they were prior to puberty and that no significant steps have been taken toward autonomy. A severely obsessional eight-year-old is likely to become a severely obsessional fifteen-year-old, although the individual has coped with some of the psychological issues of puberty and there is some recognition of body-image change. Attempts at mastery are not enough and the characterological difficulties that existed prior to puberty have prevented the development of adolescence.

An individual who suffers from childhood schizophrenia experiences such a situation. This illness typically appears prior to puberty. Such children, while attempting to cope with the psychological stresses of puberty, do not become psychologically adolescent. This is partly because they have not sufficient personality strength to tolerate the stress produced by physiological change and partly because psychological separation from parents cannot be envisaged. Other examples are some types of unipolar and bipolar affective illness in childhood and adolescence that are commonly not recognized. Children who suffer from these disorders may be diagnosed prior to puberty as only characterologically disturbed. After puberty they may become even more turbulent and the likelihood of adequate diagnosis is lessened (Perris 1966).

Lower-socioeconomic-class children who suffer in this way often are mishandled in both the mental health and correctional systems. They become increasingly developmentally damaged and develop iatrogenic difficulties similar to those of poorly treated chronic schizophrenics. Borderline children who are not successfully treated are more disturbed at fifteen than they were at five.

Another subgroup of seriously disturbed adolescents become psychologically adolescent, but for a whole variety of reasons the psychosocial processes that are required to support the continuing development of healthy adolescence do not occur. Some early adolescents repond to traumatic experiences such as parent loss, parental separation, moving, and illness by the abuse of drugs. The regressive effects of such substances as marijuana and alcohol reinforce the regressive developmental pull which is always present in early and midadolescence and become an impediment to further emotional development.

There is a current concept that an isolated nuclear family can easily offer sufficient developmental support, but in my opinion this is inaccurate. If adolescents are not exposed to a social system which provides them with meaningful and consistent relationships with emotionally significant adults and peers, serious developmental disturbance can occur even in those children who have previously been well nurtured (Miller 1970, 1974). This problem is often most clearly seen in the children of highly mobile social groups—diplomats, international businessmen, and the like.

It would appear that the severity of problem presentation in adolescents does not necessarily relate to the severity of the underlying illness. However, the psychosocial feedback secondarily produced by the adolescent's problems can reinforce those personality disorders that present mostly as behavior disturbances. Symptoms become intractable when youngsters receive so much instinctual gratification from their problems that they cannot abandon them. It may become so satisfying to smoke marijuana that there is no reason to do anything else. Similarly, adolescents may not be able to give up tormenting their parents, the emotional gratification of greed associated with theft, or the omnipotence associated with suicidal threats.

Problem presentation may also confirm a child's distorted view of the world. A central issue for the disturbed adolescent is dealing with helplessness. Most psychologically ill adolescents—whether they are depressed, schizophrenic, or suffering from characterological disturbances or psychosomatic illness—are dealing with problems of autonomy. If separation-individuation does not take place, the adolescent has to deal with a pervasive sense of helplessness. Along with this experience goes a perception that the world is tormenting and persecutory (Klein 1950). In the pubertal early adolescent, a normative attempt by parents to be benign may produce a startling persecutory response: the good intent of authority figures may be felt as highly coercive and the experience of helplessness is then reinforced in the child. The sense of helplessness and persecution is even greater for disturbed adolescents. Those adolescents who have some capacity to appraise reality may have the confused feeling that the world is not as persecutory as they sense it to be. The environment is then manipulated in order to make individuals within it really persecutory; to make others persecute is to give a bizarre sense of mastery. This issue pervades residential care, individual therapy, and family work with adolescents.

To obtain environmental consistency, disturbed adolescents usually conform to implicit environmental messages. Johnson and Szurek (1956) wrote that children and adolescents often act out the unconscious (implicit) wishes of their parents. Aichhorn (1935) pointed out that delinquent adolescents in treatment may respond to the unconscious provocation of their therapists. In almost every communication from a social system to a child there are always two messages—the overt and the covert. If these are consonant both are obeyed; if they are dissonant the implicit one is more likely to be heard. It is common for parents to shout, "Don't shout"; the child is then implicitly told that it is acceptable to shout but one must be bigger and better at it.

In family and therapeutic systems, the implicit message often represents the expression of the conflicts of significant members of the system. For example, a family who found narcotics belonging to their son in the house threw them away, did not seek to find out where they came from, and never considered involving the law. The father did not conceal the fact that he did all in his power to avoid paying income tax and the boy knew about these family attitudes. His parents, however, were incensed with him because he broke the law.

In family therapy with seriously disturbed adolescents an important clarification is to demonstrate to parents how they implicitly communicate to their children how to behave. In residential settings the same issue is relevant with the staff.

On the one hand, adolescent symptoms can be used in the service of making the world persecutory; on the other, young people may get instinctual gratification from their symptoms. Symptom presentation can then become part of a phenomenological homeostasis.

Principles of Treatment

Specific therapeutic intervention in serious disturbance requires diagnosis of etiology and assessment of the rapidity with which symptoms must be contained. Neuropharmacological approaches may not deal with the personality difficulties that have developed because of the effect of symptoms in distorting both the life space and ego development of the child. Characterologically disturbed adolescents who suffer from one or another neuroendocrine disorder will not be significantly assisted by psychotherapy or social system intervention alone. Even though these may assist the adolescent to correct a distortion of the perception of stress, they will not change the stress response. On the other hand, only to treat the neuroendocrine etiology of the disturbance will not resolve the personality distortion. If the individual has learned techniques of relating to the world through a characterological disorder, psychotherapeutic and social system interventions are required. Thus, to avoid intractable illness, the balance of neuroendocrine and psychodynamic etiology must be assessed to ensure competent decisions as to where the maximum weight of intervention should be.

Disturbed adolescents are highly intolerant of separation from emotionally significant people. Such separation appears to arouse intense persecutory anxiety and thus a resurgence of symptoms and ego disintegration. Acute schizophrenia may be understood as being a three-phase illness with prepsychotic, psychotic, and postpsychotic periods (Feinstein and Miller 1979). The illness may become chronic and intractable particularly when the effects of the postpsychotic phase are not recognized, especially on cognition (Serbang and Gidynski 1979).

When cognitive regression is created by illness, the individual is no longer as capable of abstract thought as heretofore. If the cognitive deficit is not recognized, then the adolescent may do his best to hide it, for example, by cutting classes. In the prepsychotic or, later, postpsychotic phase of the illness the adolescent may feel and be persecuted by his school environment and perhaps by his parents.

Reexposed to stress, further disintegration may occur. The adolescent may then be forced into an increasingly regressive stance and a chronic neuroendocrine illness becomes a chronic personality disorder. Chronic schizophrenia may then be created which can be as much a result of inadequate care delivery as were hebephrenia and catatonia, which should be considered neglect disorders. A failure to understand the natural history of a mental illness can produce intractable disorder as can the inability to recognize its most significant etiological determinants.

A depressive equivalent often presents itself in adolescence as monosymptomatic illness. Children whose symptomatic behavior is repetitive (for example, auto theft, stealing, drug abuse, underachievement, bed wetting), and in whom the symptoms appear intermittently, should be suspected of suffering from affective illness. Those adolescents who experience affective storms may be suffering from a bipolar illness (Miller 1978a).

Transference Problems with the Use of Medication

One particular transference problem of psychopharmacological treatment of adolescents is that associated with the projection of omnipotence onto therapists. Although the use of medication does not resolve the characterological damage produced by the neuroendocrine disorder, to some, pharmacological treatment appears to offer magical answers. The therapist needs to clarify this issue with the adolescent and his family, since a failure to deal with this is one reason why many adolescents in treatment, when psychopharmacology is used, eventually become reluctant to continue the use of medication. In many other ways omnipotence is a particular transference response in the treatment of adolescents. Disturbed adolescents who cannot bear to experience helplessness and feel externally controlled use their grandiosity as a defense. Such young people attempt to project both their own onmipotence and helplessness onto therapists. If the grandiosity is inappropriately reinforced, the youngster is left with a more pervasive feeling of helplessness and may flee from therapy. On the other hand, if the therapist refuses to accept any of the projection of omnipotence he may be perceived by the adolescent as helpless and useless, creating increased anxiety and frantic acting out in the patient. Medication at first reinforces therapeutic omnipotence if it assists the adolescent to feel calmer. Ultimately, however, the very success of the intervention may make the adolescent feel helpless, and it is at this point that the medication is likely to be refused.

Another possible reason for resisting medication is that pubertal youngsters who have never reached psychosocial adolescence before therapy may become adolescent with a combination of successful pharmacotherapy and psychotherapy. They may then use the therapist as a parental equivalent and refuse medication as a way of establishing autonomy.

Splitting in the Treatment of Adolescents

Another issue which commonly helps create intractability is a failure to deal with the psychological splitting mechanisms of the adolescent. The process of splitting—the active process of maintaining a separation between introjects of opposite qualities (the good and the bad)—exists in normal adolescence but may become a significant barrier to the successful treatment of the seriously disturbed (Kernberg 1975). Prepubertal children normatively use the nuclear family to gain emotional support against the effect of splitting. For example, the child expressing frustration may come home from a visit to the extended family and say, "I hate my grandmother." A parent who replies, "You do not hate grandmother, you love her," may only create alienation. The parent who hears the child, absorbs the concept, and returns to the child a sense of security by accepting the hatred but not reinforcing it provides a type of psychological holding which may result in a positive introject (Winnicott 1965). The child may then visit the grandparent and enjoy the experience. This is the equivalent of the process a mother uses to absorb the rageful tensions of her infant. She holds the child in a loving supportive manner, absorbs tension and anxiety, and gives the child back a feeling of nurturance. In the family, parents alleviate the anxious effects of splitting. As the child brings its hatred home, the family absorbs it and the child is then able to function.

At the beginning of adolescence, as the child once again seeks to be autonomous from parents, this mothering process is no longer possible. An adolescent who brings a split for parental absorption and resolution will seem to the self to be abandoning the attempt at autonomy. The individual can thus no longer comfortably use parents to absorb splitting. What the adolescent then does is to use a relationship with other social systems—significant adults and peers. The problem of peers receiving the individual's split-off bad feeling is that the split may be reinforced. Peers do not say, "Really, teacher is a nice guy"; they have to say, "Yes I agree with you, he is an S.O.B." Thus when adolescents can no longer use their nuclear family as a support against the split and have only peers to console them, the split is reinforced. This creates more projection and the adolescent then has to flee from his or her own intolerable feeling of hatred—a common reason for either regression or acting out. Alternatively, the system or individuals being projected onto may receive the hatred and return it in good measure, becoming primitively coercive instead of supportive. This is a common problem in adolescent wards of psychiatric hospitals which are inadequately staffed and have poorly designed treatment programs.

Social systems which treat and support adolescents may particularly find that the adolescent's family cannot tolerate not being the recipients of their child's split-off feelings. Parents may feel useless and devalued if their disturbed adolescent no longer needs them in this way, and if such parents are not assisted to understand this need they may sabotage the child's treatment.

Sometimes a therapeutic system, unable to tolerate adolescent acting out, which goes with the projection of hatred, may unconsciously deflect this onto parents. This process is enshrined in the high school system which routinely calls parents if their children behave in a way the school dislikes, even if the principal determinant of this is a teacher's behavior. Parents may return the compliment and try to buy the child's love by projecting back onto a therapeutic or educational system. This is a particularly common difficulty in the treatment of schizophrenic adolescents. One possible reason why such adolescents have so many therapists is that professionals are only too willing to accept the adolescents' and families' projections onto previous therapists.

By the time seriously disturbed adolescents come for treatment the projection of hatred may be intense. The individuals within the treatment systems often cannot tolerate being hated. The adolescents' inability to resolve splitting and to feel ambivalent means that while they are hating they cannot also love. The recipient of unambivalent hate may find it as exquisitely painful as the individual who experiences it. The more disturbed the adolescent, the more likely is the youngster to fantasize that therapeutic personnel will be cruel and vicious. The projection of his or her hatred onto staff can be so great that the adolescent cannot tolerate inaction as a response to acting out of hatred and words alone may be so interpreted. The more seriously disturbed the adolescent might be, the more punitive is his expectation of his caretakers. Unfortunately, in standard psychiatric hospital settings, commonly used techniques of isolation and restraint may allow staff to play out the child's punitive fantasy.

The treatment of a schizophrenic boy demonstrates this issue. Acutely disturbed children and adolescents who become overwhelmed with intolerable rage experience a high degree of fragmentation of personality function. All sense of self along with a perception of body boundaries may be lost. One such schizophrenic boy wanted to wear a hat at all times to stop his brain from flying out whenever he became angry. In one treatment setting he was sent to the time-out room (wearing his hat) whenever he became enraged. If he was sufficiently angry, if there was a staff shortage, or if the staff were sufficiently furious in their turn, he was placed in strap restraints. This action reinforced his destructive fantasies, which included visual imagery of skulls with knives stuck through them, and led to greater personality disintegration and increasing preoccupation with suicide.

If seriously disturbed adolescents are isolated from nurturing support which can offer appropriate controls, their psychiatric illness may worsen and inevitably they become developmentally more disturbed.

Growth and Serious Disturbance

Although in itself a highly significant developmental period, adolescence is also the end of preadulthood. A young person who cannot make the move from preadulthood to early adulthood is in difficulties similar to those of the child who cannot become adolescent (Levinson 1978). Successful mastery in adolescence precedes the move to early adulthood with all its psychological implications. Chronic mental illness in adulthood may result from a therapeutic failure in adolescence. Apart from issues such as misdiagnosis (Ford, Hudgens, and Welner 1978), poor care delivery may be due to a failure to deal with primitive narcissistic defenses, the consequent sense of persecution, and the development of external coercion.

All adolescents in treatment have nonspecific needs which are required to reinforce development (Knesper and Miller 1976). These may be subsumed as social, psychological, and biological. Social needs include the provision of a social system with mores which are normative for the patient's social

476

and ethnic groups, a caring intergenerational network, and appropriate outlets for physical and vocational productivity. Psychological needs include adequate education (cognitive, creative, and imaginative) as well as provision for appropriate external controls within the context both of social reality and interpersonal concerns. Biological needs include such issues as adequate food intake (not just in terms of calories and protein but also in availability at all times), adequate exercise, adequate cleanliness, and so on. An example of nonspecific psychological intervention is as follows.

An adolescent who is dependent on marijuana is likely to spend up to eight hours a day in this activity. The psychological complaint of such young people is often of boredom and emptiness, depressive equivalents. Such individuals, however, who have not had their capacity to be creative generally reinforced, even if they do abandon marijuana abuse, may have no ability to spend time in a way which is felt as interesting. A generally creative human experience is only possible when all staff are trained to involve the youngsters in athletic, creative, and intellectual pursuits during leisure time.

In almost all treatment settings nonspecific, generally nurturing care is the hardest to provide. Institutions may have to be persuaded that children need to snack in the evenings; in some centers this is withdrawn as a punishment even if it is offered. Funding to take children to plays and concerts is desirable. Ancillary therapists are often reluctant to share their skills with others, and compartmentalization of staff skills impedes the provision of nonspecific care. In outpatient care nonspecific needs should also be considered in the planning of treatment.

Seriously disturbed adolescents in particular are generally not offered reinforcement of their creativity in therapeutic situations. One common side effect of serious illness is the loss of imagination and creativity, a loss which will not return without special effort. The loss of creative capacity parallels the interruption in the capacity for cognitive learning and impairment of the capacity to abstract. The resolution of mental illness precedes the restoration of full ability in these areas. In therapy with disturbed adolescents educational treatment and stimulation of the senses is as necessary as psychiatric treatment.

Indications for Therapeutic Hospital Care

In seriously disturbed adolescents indications for hospital care are as follows:

1. Symptomatic behavior which is dangerous to the self or others, which appears as a response to perceived frustration. If this cannot be totally contained on the basis of an interpersonal relationship, with or without adequate pharmacotherapy, inpatient care is necessary. For potentially homicidal behavior or that which is dangerous to others complete containment is clearly necessary. A spillover of potential suicidal behavior is tolerable providing the patient can give a trustable absolute assurance that no action will be taken without first giving the opportunity to a therapist to intervene. This assurance is possible in some types of suicidal personalities; it does not seem to be observable with those who are potentially homicidal. Projection of badness onto others, as a preliminary to attempts at destruction, is harder to contain than the projection of badness onto the self.

2. Developmentally destructive behavior which cannot be contained and may include chronic drug abuse, alcoholism, and sexual promiscuity.

3. Psychic pain of such intensity, or symptomatic attempts at pain resolution, which make it impossible for the adolescent to function in an age-appropriate way. This pain cannot be attenuated by outpatient therapeutic intervention with the patient or the family.

4. A psychonoxious environment which makes the patient inaccessible to therapeutic intervention. The disturbance of the patient is so needed by the family or society that no successful treatment is possible while the patient is being stimulated or provoked, consciously or unconsciously, to disturbed behavior.

Many seriously disturbed adolescents require residential care either in a hospital or other setting. Many such care systems are psychologically depriving and result in institutionalization, which has been defined as an emotional deficiency disease (Bettelheim 1974). Alternatively, it can be looked upon as teaching its residents to lead an aberrant social life when a unit may become a justification for staff-patient noncommunication and mutual passivity (television is often used in the service of this deficiency).

Psychotherapeutic Strategies

Developmental issues and psychodynamic understanding are often omitted in the planning of psychotherapeutic programs. Group therapy, family therapy, and individual therapy have different meanings to different professionals. Different types of therapy are necessary for various syndromes. For many adolescents the traditional psychiatric hour is inappropriately long because many seriously ill adolescents cannot pay attention for more than a few minutes. In the special care unit of the adolescent treatment center of Northwestern Memorial Hospital therapists report how much time they spend with each adolescent. Generally the more disturbed the adolescent the shorter the time spent by psychotherapists. As a general rule schizophrenic adolescents are seen daily for about fifteen or twenty minutes during the acute phase of their illness; when they go into remission the therapy time span flexibly varies from thirty to forty-five minutes.

The issue of therapeutic frequency also has not been well conceptualized. In the preliminary assessment of a patient's illness in outpatient practice, therapeutic frequency cannot be predetermined. The gap between sessions is determined by: (1) the patient's capacity to make a therapeutic relationship; (2) the level of anxiety; (3) the intensity of pain inflicted on others and felt by the patient; (4) the presence of regressive symptomatology, especially drug abuse, which needs to be attenuated or no therapeutic contact is really possible; and (5) the patient's conscious motivation for treatment.

The therapist who only has time available on a once-weekly basis cannot perform an adequate therapeutic assessment and, similarly, those who are wedded to rigid concepts negate the concept that psychotherapy, its type and its frequency, is a function of adequate diagnosis and planning. Family therapy (for example) should not be automatically used unless there are clear indications for this type of intervention.

Adolescents cannot use expressive therapy if formal thinking (Piaget and Inhelder 1958) has not developed or has been interrupted by illness. The therapist is often seen by such young people as making interpretations that deny the validity of their communication. Thus for such an adolescent an interpretation may become a persecutory experience and as alienating as a parent's appearing to deny to a child the validity of its feelings. Interpretation, in which motivation is explored or unconscious feelings are brought to consciousness, should only be used by trained psychotherapists in a structured setting. If seriously disturbed adolescents are told by care workers about the meaning of their unconscious communications in a nonstructured situation, anxious confusion may develop. Therapy can be supportive, behavioral, interpretative, or a combination of these. The failure to make an adequate assessment of which type of therapy and its frequency is appropriate can convert a seriously disturbed adolescent to one who is intractably ill. There are effectively three types of psychotherapeutic intervention: those that invite bonding, those which provide developmental models for the young, and those which resolve conflict.

The Law and the Seriously Disturbed Adolescent

There are particular problems in adolescent treatment insofar as the law impinges on care delivery. In many states children are only seen as ill if they are ready to damage themselves or somebody else. One third-party carrier wrote, ''The mere fact that this boy is likely to commit matricide does not in our opinion justify his hospitalization.'' In some states, attorneys representing the child will demand of hospitals that they justify the retention of the patient. Unless there is clear agreement about the indication for hospitalization and clarification that dynamic understanding of the child's prehospital and hospital behavior is crucial to understanding his probable function in the community at large, premature discharge may occur. Conformist behavior in treatment institutions indicates little or nothing of acceptable social mastery techniques in the community at large, and professional collusion with inadequate resources is not likely to be helpful.

Conclusions

An understanding of the sociopsychobiological etiology of emotional illness to allow for maximal therapeutic intervention is essential if the seriously disturbed adolescent is not to become intractably ill. Significant aspects of nonspecific care delivery should be performed if specific interventions are to be effective at the best possible level. Apart from this, the internal pain for the professional dealing with children who constantly attempt to make him or her feel useless is a major problem in care delivery to severely disturbed young people. Society reinforces this by being generally derogatory about the role of psychiatrists.

Awareness of these issues is helpful in alleviating the possibility of creating even more seriously disturbed human beings.

REFERENCES

Aichhorn, A. 1935. *Wayward Youth*. New York: Vantage.
Bettelheim, B. 1974. *A Home for the Heart*. New York: Knopf.

Feinstein, S., and Miller, D. 1979. Psychoses of adolescence. In J. Noshpitz, ed. *Basic Handbook of Child Psychiatry*. Vol. 2. New York: Basic.

Ford, K.; Hudgens, R.; and Welner, H. 1978. Undiagnosed psychiatric illness in adolescents: a perspective study and seven year follow-up. *Archives of General Psychiatry* 35:279–288.

Johnson, A. M., and Szurek, S. A. 1956. The genesis of antisocial acting out in children and adolescents. *Psychoanalytic Quarterly* 22:323–343.

Kernberg, O. 1975. *Borderline Conditions and Pathological Narcissism*. New York: Aronson.

Klein, M. 1950. *The Psychoanalysis of Children*. London: Hogarth.

Knesper, D., and Miller, D. 1976. Treatment plans for mental health care. *American Journal of Psychiatry* 133(1): 65–80.

Levinson, D. 1978. *The Seasons of a Man's Life*. New York: Knopf.

Mahler, M. D. 1972. A study of the separation-individuation process and its possible application to borderline phenomena in a psychoanalytic situation. *Psychoanalytic Study of the Child* 26:403–424.

Miller, D. 1970. Parental responsibility for adolescent maturity. In K. Elliott, ed. *The Family and Its Future*. London: Churchill.

Miller, D. 1974. *Adolescence: Psychology, Psychopathology and Psychotherapy*. New York: Aronson.

Miller, D. 1978a. Affective disorders in adolescence, and the differential diagnosis of violent behavior. In F. J. Ayd, ed. *Mood Disorders: The World's Major Public Health Problem*. Baltimore: Ayd.

Miller, D. 1978b. Early adolescence: its psychology, psychopathology and implications for therapy. *Adolescent Psychiatry* 6:434–447.

Perris, C. 1966. A study of bipolar and unipolar recurrent depressive psychosis. *Acta Psychiatrica Scandanavia* 162 (suppl.): 45–51.

Piaget, J., and Inhelder, B. 1958. *The Growth of Logical Thinking*. New York: Basic.

Serban, G., and Gidynski, C. 1979. Relationship between cognitive defect, affect response and community adjustment in chronic schizophrenia. *British Journal of Psychiatry* 134:602–608.

Winnicott, D. 1965. *Maturational Processes and the Facilitating Environment*. New York: International Universities Press.

37   THE CHANGING NEEDS OF FEMALE
ADOLESCENTS

JUDITH A. ASHWAY

> I am a Person like everyone else
> yet different in my own light.
> I am lonely, surrounded by a
> faceless world.
> I am a young girl caught in a
> deeply changing world.[1]

The adolescent years have always been filled with intense emotional conflict and change (Freud 1936, 1958). Adolescents in America, both males and females, are developing in a society where social and sexual roles are undergoing rapid modifications. What are some of the effects of these changes on the emotional growth of the adolescent of this decade, and in particular on the female adolescent? What are her needs today? Who is she becoming?

The Changing Roles of Women

In this decade American women are in a position never before held by their predecessors. Women are freer now to choose whomever or whatever they wish to be than ever before. Stereotyped ideas about male and female occupations, natures, roles, and abilities are dissolving. Women are no longer expected to function as wives and mothers only, and they are exploring alternative life-styles and expanded roles. In the past more cultural pressures had been brought to bear on women than on men to be polite, attractive, submissive, kind, and other-oriented. Such limited behavioral expectations suppressed women's spontaneity, freedom of thought, and expression of genuine feelings to a large extent (Marmor 1968). Today people are questioning the validity of such past expectations and ideas. Traditional notions of innate "female masochism" and "female passivity" are being dispelled by prominent authors and social scientists. For example, Marmor states, "The assumption that normal men are naturally dominant and aggressive, while normal women are naturally submissive and masochistic, is another myth that the changing patterns of relationships between the sexes has begun to dispel." Also Horney (1935) argued for an appropriate examination of cultural influences as well as biological facts in the study of females today.

Change of any kind holds both promise and burdens. On the positive side, the increasing availability of options and freedoms for women is growth promoting and creates opportunities for women to fulfill their potentials. Freedom, however, also means responsibility to choose and to become. Sometimes the more choices one has, the more difficult and painful are the struggles in making decisions. With social and sexual roles less delineated today, it is not unusual for normal, healthy female adults to be in conflict about who they are. Given the fact that adult women are currently struggling with their roles and identities, it is no wonder that the problem is exacerbated for female adolescents, who at that stage of development normally are grappling with identity conflicts (Duetsch 1967; Greenacre 1975; Seiden 1975).

Adolescent Developmental Tasks

The accomplishment of certain universal tasks that characterize healthy emotional development during the middle to late adolescent periods include some of the following issues: separation and individuation, development of the capacity for lasting relationships with the opposite sex, establishment of a sound sexual identity, development of a personal moral value system, and the establishment of one's productivity in society (Group for the Advancement of Psychiatry [G.A.P.] 1968). During adolescence we see the roots of an individual's sexual life, capacity for love, and general character formation (Freud 1936). These tasks, which are continually being worked on and established throughout one's adult life, are today made more difficult by current sociocultural sex-role conflicts and value redefinitions. Adolescents are enormously aware of social realities around them, partly because one of their major tasks is to identify with, reject, or partially integrate what they perceive (G.A.P. 1968). The degree of consistency and the clarity of values, roles, and expectations passed on to them greatly affect the emotional adjustment of young people.

Today female adolescents particularly receive conflicting messages and are aware of the many inconsistencies concerning who they are expected to be and to become. They are told they should be mothers and wives, and yet now there are expectations that they establish careers as well. Premarital sexual involvement is still unacceptable to many parents, especially where their daughters are concerned, and yet peer pressures to become sexually involved are rapidly increasing. Heterosexuality is still the overt norm within our society, and yet adolescents come in contact daily with issues of homosexuality, lesbianism, and bisexuality through both personal experiences and the media. These ambivalent messages are confusing and anxiety provoking for adolescents, especially when they are wrestling with the establishment of their own identities.

Thompson (1964) points out that "inconsistencies and conflicts arising when a cultural situation is in a state of rapid transition become a part of the neurotic conflict of the individual." Because today's adolescent females are both bearing the pain and sharing in the opportunities created by the women's liberation movement which began in the sixties, they are feeling intensified emotional and identity conflicts. There exists within this crisis situation, however, a great deal of potential for growth and development.

To illustrate adolescent developmental tasks and ways in which the needs of young women are changing in relation to these tasks, excerpts from long-term cases (in individual treatment anywhere from four to twenty-four months, on a once-a-week basis) and crisis cases will be cited. Also included are observations from five different adolescent women's groups, made up of a total of approximately fifty-two members, aged fifteen to twenty years, who met weekly or twice weekly over periods of two to five months. The groups had one or two female professional leaders, and they functioned as combined high school classes for academic credit and as young women's personal-issues groups. Clients' identities are appropriately disguised to preserve confidentiality. Although adolescent issues overlap, they have been divided into four major areas for the purpose of discussion: (1) family relationships, (2) peer relations, (3) sexuality, and (4) self-esteem, and all are related to the central one of identity formation.

Family Relationships

The adolescent's psychodynamic task of separation from the family and of establishing one's identity as an individual is becoming increasingly complex, especially for females. This particular adolescent population is growing up in a fairly well-educated suburb where woman's role within the family is greatly in flux. As a result of changing expectations in the roles and behaviors of men and women, parents are finding it increasingly difficult to balance adequately and maintain their marital relationships. These communities, not unlike many others, have been experiencing a rise in the divorce rate, an increase in the number of working housewives and career women, an increase in father absenteeism, and an expansion of the number of single parents.

Many of the adolescents seen from these communities were finding such changes overwhelming and disorienting. It was not uncommon to find a young woman seeking help for herself when her parents were in the process of separating or divorcing (Kalter 1977). She would often complain, directly or indirectly, that her needs for stability and guidance at home were not being satisfied. The grief work around the loss of her formerly intact nuclear family was painful and lengthy. Feelings of sadness and loss, anger and bitterness, or confusion and anxiety were common. The frequent remarriage of one or both parents and the adolescent's task of accepting or rejecting the new stepparent were additional painful issues.

The establishment of a sexual identity, another task of adolescence, is strongly influenced by the young person's relationship to the family. In order for a young woman to establish a sound sexual identity and self-acceptance, it is important for her to identify positively with her mother. Identification is not necessarily total imitation but may include a process of working through ambivalent feelings about that parent, so that an adapting and incorporating of the mother's positive qualities can occur. A mother's feelings about herself as a worthwhile and fulfilled person are crucial to the development of healthy esteem and self-respect in the adolescent female daughter. Because of the reality of changing role expectations for women today, however, the effects of these changes upon mother, daughter, and mother-daughter relationships must be surveyed.

Many of the individual clients and group members sensed and knew that their mothers were increasingly frustrated and unfulfilled emotionally as wives and mothers.[2] They often watched their mothers going through intense role conflicts and identity changes. Their mothers' frustration levels, interestingly enough, often seemed to peak around the time of their daughters' adolescence. It was a rare young woman who described having a respecting and relatively conflict-free relationship with her mother. Although the adolescent stage is characterized by increasing disillusionment, conflict, and tension between the adolescent and parents, the majority of these clients felt what might be considered exacerbated hostility, conflict, and disappointment. They mentioned frequently that there were discrepancies between their life ambitions and aspirations and those of their mothers. Many perceived their mothers as weak and with little sense of self-worth, and this, in turn, caused them to feel angry and critical. Many verbalized a fear of becoming like their mothers. For those who saw their mothers as unable to cope well or as dependent, they felt an obligation to protect and take care of their mothers. Similarly, some complained of feeling like the mother of the household, or like the marriage counselor, and several felt that their mother was really more the child in the family. What emerged, as a result, was a resentment for this burdensome responsibility and situation of reversed roles.

They needed and wanted nurturing which they felt they lacked because of having emotionally inadequate mothers. Some of these perceptions of their mothers were based on a fear of narcissistic fusion, secondary to the identification process. In addition, much of the expression of hostility may have been due to these adolescents' increased cognitive and emotional development, including an increased ability to verbalize perceptions and feelings. These factors, however, do not deny the fact that their perceptions of their mothers were, on the whole, often rooted in reality.

Beneath the feelings of hostility and hurt which adolescent girls often felt with regard to their mothers there were indeed positive feelings expressed as well. At times they indicated that they admired qualities such as family devotion and loyalty, warmth and understanding, and that they wanted very much to identify with them. Nonetheless, mother-daughter relationships today seem to be filled with intensified and augmenting conflicts in a new context that condemns roles and behaviors which were once easily accepted for women. The result is increasing turmoil and competition for both. With adolescent women and their mothers now questioning the paths which previously have been taken by women, there is a magnified threat to the stability of both their identities.

Adolescence is a period of increasing instinctual drives and accompanying anxiety. It is a time of tremendous inner turmoil between a weakened ego (with a changing superego) and a surging increase in libidinal wishes and processes (Freud 1936). External social and familial instabilities only heighten the internal instability the adolescent feels. Situations where an adolescent girl lives with a newly divorced mother who dates, who becomes a lesbian, or who turns against men are not unusual. Each one of these possible solutions of a mother to a life crisis provokes anxiety and often produces acting-out behavior in the adolescent girl who is struggling with her own age-appropriate but confused sexual feelings.

486

When roles and behavioral expectations of women alter, the corresponding characterizations of men are inevitably affected as well. Clients, on the whole, had ambivalent impressions of their fathers and diverse relationships with them. One overriding theme was found: the majority were very sensitive to and aware of their fathers' relative absences due to choice of occupations which demanded large portions of time spent away from home and family. Paternal uninvolvement was found in physical distance from the family, in emotional aloofness or unrelatedness, and in passive-aggressive behaviors such as are seen in the alcoholic or abusive father. Clients verbalized resentment and hurt for emotional deprivation caused by these areas of lack of adequate fathering. Just as these young women did not feel satisfied with or respect the roles their mothers had adopted, they were similarly dissatisfied with the counterpart of those roles as seen in their fathers.

Increasing numbers of adolescent females are having little or no contact with fathers following parental separations and divorces. This issue of adolescent object loss of the parent of the opposite sex may have a detrimental effect on the adolescent female's future ability to establish a sound heterosexual relationship.

One last family theme frequently raised by adolescent females concerned their male siblings. Many young women felt angry because their brothers were treated as the favored ones in their families. They gave evidence that their parents often supported their brothers' ambitions and achievements at the expense of their own. Male siblings were frequently allowed greater freedoms and privileges. Many of the clients felt inferior because of the reality of the double standard which they believe operated in their own homes as well as in society.

Peer Relations

During the adolescent period of development there exist intensified needs to be accepted by one's peer group as well as an increased and appropriate drive to move away from one's parents and family. Although an increase in relating with the opposite sex is normal and healthy in adolescence for the development of a sound sexual identity, there has existed, to date, a pathological degree of conflict between females. According to Thompson (1964), ''Women who cannot have a good relationship with their own sex cannot have a satisfying relationship with men either. Capacity for genuine affection for members of one's own sex is essential for healthy human relationships in general." As changing attitudes stress women's needs for more independence from men, more adolescent women are realizing the need for satisfying relationships with their female peers.

The documentary movie *Growing Up Female* (Reichert and Klein 1971) encourages viewers to note both the typical withdrawal from activities with one's own sex which occurs among females around the ages of eleven to fourteen years and the augmenting feelings of competition with and mistrust of same-sex peers by older adolescent females. A theme frequently raised in the adolescent women's groups was a lack of trust members felt toward their own sex. They talked of feeling suspicious of other females, and many related past experiences of having been betrayed or hurt by females. The groups enabled these young women, over a period of time, to perceive members of their own sex in a different light. The theme of "girls gossip" and "hurt each other" was gradually replaced by one of mutual respect and caring. The group atmospheres became ones of encouragement, sensitive listening, and support for each other.

One can see these issues of inadequate peer relationships with other females not just in groups but in listening to individual clients as well. One adolescent spoke of her recent placement of her boyfriend's demands and needs above her own, to the point where she was excluding herself from female peer friendships completely. Through the exploration of her feelings about these unconscious decisions and priorities she came to realize that she did have emotional and social needs for girl friends and that she was denying herself the fulfillment of these needs. She became increasingly aware of the fact that she was missing out on something she used to enjoy and value—closeness with other girls. Her needs for female companionship had become buried over the last few years by commonly held beliefs that all her needs would be taken care of when she found a boyfriend.

Young women are beginning to value themselves to a greater extent as they are beginning to feel less dependent on males for self-acceptance, security, or validation. Although the social pressures for females to define their worth and identity based on male approval is still a powerful influence, adolescent women are becoming more aware of their own needs for emotional and intellectual growth, and they are concentrating less on functioning for the mere purpose of "finding a man." Many of the clients in the young women's groups testified at the termination stage that they were pleasantly surprised to have found a great deal of support, as well as emotional and intellectual companionship, in relating to their female peers in the groups.

Sexuality

Adolescent women's needs are changing tremendously in the area of sexuality. The young woman of the seventies and eighties must make choices about the prevailing realities relating to sexuality. Some of these realities are the dissolution of social and religious mores condemning premarital sex, increasing pressures for sexual activity at earlier ages than ever before, the increasing availability of birth control information and methods, and the accessibility of abortion to teenagers. These choices involve emotionally laden responsibilities and life-death issues which never before have faced the female adolescent as they do today.

Adolescents today feel enormous pressures, both from within themselves and from their peer group, to become sexually active; in particular, to have sexual intercourse. A recent survey of 2,193 adolescent females by Zelnik and Kanter (1977) revealed that approximately 35–40 percent of all female teenagers between the ages of fiteen and nineteen years were sexually active. A further breakdown of statistics showed that the rate of premarital sexual relations for white female teens in 1976 was 37 percent and for blacks was 64 percent. Of these sexually active teens, approximately 60 percent did not use birth control procedures of any kind; the percentage using them did rise from 20 to 40 percent from 1971 to 1976. They also reported that although teenage pregnancy is on the increase, out-of-wedlock births are on the decrease. The percentage of adolescent females seeking abortions has risen considerably. In 1976, for white female teenagers, nearly half (45 percent) of first pregnancies ended in abortion as compared with 33 percent in 1971.

Puberty is the first recapitulation of the infantile sexual period, and genitality acquires an increased psychic importance during adolescence (Freud 1936). The normal breakdown of superego and ego ideals in adolescence is a problem which today is amplified by changing mores. Conservative sexual mores have been breaking down quickly, and there are no longer clear-cut paths to follow. Due to this confusing situation, an increase in sexual activity and freedom among the adolescent female population does not always promote enjoyment of these new intimacies, nor does it guarantee freedom from inhibition.

What does having sexual relations mean to the female adolescent today? Many young women revealed that they often did not really enjoy sex, and many were unable to have orgasms. Many of the clients seen felt that they were pressured into having sex by their boyfriends. In spite of the fact that many adolescent women seemed to be involved sexually with only one male at any one time and usually for a length of time, they often overlooked their own needs and feelings in the relationship. It was not unusual to hear girls mentioning that they felt used sexually, and that they perceived the males as the aggressors in the relationship and themselves as objects.

It is true that these clients were unable to accept a more active, responsible part in recognizing their sexual drives because they had to deny feelings of guilt associated with increasing libidinal drives of the adolescent period. The use of such a defense mechanism (denial) is facilitated by a socialization process that encourages females to assume passive roles and feelings in relationships in general. Powerlessness and inferiority in any relationship can lead to feelings of humiliation and dissatisfaction (Boston Women's Health Collective 1971). It seems as if, due to ambivalence and guilt about sexual involvement, many young women are having difficulty in recognizing, respecting, and accepting their own needs for intimacy and sexual expression.

Ambivalence and guilt about sexuality are contributed to by the still-prevalent idea that "nice girls don't do it," which is in contrast to the adolescent's heightened feelings of sexual intensity within a current peer cultural context which advocates sexual involvement. Learned attitudes toward menstruation, female reproductive and sexual organs, and sexuality and birth control greatly influence an adolescent's attitude toward her own body and sexuality (Thompson 1964). Embarrassment and denial breed shame, anxiety, and self-abnegation. Many young women said they were taught by their parents to be the limit setters in sexual activity, and that they learned to see premarital sex as wrong or dirty. Helping the adolescent to learn to set limits in sexual behavior is often healthy and useful in terms of developing adequate superego functioning. When the restriction of sexual behavior, however, is accompanied by the attitude that sexual behavior itself is unclean, then a healthy acceptance of and comfort with one's own body and sexuality is not promoted. For those who did have sex, such attitudes often led to a lack of enjoyment of sex, or to feelings of worthlessness, depression, guilt, conflicts, and to unconscious needs to punish oneself (often through unwanted pregnancy and/or abortion). Others reacted by becoming indiscriminate about sexual involvement and became promiscuous. Still others withdrew from normal adolescent heterosexual relationships, and some became bisexual, lesbian, or totally uninterested in sex.

The integration of the old and the new sexual mores is conflict producing, painful, and anxiety filled even for the adolescent female who is reared with fairly healthy and open attitudes about sexuality. As one insightful seventeen-year-old so poignantly expressed it after she'd lost her virginity and was feeling conflicted and depressed, "A loss of innocence means death. . . ." She was aware, at some level, of her lost childhood status never to be regained, and she was experiencing very real grief feelings. This client, in spite of this fact, was an exception in the sense that she waited to have sex until she felt she was "secure and ready." She had known her boyfriend for nearly two years, and they used birth control. She took an active role in responsibly accepting her sexuality, her feelings of closeness and love for her boyfriend, and her desire for protection against unwanted pregnancy.

Perhaps more typical, however, is the adolescent woman who incorrectly uses birth control or who does not protect herself at all. Hundreds of young women seen at the agencies sought birth control after several months of having already been sexually active, or after a pregnancy scare. Many of them, in fact, did become pregnant. A young woman's failure to take necessary precautions against unwanted pregnancy is often symbolic of deeper emotional conflicts she may be experiencing. She may want to be a mother in order to feel useful, loved, and completed as a female. Early and irresponsibly handled sexual involvement can also be an acting out of guilt, loneliness, identity struggles, parent-child conflicts, unresolved loss or grief, insecurity in a male-female relationship, or feelings of worthlessness (Lowry 1971). Correct use of contraceptives is undeniably an open admission that one is sexually active and is responsible for one's own actions. This is an admission that is difficult, and sometimes impossible, for the adolescent woman who is in conflict about her sexuality. Contraceptive use also involves certain cognitive demands that often oppose other pressures (Mudd et al. 1978). Birth control information may be difficult to obtain, and there are still many misperceptions about reproduction and pregnancy, even among intelligent and educated adolescents. Our society, as a whole, does not promote adolescent contraceptive use or education, despite the statistics available on adolescent sexuality.

Unwanted pregnancy is always an emotional crisis for an adolescent. Today more and more young women are being faced with this crisis, and partly because of the increased availability of a last-minute option, abortion. Rather than choose adoption or keeping the baby, most clients who came to the agencies selected abortion as the solution to their unwanted pregnancies. Reasons such as the following were often given: "I'm not ready to have a child"; "I want to go to college and have a career"; "My parents would kill me if they knew"; "I'm financially not able to yet"; or 'I want the baby to have a father." The adolescent female is not emotionally equipped to cope with the reality or the emotional aspects of either a pregnancy or an abortion (Kremer 1973). Perceiving an abortion as similar to "having a tooth pulled," many adolescent females tried to deny their feelings about the reality of what they were actually doing in terminating pregnancies. Repressed or unresolved feelings about an abortion later resulted in feelings of guilt, depression, self-hatred, worthlessness, and isolation. In some cases suicidal gesturing, repeated pregnancies, and abortions were noted. Many of the young women seen had second and even third abortions. One can only postulate that these adolescents were only repeating unresolved, unconscious conflicts which led to their first pregnancies, and that these unfortunate repetitions were destructive attempts to master their previous situations and conflicts. We still do not know the long-range psychological effects for these young women of their decisions to terminate pregnancies in adolescence.

The emotional burdens of being an adolescent female in today's world of greater freedoms can be enormous. No other female generation to date has had to pay such a price during its teenage years.

Self-Esteem

The development of a sound sexual identity and capacity for productive adult functioning is rooted in a foundation of positive self-worth. Even with greater opportunities and supports presently available to women, the development of positive self-esteem is still a formidable task for adolescent females today. Women, young and old alike, have difficulty in freeing themselves from the idea of innate inferiority which has been part of their conditioning for so long (Thompson 1964).

Coupled with this fact is that the adolescent's sense of self-worth is not yet well established, and it often fluctuates greatly from day to day, or from one week to another. Normally during the adolescent period of development a relatively strong id confronts a relatively weak ego (Freud 1936). In a society where role confusion and value conflicts comprise the present-day norm, it is no wonder that adolescents find it astoundingly hard to find themselves, not to mention feeling good about whom they do find. The formation of a sound ego ideal is next to impossible when there are no well-defined roles for women today.

Society, particularly through the medium of the family unit, has taught women to repress aggression and self-assertiveness. Women have been reared largely with a sense of self-abasement about their needs and feelings. Horney (1935) refers to "adequate aggressiveness" as a healthy and desirable trait: "One sees that the deterioration of self-esteem lies rooted in the paralysis of what may be termed 'adequate aggressiveness.' By this I mean the capacities for work, including the following attributes: taking initiative; making efforts; carrying things through to completion; attaining success; insisting on one's rights; defending oneself when attacked; forming and expressing autonomous views; recognizing one's goals and being able to plan one's life according to them."

Adolescents, including females, normally experience a surge in aggressive as well as sexual impulses and feelings. For females, what to do with their aggressive urges is a key question. Clients often spoke of never having learned how to be assertive. "I've been taught only how to be nice and sweet," one young woman stated. Anger turned inward often results in depression, worthlessness, and masochistic tendencies. These adolescent women usually dealt with intense anger feelings by acting out in a self-destructive manner: alienation and isolation, drug or alcohol abuse, delinquency, truancy, pregnancy, suicidal gesturing, weight gain or loss, and frequent illness were common expressions of anger. They spoke of their difficulties in expressing anger directly and of their fear that they would, as a result, "hurt someone," "ruin a friendship," "be rejected," or "go out of control" if they did get angry openly. Adolescents, who are normally experiencing increased sexual and aggressive drives, are frightened by these intense feelings. This compounds the task of learning to cope adequately with these feelings of emerging anger and sexuality. Those young women who began to reconignize their needs for assertiveness and the expression of aggression, and who constructively found realistic ways to act on their feelings, were surprised by the sense of strength and self-acceptance they felt within as a result. They also found an accompanying ability to work through problems in interpersonal relationships as they became more constructively assertive. These were positive corrective emotional experiences for them.

Many of these adolescents, despite feelings of low self-worth, were able to muster needed support systems for themselves and to succeed in attempted endeavors. Whether it was having close friends, doing well in school or on a job, organizing a club, writing poetry, or getting accepted onto a school's athletic team, young women were proud of and felt good about their achievements and areas of mastery. Maslow, a personality-actualization theorist, writes about three higher needs of human beings for healthy survival: (1) esteem needs, (2) the need for self-actualization of one's capabilities, and (3) the need for cognitive understanding (information and stimulation need) (Maddi 1968). Although adolescent females have always possessed these needs, they are currently becoming increasingly aware of the importance of recognizing and fulfilling them, which results in gaining more control over their own lives and in achieving greater feelings of self-worth.

493

It might be interesting to mention some of the personal and career aspirations of some of the adolescent female clients. Increasing numbers of them were interested in pursuing traditionally nonfeminine careers such as law, medicine, or restaurant management. Only a few considered the idea of being married and having no career. Some thought they might pursue careers only and remain single. The remaining majority wanted to combine both having a career and a family. Many were undecided about whether or not they would have children. Clearly the women's movement has affected today's adolescent females' career and family aspirations. In addition, one study argues that the current dissolution of the nuclear family unit is especially painful and upsetting for females, especially those who identify more closely with the need for a settled family in which they can envision their future and their role in it as mothers and wives (Offord, Abrams, Allen, and Poushinsky 1979). What still remains to be seen is exactly who and what these adolescent women will become.

Implication for Practice

Today's adolescent female is painfully and courageously carving out her own role in a changing society. Although this chapter examines the needs and problems of a few specific populations, psychodynamic similarities probably do exist among other socioeconomic female groups. It is, therefore, of paramount importance for the psychotherapist involved in helping female adolescents to be aware of both the changing psychosocial realities currently affecting women of all ages as well as the psychological conditioning influencing the development of women. A sound knowledge of adolescent development is, of course, mandatory as well. The psychotherapist's expectations of and attitudes toward clients greatly influence the emotional growth and maturation of that person. Knowledge, understanding, and attitudes are intrinsically related.

Working with adolescent women is an exciting and difficult challenge. The role of the therapist requires patience and a sense of humor as well as sound diagnostic skills and clinical understanding. It is important for anyone working with an adolescent to encourage autonomy and growth and yet to respect the adolecent's mood swings, defenses, frequent regressions, and fluctuating dependency needs. Adolescent defenses can be stubbornly immutable because the ego is redoubling its defensive activities whenever instinctual demands are more urgent, as during this developmental stage. The therapist should also be aware of trying to build the adolescent's sense of self-respect through

494

supporting her individual ego strengths and by increasing her capacity for verbalization, decision making, and reality testing (Bracken, Klerman, and Bracken 1978). Helping the adolescent to have an increased awareness of conflicts and feelings, through building insight capacity, is necessary as well. Adolescents feel most comfortable with adults who are informal and warm, who enjoy them and are genuinely concerned for them, and who are not afraid to be tactfully honest and direct with them.

The adolescent female needs help in developing corrective, positive, and realistic expectations for herself. In addition, because the female adolescent today experiences exacerbated psychosocial conflicts, she is more often in crisis. It is, therefore, necessary for the therapist to be flexible and readily available to the adolescent in need. Psychotherapy on a regular weekly or twice weekly basis is not always feasible with the adolescent client, though ideally, regular sessions should be set up.

Respecting the adolescent's struggles for autonomy and identity formation also involves a respect for her needs for confidentiality and privacy. Particularly in working with the older adolescent female, parents need not necessarily be involved in the therapeutic process. There is a fine line to be delicately balanced in this area. Often adolescents yearn for parents to be involved with them, but they cannot openly admit this to themselves, let alone to anyone else. Building the therapeutic alliance may take considerable time, patience, and testing of the therapist, but eventually trust can be established.

Because today's adolescent client is more sophisticated and more involved sexually than previously, therapists can be useful to clients if they are knowledgeable about female anatomy, reproduction, birth control, and the emotional and physical aspects of pregnancy and abortion (Bracken et al. 1978). This enables the therapist to have a more holistic approach to the client. Also, the process of referring a client to another counselor, a specialist in the area of sexuality, only conveys the message to the adolescent that the therapist feels unable to cope with the client's sexuality, just as she herself and her parents are usually already feeling. The problems which are associated with adolescent sexuality and pregnancy demand the attention of clinicians, researchers, and social policymakers (Schinke, Gilchrist, and Small 1979).

Conclusions

The therapist, male or female, can provide a desperately needed adult role model for the adolescent female in conflict. Adolescents are seeking new

495

nonincestuous role models to identify with while they are emotionally separating themselves from their parents. Complete emotional dependence on parents ceases during puberty, and identification begins to take the place of object love (Freud 1936). Female psychotherapists have the advantage of providing adolescent females with a same-sex role model, as is often needed at this critical period of identity formation. The therapist can be a model of strength and humanness, competence and sensitivity. Females have not been taught to take themselves and their abilities seriously. The therapist, therefore, can also be a person who encourages the client to respect her own needs, feelings, and ambitions, and who takes them to heart.

In addition to the utilization of the individual psychotherapy approach, the group-work modality is extremely effective with adolescents and can be helpful to females in need of learning to better relate to peers of their own sex. Women have been taught largely to compete with one another for male attention rather than to cooperate and learn from one another. A women's support group can promote sharing, honesty, friendships, and self-respect for adolescent females.

The critical process of helping a female adolescent grow from childhood to adulthood in today's rapidly changing world is no easy task. The rewards are immeasurable, however, when a young woman begins to emerge as a more secure, self-respecting, and productive person.

NOTES

The author would like to express gratitude and acknowledgment to Mel Glenn, M.D.; Jules Glenn, M.D.; and Howard Wolf, M.S.W. for their critical comments and helpful suggestions.

1. This quote was taken from Konopka's book, *The Adolescent Girl in Conflict* (1966, p. 118). It is part of an original poem written by an adolescent female.

2. This study's findings (Newberry, Weissman, and Myers 1979) suggest differences in the roles themselves between working women and housewives and differences in the intrinsic satisfaction provided by these roles. They found that working women derived considerably more satisfaction from their outside jobs than either they or the housewives did from their work in the home (pp. 287–288).

496

REFERENCES

Boston Women's Health Collective. 1971. *Our Bodies, Ourselves*. New York: Simon & Schuster.

Bracken, M.; Klerman, L.; and Bracken, M. 1978. Coping with pregnancy resolution among never-married women. *American Journal of Orthopsychiatry* 48(2): 331–332.

Deutsch, H. 1967. *Selected Problems of Adolescence*. New York: International Universities Press.

Freud, A. 1936. *The Ego and the Mechanisms of Defense*. New York: International Universities Press.

Freud, A. 1958. Adolescence. *The Psychoanalytic Study of the Child* 13:255–278.

Greenacre, P. 1975. Differences between male and female adolescent sexual development as seen from longitudinal studies. *Adolescent Psychiatry* 4:106–119.

Group for the Advancement of Psychiatry (Committee on Adolescence). 1968. *Normal Adolescence*. New York: Scribner's.

Horney, K. 1935. The problem of feminine masochism. *Psychoanalytic Review* 22:241–257. Reprinted in Jean Baker Miller, ed. *Psychoanalysis and Women*. Baltimore: Penguin, 1973.

Kalter, N. 1977. Children of divorce. *American Journal of Orthopsychiatry* 47:1–50.

Konopka, G. 1966. *The Adolescent Girl in Conflict*. Englewood Cliffs, N.J.: Prentice-Hall.

Kremer, M. W. 1973. The adolescent sexual revolution. Introduction. *Adolescent Psychiatry* 2:160–162.

Lowry, P. 1971. Unwanted pregnancy—why? *Harvard Crimson* (August 10, 1971), pp. 2–4.

Maddi, S. R. 1968. *Personality Theories: A Comparative Analysis*. Homewood, Ill.: Dorsey.

Marmor, J. 1968. Changing patterns of femininity: psychoanalytic implications. In S. Rosenbaum and I. Alger, eds. *The Marriage Relationship*. New York: Basic.

Mudd, E.; Dickens, H. O.; Garcia, C.; Rickels, K.; Freeman, E.; Huggins, G. R.; and Logan, J. 1978. Adolescent health services and contraceptive use. *American Journal of Orthopsychiatry* 48(3): 501–503.

Newberry, P.; Weissman, M.; and Myers, J. K. 1979. Working wives and housewives: do they differ in mental status and social adjustment? *American Journal of Orthopsychiatry* 49(2): 287–288.

Offord, D.; Abrams, N.; Allen, N.; and Poushinsky, M. 1979. Broken homes, parental psychiatric illness, and female delinquency. *American Journal of Orthopsychiatry* 49(2): 261–262.

Reichert, J., and Klein, J. 1971. *Growing Up Female.* Franklin Lake, N.J.: New Day Films (distributor).

Schinke, S.; Gilchrist, L. D.; and Small, R. W. 1979. Preventing unwanted adolescent pregnancy: a cognitive-behavioral approach. *American Journal of Orthopsychiatry* 49:1–87.

Seiden, A. M. 1975. Sex roles, sexuality, and the adolescent peer group. *Adolescent Psychiatry* 4:213–215.

Thompson, C. 1964. *On Women.* New York: Mentor Books, New American Library.

Zelnik, M., and Kanter, J. 1977. Sexual and contraceptive experience of young women in the United States, 1971 and 1976. *Family Planning Perspectives.* New York: Alan Guttmacher Institute.

38 A FAMILY-SYSTEMS MODEL FOR INPATIENT TREATMENT OF ADOLESCENTS

JOHN G. LOONEY, MARK J. BLOTCKY, DOYLE I. CARSON,
AND JOHN T. GOSSETT

Truax and Carkhuff (1967) have illustrated convincingly that psychotherapy is a powerful tool, but that, because of its power, it can produce either a positive or deleterious effect. The same is true with regard to the potential effect of hospitalization upon an adolescent. A skillfully managed inpatient treatment setting can lead to patients' restructuring of long-standing conflicts, growth, mastery, and movement toward autonomy. However, a poorly managed program may produce nothing but diminution of self-esteem, regression, and dependency. One way of determining the quality of a treatment program is to construct a model that may be clearly conceptualized, that is appropriate to the developmental needs of teenagers, and that has heuristic value in assessing how the real impact of the treatment unit approaches the ideal effect that could be predicted by the model (Beavers 1977). In this chapter we suggest that the model of a well-functioning family can offer useful guidelines against which to weigh the quality of care provided by a hospital program for adolescents.

Systematic investigation of models of social systems is of relatively recent origin, and we owe much to modern statisticians who have taught us to conceptualize and to measure the impact of multiple variables operative in a system. In addition, the seminal concepts of von Bertalanffy (1968) have spawned large numbers of systems theoreticians who attempt to help us to understand the underlying forces operative in evolving systems. An example of our increased ability to conceptualize models of complex systems in our field is illustrated in a recent study by Wright[1] which views an inpatient unit through general systems theory.

Even though intense interest in model building is recent, a selective historical review of inpatient treatment practices suggests that some types of models have been the basis for many important past contributions, even though the models may have not been delineated explicitly. The "moral treatment" of the mid-nineteenth century seems to have been built on an implicit model of psychiatric illness as caused by a demeaning environment, irregular work, and religious and personal habits. It was proposed that emotional disturbance could be corrected by placing the patient in an environment in which he or she was treated with respect and given useful duties to perform. Simmel's (1929) paper, "Psycho-Analytic Treatment in a Sanatorium," is based on a model of a patient's unconscious conflicts being restructured through the transference to the analyst, but extends that model to encompass dealing with the projection of the patient's transference feelings onto other therapeutic personnel. Approximately a decade later, William Menninger (1936, 1937) elaborated on Simmel's concept and built a more complex model which viewed the patient and hospital as interacting in ways beneficial to the general social as well as unconscious needs of the patient. Stanton and Schwartz (1954) further elaborated on the effects of interaction between the patient and a psychoanalytically oriented hospital. They demonstrated the complexity of the interaction by illustrating, for example, how covert power conflicts between key staff members could increase the floridity of a patient's symptoms.

A model of an optimal hospital milieu for adolescents must carefully focus on three important elements that are not particularly emphasized in reports of treatment of adults. These are: (1) adolescents demonstrate a great propensity to act out their conflicts and needs through troublesome behavior; (2) adolescents have primary families with whom conflicts may be very serious; and (3) adolescents have developmental needs, in particular the evolution of social skills, which must be met.

With these three important elements in mind, one can collate a growing body of literature from which assumptions about a model of hospital treatment begin to emerge. Reports by Blotcky, Offutt, Hagebak, and Stewart (1975), Curran (1939), Easson (1969), Falstein, Feinstein, and Cohen (1966), Hendrickson and Holmes (1959), King (1974), Krohn, Miller, and Looney (1974), Levy (1969), Lewis (1967, 1969, 1970), Lewis, Gossett, King, and Carson (1973), Looney, Miller, and Zinn (1977), Masterson (1972), Miller (1957, 1973, 1974), Noshpitz (1957), and Rinsley (1961, 1968) in differing foci, cumulatively elaborate basic aspects of a model of an optimally functioning adolescent unit. Some of the basic assumptions of such a model, based on this literature, are as follows.

1. Adolescents seriously disturbed enough to be admitted to a hospital often will use ego syntonic, action-oriented defenses which, as well as in-

dicating the psychodynamics of long-standing unconscious conflicts, seriously provoke other people. These alloplastic defenses may provide the patient instinctual gratification, prolonging the initial phase in which these maneuvers predominate. This behavior, which distorts all object relationships, must be brought within manageable limits through the use of reasonable controls, confrontation, and clarification before a treatment alliance can develop.

2. Individual psychotherapy is usually necessary to change the expression of conflicts from behavior into verbal expression of feelings.

3. Adolescents seek major support from peers, and thus the development of protreatment group process is a powerful treatment technique.

4. Distorted relationships with families—most often the results of conflicts over dependency, or more primitive, nurturant conflicts—must be reworked. Such change is usually accomplished by initial separation, transference of the patient's familial conflicts to the new pseudofamily represented by the treatment unit, and, lastly, gradual increase and monitoring of interactions with the family of origin to achieve reunion or emancipation, depending on the developmental level of the patient.

5. Members of the treatment team must have clearly defined roles and healthy interactions among themselves. Since staff have a major impact on patients by providing models for identification, they must function in a way which indicates that achieving maturity and autonomy is more gratifying than being dependent and immature. Team members higher in the social power hierarchy must be supportive of less powerful staff, but unhealthy dependency must not be fostered.

6. Adolescents are in the process of growing up, and their evolving educational, cultural, social, vocational, and physical needs must be attended to.

7. Finally, there is a temporal assumption in the model which dictates that fostering abiding psychological change cannot be rushed.

These assumptions, while being of time-proven importance, are difficult to synthesize into a holistic and simply conceptualized model in which key variables can be identified and measured in a systematic way. Yet such conceptualization seems important if one is to assess how closely the real functioning of a treatment unit approaches its potential effectiveness. Perhaps it would be helpful to think of a treatment unit in terms of some other type of well-studied social system, the variables of which have been delineated. In the search for a conceptually similar social system, one might first look for one in which primary tasks are similar to those of an adolescent inpatient unit. Basically, what do we try to achieve with inpatient treatment? Two results are elemental. The first is that we help young people grow up. The second (serendipitous) effect is that we, ourselves, find gratification, grow, learn, and stabilize a sense of our own life directions. We agree, therefore, with Rinsley (1961), who states, "Finally it must be remembered that psychiatric treatment in the general sense should constitute a growth experience for both the patient and those who essay to treat him."

What social systems most closely approximate these two effects? One whose similarity is clear is the family system. Parsons and Bales (1955) describe the family as having two primary functions: (1) the stabilization and maturation of parental personalities, and (2) the production of autonomous children. If the primary tasks of these two systems are so similar, the next question is whether there are other similarities between them. Certainly some members of the team serve the patients as surrogates for parents and other older relatives. Other team members, lower in the hierarchy and often younger, serve as older sibling or cousin-like surrogates. The patients resemble a sibling system. Day-to-day activities—such as getting up, getting to school, shared meals, shared fun activities, bedtime rituals, and even squabbles—all extend the family simile. Other examples could be offered, but, in brief, the point is that there are structural as well as functional parallels.

The next important question is whether or not family-systems variables have been defined and measured in such a way as to allow their use in assessing process in a treatment unit. Lewis, Beavers, Gossett, and Phillips (1976) have defined thirteen family interactional process variables[2] to describe how well families accomplish the two tasks elaborated by Parsons. That body of research suggests that a continuum of family competence can be established, with "optimally functioning" families at one end and "chaotic" at the other (see fig. 1). Between these extremes it is possible to describe "competent but pained," "dominant-submissive," and "conflicted" families. To some degree, the severity and type of psychopathology of an adolescent patient can be predicted by the point on the continuum at which his or her family functions. For example, severely dysfunctional, chaotic families tend to produce profoundly borderline or process psychotic youngsters. The children of optimally functioning families, by contrast, move toward autonomy with little difficulty.

It is beyond the scope of this chapter to explain the relevance and method of quantifying all of the variables used in measuring family interaction, and it is similarly not possible to illustrate the use of all of them in assessing interactional process on an inpatient unit. However, it is possible to demonstrate how some of these variables can be used through illustration with vignettes of our experiences. First, however, it is necessary to describe the

502

process of functioning of optimal families, our stated ideal (see also Lewis 1978).

In Lewis's (1980) terms,

Optimal families demonstrate clear structure with flexibility. The parents share power, demonstrate a strong coalition, and provide clear leadership to the family. Such families encourage clear ego boundaries, high levels of interpersonal closeness, and they communicate clearly. They negotiate effectively to reach solutions to problems. Family members are encouraged to communicate feelings and thoughts clearly, to take responsibility for their own actions, to be responsive to each others' communications, and they do not invade each other's minds. Such families are open with feelings; warm, affectionate, and humorous in mood; low in conflict; and high in empathy.

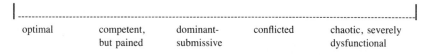

| optimal | competent, but pained | dominant-submissive | conflicted | chaotic, severely dysfunctional |

FIG. 1.—Continuum of family competence

For purposes of illustration, we will use five variables from the family-systems research to demonstrate their utility in conceptualizing treatment process. Of central importance is the strength of the parental coalition. In optimal families, the parental coalition is strong, and there is an absence of covert coalitions between either parent and a child. On a treatment unit in which power is shared between the unit director and the head nurse (also an optimal condition predicted by the family research), the doctor and nurse assume parental surrogate roles for the patients. Thus, these key people must monitor the strength of their working alliance closely. It is also important for these two people to check with each other frequently to make sure that neither unintentionally establishes a covert favorite-patient coalition which would be massively destructive to the integrity of the system. Many patients will have had past family experience and skill in splitting parents and establishing covert parent-child coalitions and unconsciously maneuver to achieve the same situation in the treatment milieu. In treatment units in which two mental health professionals, for some selected patients, may fill the roles of therapist

503

and administrator, the potential for parental surrogation and covert coalition between one professional and the patient is also present and must be monitored.

Optimal families negotiate the solution to problems efficiently. In a treatment unit, staff members need to provide effective models of the ability to negotiate. The efficiency of negotiation should be monitored in intrastaff interactions (both in the presence and in the absence of the patients' observation), in interactions between patients, and in negotiations between staff members and patients. The following vignette illustrates recognition of a problem with regard to the latter.

Case Example 1

A sixteen-year-old girl seemed overly compliant with her psychiatrist's denial of a request to visit off grounds. Previously the psychiatrist consistently had been willing to explain any such refusals and had been amenable to changing his mind when presented with additional information. Reminded of this fact, the girl became aware she needed to see him as arbitrary rather than reasonable. This realization of his willingness to negotiate led her to express a great deal of emotionally laden material concerning transference distortions about fear of autonomy. She became more aware of her feelings of helplessness and her wish to transfer power to an omnipotent other.

Both patients and staff easily can slip into roles reflective of the patient's previous pathological experiences, and one of the early signs of this regression may be a lack of emphasis upon negotiating decisions.

In the more competent families, individuals assume responsibility for their own actions. Disturbed adolescents are very rarely able to achieve this responsibility early in treatment, and staff must provide adequate modeling. The unit director must begin the modeling process by being very honest about mistakes he or she may have made and by not placing the problem on other staff or on patients. Moving down the hierarchy, it is important for each staff member to be aware of how he or she utilizes both affective and cognitive components in making a decision and to take personal responsibility for that decision. Problems in staff modeling may be most apparent when various staff members differ about a provocative situation, as in the following vignette.

Case Example 2

A seventeen-year-old girl had been in the hospital for two years. Whenever she was given more responsibility she acted out dangerously. She was discussed intensively in a staff meeting and subsequently in a patient group meeting. Staff members had various feelings from rage to fatigue and pity. A number of team members felt like giving up. Others felt like protecting her and continuing. It was important that these affects were shared, and that each individual team member took responsibility for articulating clearly his or her personal position.

The mood and tone in a competent family is usually warm, affectionate, humorous, and optimistic. A similar feeling is experienced on a treatment unit when treatment is progressing well. The following illustrates the feelings of hostility, depression, and cynicism which are present when a unit is floundering.

Case Example 3

The adolescent boys' unit became quite dull during group meetings. There was little discussed, and several patients had run away. It slowly became apparent that the group was depressed, empty, and needy, and that prodding them to discuss their feelings was a dead end. The unit director began some added recreational programs, including competitive physical activities, group lunches, and a small picnic. Slowly the energy level of the group was raised, with increased optimism on the part of both the patients and the staff.

Competent families are able to empathize with consistent effectiveness. If one family member is distressed, he or she is blessed with the support of knowing that other family members can understand his or her feelings in a nonjudgmental manner. Since most disturbed adolescents have little capacity to be empathic, key staff members must demonstrate continually the capacity for empathy, as illustrated in the following vignette.

Case Example 4

Several girls became sullen, provocative, and obstinate after an important holiday. At first their peers attacked them for their grouchy, disruptive behavior. Several staff members who had worked on that holiday and missed their own families suggested there might be some shared underlying feelings of loneliness. The attacking girls were then able to share their own pain and made empathic contact with the provocateurs.

If a treatment team chooses to use concepts extracted from family-systems research, there are several preparatory steps. The first step is to understand the impact of the key process variables. Several authors have noted that many psychiatrists' childhood family experiences were in dysfunctional families (Burton 1972; Henry, Sims, and Saray 1971) and the same is probably true of others attracted to mental health work. Understanding the importance of these variables, therefore, often does not evolve naturally from past experiences. Second, staff members must learn to monitor themselves with regard to how effectively they are being empathic, sharing power, avoiding covert alliances, negotiating, and the like. Vigilant self-monitoring is crucial because staff members are constantly providing models for identification. Finally, the unit director must monitor the cumulative functioning of staff and patients along the different dimensions described. Dysfunctional operation with regard to one key variable often foreshadows problems with many.

Several disclaimers and qualifiers are germane. One important disclaimer is that the family-systems research with optimally functioning families has been predominately with urban, Caucasian, middle- or upper-middle-class families. It is not certain that competent families of different socioeconomic and ethnic backgrounds function in the same manner. For example, an optimal, lower-income, minority family may not be able to share power in an egalitarian fashion, but rather may need to be led by one very strong parent. One should be cautious, therefore, in applying the principles we have outlined to an inpatient unit serving economically distressed, minority adolescents.

We must also remind ourselves that distortions and misjudgments may take place if one social system is compared too closely with another. Useful parallels exist, certainly. However, various factors—the complexity of an inpatient unit resulting from the admixture of such elements as patients with severe psychopathology; the incredible role complexity engendered by the presence of unit administrators, nurses, adolescent care workers, teachers, activities specialists, family members, consultants, psychotherapists, and others; medical-legal and third-party payor demands; the complexity of the greater hospital system; and inherent intrastaff competition—combine to create a more complicated and more highly stressed system than that of a family. In addition, moving from this theoretical statement about increased complexity to an empirical focus based on our cumulative forty years of experience, it is uncommon to see any treatment team function consistently at the same level of competence as the previously described optimal research families. In using the five-level system we have described (optimal, competent but pained, dominant-submissive, conflicted, and chaotic), most treatment teams in reality fluctuate in function between the levels of competent but pained, dominant-submissive, conflicted, and chaotic. In practice, the judicious use of authority as seen in benevolent and humane dominant-submissive systems may be the best we can hope to sustain over an extended period of time. Brief and perilous excursions into chaos do occur. Those rare occasions during which the unit functions in the optimal range should be savored. The statement that a treatment team does not usually function for prolonged periods at the optimal end of the continua of the various interactional process variables in no way, however, minimizes their utility as ideals against which to assess quality of functioning.

Another important caution is that a myopic focus on any single model can lead to the unfortunate situation in which a treatment unit becomes a self-contained microcosm. Optimal families, after all, are open systems—family members actively engage in activities in the world at large. It is the supportive nature of the family that allows and encourages them to do so. Similarly, an effective treatment unit is one which has patients as engaged in the outside world as their abilities will allow.

Conclusions

The task of assessing the quality of care provided to hospitalized adolescents is difficult, and the search for newer methods is warranted. One way of assessing how the real quality of care approaches an ideal is to conceptualize a model whose multiple variables can be defined and quantified, and to strive to achieve maximal effectiveness with regard to the defined variables. A family-systems model seems relevant because of the similarity of the structural and task attributes of families and of hospital treatment units for adolescents. As with all models, expansion and redefinition must be carried out in a process of refining the model. The true test of the effectiveness of inpatient treatment is the degree and permanence of improvement in patients, over time, after discharge. It is imperative, therefore, that any theoretical concept, such as the one we outline, be subjected to the rigorous test of follow-up research (Gossett, Barnhart, Lewis, and Phillips 1977; Gossett, Lewis, Barnhart, and Phillips 1976; Gossett, Meeks, Barnhart, and Phillips 1976). Otherwise, as Eysenck (1960) has noted, anything we devise can be a wondrous cure, and we can deceive ourselves with wondrous nonsense like our ancient predecessor Galen, who stated, "All who drink this remedy recover in a short time, except for those whom it does not help, who all die and have no relief from any other medicine. Therefore it is obvious it fails only in incurable cases."

NOTES

1. J. G. Wright, "The Psychiatric Hospital in an Era of Accelerated Change: Application of the General Systems Approach," unpublished manuscript (Louisville, Ky.: University of Louisville, 1979).
2. These variables are: overt power, strength of parental coalition, closeness, family mythology, goal-directed negotiation, clarity of expression, responsibility for one's own feelings and behavior, invasiveness, permeability, range of feelings, mood and tone, degree of unresolvable conflict, and empathy.

REFERENCES

Beavers, W. R. 1977. *Psychotherapy and Growth: A Family Systems Perspective*. New York: Brunner/Mazel.
Blotcky, M. J.; Offutt, D. N.; Hagebak, R. W.; and Stewart, R. P. 1975. A developmental model for inpatient management. *Bulletin of the Menninger Clinic* 39:183–188.

Burton, A., et al. 1972. *Twelve Therapists*. San Francisco: Jossey-Bass.

Curran, F. J. 1939. Organization of a ward for adolescents in Bellevue Psychiatric Hospital. *American Journal of Psychiatry* 95:1365–1388.

Easson, W. M. 1969. *The Severely Disturbed Adolescent*. New York: International Universities Press.

Eysenck, H. J. 1960. *Behavior Therapy and the Neuroses*. New York: Pergamon.

Falstein, E.; Feinstein, S.; and Cohen, W. P. 1966. An integrated adolescent care program in a general psychiatric hospital. *American Journal of Orthopsychiatry* 30:276–291.

Gossett, J. T.; Barnhart, F. D.; Lewis, J. M.; and Phillips, V. A. 1977. Follow-up of adolescents treated in a psychiatric hospital: predictors of outcome. *Archives of General Psychiatry* 34:1037–1042.

Gossett, J. T.; Lewis, J. M.; Barnhart, F. D.; and Phillips, V. A. 1976. The adolescent treatment assessment project: lessons learned in process. *Journal of the National Association of Private Psychiatric Hospitals* 8:26–30.

Gossett, J. T.; Meeks, J. E.; Barnhart, F. D.; and Phillips, V. A. 1976. Follow-up of adolescents treated in a psychiatric hospital: onset of symptomatology scale. *Adolescence* 1:195–211.

Hendrickson, W. J., and Holmes, D. J. 1959. Control of behavior as a crucial factor in intensive adolescent treatment in an all adolescent ward. *American Journal of Psychiatry* 115:967–973.

Henry, W. E.; Sims, J. H.; and Saray, S. L. 1971. *The Fifth Profession*. San Francisco: Jossey-Bass.

King, J. W. 1974. Teaching goals and techniques in hospital schools. *Adolescent Psychiatry* 3:419–421.

Krohn, A.; Miller, D.; and Looney, J. 1974. Flight from autonomy: problems of social change on an adolescent inpatient unit. *Psychiatry* 37:360–371.

Levy, E. D. 1969. On the residential treatment of adolescent girls. *Seminars in Psychiatry* 1:3–14.

Lewis, J. M. 1967. Unsolved problems of milieu therapy. *Hospital and Community Psychiatry* 18:39–40.

Lewis, J. M. 1969. The organizational structure of the therapeutic team. *Hospital and Community Psychiatry* 20(7): 206–208.

Lewis, J. M. 1970. Development of an inpatient adolescent service. *Adolescence* 5:303–312.

Lewis, J. M. 1978. The adolescent and the healthy family. *Adolescent Psychiatry* 6:156–170.

Lewis, J. M. 1979. Interfaces in schizophrenia research: the family interaction/psychopharmacology interface. Paper presented before the Group for the Advancement of Psychiatry, Philadelphia, April.

Lewis, J. M. 1980. The family in the matrix of health and illness. In C. K. Hofling and J. M. Lewis, eds. *The Family: Evaluation and Treatment.* New York: Brunner/Mazel.

Lewis, J. M.; Beavers, W. R.; Gossett, J. T.; and Phillips, V. A. 1976. *No Single Thread: Psychological Health in Family Systems.* New York: Brunner/Mazel.

Lewis, J. M.; Gossett, J. T.; King, J. W.; and Carson, D. I. 1973. Development of a protreatment group process among hospitalized adolescents. *Adolescent Psychiatry* 2:351–362.

Looney, J. G.; Miller, D. H.; and Zinn, L. D. 1977. The management of pathological peer relationships in the treatment of hospitalized borderline adolescents. *Diseases of the Nervous System* 38:738–741.

Masterson, J. F. 1972. *Treatment of the Borderline Adolescent: A Developmental Approach.* New York: Wiley.

Menninger, W. C. 1936. Psychiatric hospital therapy designed to meet unconscious needs. *American Journal of Psychiatry* 93:347–360.

Menninger, W. C. 1937. Psychoanalytic principles applied to the treatment of hospitalized patients. *Bulletin of the Menninger Clinic* 1:35–43.

Miller, D. H. 1957. Treatment of adolescents in an adult hospital. *Bulletin of the Menninger Clinic* 21:189–198.

Miller, D. H. 1973. The development of psychiatric treatment services for adolescents. In J. C. Schoolar, ed. *Current Issues in Adolescent Psychiatry.* New York: Brunner/Mazel.

Miller, D. H. 1974. *Adolescence: Psychology, Psychopathology, and Psychotherapy.* New York: Aronson.

Noshpitz, J. D. 1957. Opening phase in the psychotherapy of adolescents with character disorders. *Bulletin of the Menninger Clinic* 21:153–164.

Parsons, T., and Bales, R. 1955. *Family, Socialization and Interaction Process.* Glencoe, Ill.: Free Press.

Rinsley, D. B. 1961. Psychiatric hospital treatment of adolescents: verbal and non-verbal resistance to treatment. *Bulletin of the Menninger Clinic* 25:249–263.

Rinsley, D. B. 1968. Theory and practice of intensive residential treatment of adolescents. *Psychiatric Quarterly* 42:612–638.

Simmel, E. 1929. Psychoanalytic treatment in a sanatorium. *International Journal of Psycho-Analysis* 10:70–89.

Stanton, A. H., and Schwartz, M. S. 1954. *The Mental Hospital: A Study of Institutional Participation in Psychiatric Illness and Treatment.* New York: Basic.

Truax, C. B., and Carkhuff, R. R. 1967. *Toward Effective Counseling and Psychotherapy.* Chicago: Aldine.

von Bertalanffy, L. 1968. *General Systems Theory.* New York: Braziller.

Warren, W. 1952. Inpatient treatment of adolescents and psychological illnesses. *Lancet* 1:147–150.

39 RECURRENT LARGE-GROUP PHENOMENA: STUDIES OF AN ADOLESCENT THERAPEUTIC COMMUNITY

LOREN H. CRABTEE, JR., AND DOUGLAS F. LEVINSON

Many therapists find it difficult to work in large group settings. The more or less unstructured sequences and processes, such as community meetings, are more difficult to conceptualize as systems than those of the dyad, family, or small group. The complex tensions of larger community life also tend to bring out some of our least admirable qualities, both personal and bureaucratic. It is probably for these reasons that there has been relatively little written on social processes since the pioneering studies of the 1950s (Caudill 1958; Henry 1957; Jones 1953; Miller 1957; Stanton and Schwartz 1954).

In our work in a community of hospitalized adolescents, we have found two concepts to be particularly helpful toward understanding development, management, and leadership issues at the level of the therapeutic community as a system. (1) There are stages of organizational development which describe a community's struggle to balance the potential for spontaneous experience with the need for routine and structure (Crabtree and Cox 1972). (2) Large groups undergo recurrent, more frequent oscillations of tension, whose recognition and management are central challenges to the efficacy of a community (Rapoport 1960; Levinson and Crabtree 1979). We will discuss the events which occurred during two such discrete cycles of oscillatory tension and point out some issues of leadership and management which have become evident from this analysis.

Description of the Setting

The adolescent treatment unit included twenty-four male and female patients aged fourteen to eighteen, most of them high school students from middle- and upper-middle-income families. There were patients of all diagnoses except those with significant organic impairment, who were excluded because of the emphasis on verbal interaction and learning. The average stay was three to four months, covering a period of two months to two years. At any given time there were acutely disturbed, high-risk patients as well as others who were over the storm which led to admission. The unit was in the closed section of a private psychiatric hospital, but since 1972 there had been an open-door policy (Crabtree and Grossman 1974). All patients were in treatment with private psychiatrists. The unit staff included salaried psychiatrists, resident physicians, and representatives of each therapeutic activity program. The unit was part of an adolescent treatment center which included a school, day hospital, activities programs, programs for parents and families, and the psychotherapies programs.

Stages of Organizational Development

We have identified three stages in the development of the therapeutic community as a whole. This process also can be observed in the smaller elements of the community: activities programs, community meetings, shorter-term group experiences such as classes and drug groups, and even smaller more discrete entities as experiences with a particular rule or policy.

Oscillatory Cycles of Tension

Group oscillatory cycles can be distinguished from organizational stage changes primarily by their shorter-termed nature and cause. They arise from fluctuations in relationship patterns among patients and staff leading to cycles of tension interaction in the group.

We first became aware of these short-termed cycles as a seasonal phenomenon when we realized that there were recurrent cycles of collective conflict, epidemics, or contagions of behavior. In the fall, at the start of the school year, a sense of creative energy and heightened tension pervaded the group. During winter, a general sense of monotony and depression developed around the Christmas holidays. By spring, the community polarized into a staff-patients split. Conflicts emerged which would, in turn, lead to a cathartic crisis followed by an easing of tension. During the summer, there tended to be an atmosphere of relaxation, both of programs and of spirit, and a sense of discontinuity and fragmentation.

When we observed that the springtime crisis was recurrent, we began to evolve methods of dealing with it. More recently, we have come to see that all the recurrent cycles throughout the year have a predictable course, apparently influenced by a number of variables besides the season such as the clustering of admissions and discharges, vacations of staff and leaders, and intervention in response to these disturbances—or lack of it—at the level of the total living group.

Using Rapoport's (1960) description of a four-phased cycle, each of which in our experience lasts from two to four months, we define the cycle phases to include the following.

1. Stage 1. Open opportunity functioning, random in nature, is most evident during the initial organization of the community. Later a sense of drama and intensity develops as the participants feel relief from their anxieties and create an aura of naiveté and exploration. A need and an opportunity for spontaneous charismatic leadership emerges, and the moment that epitomizes this stage is the dramatic and unscheduled encounter that galvanizes the emotions of everyone involved into a feeling of belonging to the community.

2. Stage 2. The ordering of group life emerges. The group members begin to desire a sense of mastery and improvement as experiences become familiar and their outcomes more predictable. Leadership is required in articulating strategies, organizing structures, and identifying workable sequences, for example, the elaboration of a privilege system, the establishment of multi-disciplinary teams, and the holding of meetings for specific planning and task functions. During this stage the therapeutic community as a whole, and each of its parts, goes through a progression from newness and drama to structuralization, which offers a sense of order, predictability, expertise, and mastery.

3. Stage 3. At first imperceptible, a feeling of routine, monotony, and lowered energy level develops which characterizes this stage of bureaucracy and institutionalization. There is always a need for institutional functioning in certain areas, such as administration, scheduling, and payrolling. However, in the therapeutically relevant relationships between patients and staff and

of staff to staff, this type of functioning leads to withdrawal, isolation, fragmentation, and frequently to staff-patients splits and the polarization of community attitudes.

These three stages describe the development, elaboration, and deterioration of a group experience (see table 1). We have become aware, however, through our experiences with our community and its parts, that this need not be inevitable. What is required is a leadership thrust that overthrows or replaces the debilitating rituals and returns to new open possibilities; redesigns new structures, strategies, and arenas for relationship encounters and learning; and revitalizes existing structures of program elements by the reinvestment of personal energies and enthusiasm.

The management of this organic flow requires both charismatic and strategic-organizing leadership abilities. The program and leadership must provide inspiration, creativity, and energizing effects as well as order, consistency, and greater involvement of more participants. The presence of both offsets the tendency to counterproductive excess—the charismatic toward discontinuity, chaos, and emotionality, and the strategic-organizer toward dehumanization and institutionalization of group life. It is essential that the leaders have direct, ongoing, working contact with the patients. For example, the director of the school must be in the classroom and at community meetings to offset the human tendency in all of us toward dehumanizing and routinizing educational functions.

We have found it useful to approach the problems of stage progression and deterioration not only in considering the community as a whole, but in

TABLE 1
THREE STAGES OF ORGANIZATIONAL AND GROUP DEVELOPMENT

Stage 1 (Charismatic)	Stage 2 (Strategic-Organizing)	Stage 3 (Bureaucratic)
Spontaneous experience	Organized structure	Routine
Personal encounter	Order	Monotony
Newness	Sense of knowing	Bureaucracy
Drama	Perspective	Low energy
Intensity	Consistency	Dehumanization
Creative ferment	Continuity	Withdrawal
Naivete	Expertise	Fragmentation
The unexplored	Strategies, programs,	Staff-patient split
Discontinuity	objectives become	Polarization
Fragmentation	concrete	Stereotyped thinking
Chaos		
Emotionality		

Note.—Leadership style shown in parentheses.

its discrete parts as well. Various aspects of the total program, though interrelated and interdependent, develop and progress with great divergence. The school, the community meetings, the activities program are at times at different stages, out of phase or synchrony with one another. Certain policies also clearly have longer half-lives than others. Precedures, strategies, and approaches follow a similar stage functioning, becoming ultimately routine, monotonous, and, thereby, ineffective.

We gradually became aware that these various aspects of the community life would deteriorate and were able to redesign and revitalize structures and strategies and to reformulate new areas for relationships, fruitful encounters, and learning experiences.

1. Phase A, harmony. The community is working toward its goals. The atmosphere is permissive, in keeping with the community ideals of self-responsibility and learning. Closeness, contact, and sharing are experienced in both structured and informal settings. Effective confrontations regarding shortcomings of staff and patients are possible; they are experienced not as divisive, but as concerned, helpful efforts in the pursuits of self-improvement.

2. Phase B, rise in tension. There is increasing withdrawl of staff and patients. Cliques form and deviancy mounts in the form of acting out, particularly at night (sex, drugs, AWOLS, destruction of property). The normal sequences of community life begin to seem empty and repetitive. Leader's continued espousal of community ideals is countered by cynicism on the part of both patients and staff.

3. Phase C, peak of tension. Deviancy erupts, often in the form of collective disturbance. The top staff leadership is isolated and pitted against the leader(s) and followers. The top leadership begins to assert community ideals over the needs of the individual patient, accompanied by an explicit threat of expulsion to a number of patients. Making this threat, and sometimes carrying it out, epitomizes the staff's attempts to preserve the community at all costs.

4. Phase D, resolution (abating tension). A communal mood begins to emerge again. Tension remains, but there is a "strain to conform." This is a period of renewal and reconstruction, often in the form of changes in policy, structure, or activities. We have used therapeutic contracts, for example, with the patients threatened with expulsion. Individual staff members strive to make contact with them along with those isolated, schizophrenic, and depressed patients who withdrew during the period of action. The emergence of new community projects and plans and the marked improvement in the mood and interaction at community meetings herald a new phase (see table 2).

TABLE 2
CYCLES OF COMMUNITY TENSION
(Adapted from Rapoport, with Additions)

Phase A, Harmony	Phase B, Rising Tension	Phase C, Peak of Tension	Phase D, Resolution
Work toward goals	Cliques form	Deviancy erupts	Tension abates
Community ideals	More deviance,	Collective	Communal mood
People moving	"bad action"	disturbance may	renewed
toward each other	Ideals less tenable	occur	Recommitment
Relationships develop	Withdrawal and	Setting firm limits	Social reconstruction
Relative community	cynicism	Clear authority	Lasting changes of
stability		Isolation of top	policy, structure,
Closeness, contact,		leadership and	activities
sharing		"outlaw leaders"	
Confrontations		Exclusion of	
effective		disruptive leaders	
		or renegotiation	
		Assertion of	
		community ideals	
		over individual	

This conception of cycles of tension first emerged from a series of studies in the 1950s. Although Stanton and Schwartz (1954) are better known for their analysis of covert disagreements among staff members as the cause of pathological excitement of individual patients, in the same study they relate a collective disturbance on a ward to a period of lowered morale and lack of integration within the staff. Boyd, Kageles, and Greenblatt (1954) and Miller (1957) also traced episodes of collective disturbances to the influence of staff problems on ward process. Caudill (1958) used interaction process analysis as well as observational data to trace phases of increasing staff withdrawal and polarization leading to a collective disturbance. Rapoport (1960) conceptualized the four-phase cycle of ward tension, taking as its focus not the occasional collective disturbance but the unusual phenomenon of predictable, oscillatory processes.

In our experience, the occurrence and timing of these oscillations appear to be related to a number of factors: (a) the permissiveness and intensified interaction and communication of the therapeutic community; (b) the season; (c) staff turnover of individuals or of groups; (d) cluster discharge of patients with the loss of constructive patient leaders; (e) patient population containing a large proportion of character disorders; and (f) staff withdrawal as a reaction to difficult new patients, vacations or departures, external forces in their personal lives, or to the larger hospital system.

517

We believe that oscillations of tension are an inevitable outgrowth of a ward culture which permits sufficient interaction and acting out to provide opportunities for therapeutic confrontation. The goal of effective ward administration and leadership is to manage these cycles optimally rather than trying to repress them altogether. Rapoport described two broad possibilities of mismanagement: ''collusive anxiety,'' or the collusion of staff in stifling tension too early and thereby destroying potential opportunities for treatment (as often happens in more traditional units and also in short-term units concerned with rapid discharges); and ''collusive denial,'' or the collusion of staff in permitting so much tension as to threaten individual treatment and community survival.

We examine two episodes from our initial efforts of the mid-1970s to manage oscillatory cycles that illustrate the shape and outcome of recurrent cycles of tension, with a collusive trend toward permissiveness one year and a collusive trend toward stifling the next. We have found that our recognition of these cycles is an important step in our efforts to guide the community and to diagnose and manage its recurrent impasses.

The first sequence, which occurred during the summer months, was marked by a prolonged rise of tension as the community and its leaders resisted the necessary shift from a commitment to the understanding of individual patients to the use of authority with the large group in the face of a major collective disturbance. The second sequence, during the spring of the following year, developed after the staff responded to more minor incidents, early and strongly, leading to some reduction in tension. The final resolution, however, did not come about until there was a more serious incident after which six patients were threatened with expulsion.

EPISODE 1

Phase A. When we first began to think in terms of phases, the community had just gone through a classic cycle. It began in June after the usual spring disturbance had quieted down, the regular school term had ended, and a number of key patients had been discharged. For a few weeks there was a warm, close feeling on the unit. Morning meetings had energy and contact. We could talk about what individual people were going through. Others would join in to relate their own experiences or to give significant feedback. Acting out was minimal and isolated.

Phase B. Slowly, tension started to mount. There was a camping trip during which cliques and rivalries began to form. There were a number of thefts, and we suspected an extremely disturbed sociopathic boy whom we had made great efforts to help. The nursing staff had become dubious about our ability to help him, but our efforts continued. There was another negative leader, a boy, who had been referred by the courts after a drug-related arrest. He stayed cool and detached, seemingly untouched, and, along with others, broke the rules, usually without detection. Perhaps more significant during this period was the fact that our staff was becoming less and less involved, a hallmark of periods of increasing tension. It was summer. The psychiatric residents were about to rotate off the unit, some staff were about to move into new jobs or go on vacation while others wished they could. Morning meetings became increasingly focused on the previous day's trouble, while the staff attitude was the kind of impotent anger we have come to recognize as characteristic of the phase of rising tension.

Phase C. Finally, on a weekend when the staff as a whole was engaged in a personal-growth workshop, there was a collective disturbance on the unit. Four patients were caught smoking marijuana, and six patients (with one overlap) became engaged in a raucous protest against the night staff, barricading themselves in a room all night and disturbing the whole floor with loud music and talk. Another sizable group, mostly of older patients, was incensed at the disturbance. The next morning there was a sense of quiet after the storm, with many patients fearing punishment and others (especially, of course, those who had not been involved) hoping the staff would react. Our response was to place all those involved on administrative floor confinement. The "cool" troublemaker was discharged as previously scheduled, and the more disturbed one was transferred to another unit in the hospital after he became agitated and hit a nurse. We delayed dealing with the others for part of a day to assess the mood of the unit, but when more acting out was in the wind, the director met with the troublemakers and told them to arrange through their individual therapists for transfer. He confronted them for having acted against the unit and refused to listen to any appeals to his usual conciliatory nature. These patients all responded with strong desire to remain on the unit.

Phase D. Only after several days of this unrelenting tension did we agree to sit down and negotiate therapeutic contracts which specified conditions under which each person could stay. The agreements clarified such issues as attendence at school, participating in morning meetings, and work to change specific kinds of behavior. For several patients this experience seemed to be an important step in learning to confront, realistically, the consequences of impulsive action. On others there was no discernible effect. One depressed, alcoholic young adult became upset at our failure to punish the troublemakers, and his faith in us may have been damaged. Another, a schizophrenic boy, became acutely agitated in the weeks that followed. This may have been, in part, a response to the community disorganization. At the same time we also found that now, in the postcrisis period, the community could respond to problems such as this with caring, support, and confrontation. As a staff we tried to focus less on ward problems and more on working with individual patients. Within a few weeks we felt we were beginning a new cycle in a spirit of relative harmony and commitment to our therapeutic goals. In the process, several newer patients became involved in positions of leadership in a project to refurbish the unit.

Comment. We thought we might have engaged in some collusive denial by failing to diagnose our staff withdrawal earlier and perhaps by putting off a decision about the disturbed sociopath whom we finally transferred elsewhere. But we also felt that, had tension-curbing action been taken earlier, most of the patients who ultimately participated in the reconstruction period would not have felt involved or moved. The negotiation process and the redecoration project are examples of the kinds of lasting changes which arise out of such crisis.

EPISODE 2

Phase A. The unit was quiet after a disruptive period which had ended with the transfer of a sociopathic patient. For a while there was the comfortable feeling, typical of this phase, with considerable contact, closeness, and constructive confrontations privately and publicly. During a period of several weeks, there were active discussions in morning meetings about the departure of several popular and constructive patients.

Phase B. There were several acts of vandalism. Soon thereafter, controversy arose between patients and staff about a recently inaugurated policy of locking the door during morning school hours to prevent patients from returning to the unit in order to withdraw. Several boys tried to recruit a following and seemed to be ready for a blowup. Our staff leaders felt, however, that some staff were becoming trapped in a fruitless law-and-order position because of the door and that the ensuing polarization was not constructive. We called a special floor meeting and combined a new appeal for an understanding of the issue of withdrawal, which locking the door was designed to prevent. Despite this brief crisis intervention, tension continued to mount. There was an increase in acting out at night, and the staff's impotent anger toward disruptive, unreachable patients also increased. The prevailing sentiment was exemplified by several patients who had the potential to become positive leaders but did not, feeling that no one else was interested in constructive work. Other patients became disruptive during official excursions away from the hospital, exploiting what was then a policy of not punishing patients for isolated transgressions off hospital grounds. There was a week-long hiatus for a school vacation with special activities. A strong mood of fragmentation and apathy ensued. The director confronted the increasing mess in the lounge and the apathy during the morning meetings. He offered to transfer "those who just want to watch." The evening staff carried through a two-hour crisis meeting. Patients reported that this was a particularly valuable experience, but there was a growing split between private hopes for communality and polarization between staff and patients during the day.

Phase C. The weekend after the crisis meeting, thirteen of our twenty-four patients were involved (singly or in small groups) in vandalism, running away, drug abuse, or defiance. When the vandalism persisted during the week, the director spoke out against the violation and humiliation of other patients that had resulted from some of the patients' actions. He threatened administrative action if his sense of mistrust of the community did not abate. There were several good discussions in the morning meeting following this, including one that began as a hostile challenge by patients toward an individual staff member and ended as a meaningful exchange among a large group of staff and patients. But the feeling of resolution did not develop. The next weekend (now two months into the cycle), five patients ran away and became involved in sexually promiscuous activity at a friend's apartment. When they came back they were handled individually, so that their feelings about sex and intimacy could be approached sensitively. At this point most of the unit physicians went away for a week of meetings. Morning meetings became empty, apathetic, and almost intolerable, although several potential patient leaders began talking about their desire to bring the ward together and their uncertainty as to how to do it. Following another run-away episode, the nurse coordinator took action by temporarily locking the unit door.

Having returned to the unit, the director sat with the outside circle of uninvolved patients at the morning meeting. There he articulated what it felt like to be outside. He literally could not hear what was being discussed; he had no way to connect. He proposed giving outsiders a "clearer choice" by demanding that they sit inside the main circle during morning meetings or be considered absent. (Ordinarily we allow withdrawn patients to express their mood by coming but sitting outside the group. We then find ways to invite them in.) That night, six of the most disruptive patients were caught, in separate groups, using drugs. They were threatened with expulsion.

Phase D. This episode provided the final release of tension. Each of the patients involved reacted with more seriousness than before. They expressed a desire to stay and to negotiate a therapeutic contract. Morning meetings improved, several of the patients who has expressed a desire to help the community, and several of those who had been disruptive, now took an active part in more constructive discussions. Again it became possible to confront individual problems with a sense of a desire to help rather than with a sense of polarization and defensiveness. As the feeling of comfort, contact, and person-oriented energy returned, the community appeared ready to begin a new cycle.

Comment. This cycle included several bursts of conflict without a feeling of resolution or renewal among them. The director reacted forcefully to each outburst of anticommunity action in contrast to the delayed response described in the first episode. The advantages of these forceful interventions seemed to be that several patients who were in trouble reacted with guilt and may have been prevented from further action. The nursing leadership perceived the director's behavior as a show of support for their own attempts to use reality confrontation as a therapeutic tool. The director in turn felt that nursing efforts to follow through on his intervention supported what he was doing. This feeling of teamwork was a source of satisfaction for the leadership group (see fig. 1).

Discussion

Rapoport (1960) offered the subjective conclusion that some patients were benefited by the period of social reconstruction that followed oscillation of tension while others were hurt by the chaos, especially at the peaks of community tension. He also studied the interrelations of patient adaptation to ward norms, staff evaluation of patients, and long-term improvement. Patients who adopted ward norms received better evaluations from staff but did not necessarily do well in the long run. Those who failed to adopt ward norms received worse evaluations and also did more poorly after discharge. The only factor significantly related to long-term improvement was length of stay of six months or greater.

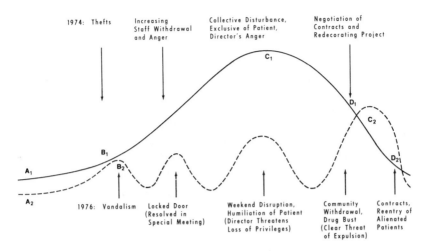

FIG. 1—Two cycles of community tension. Solid line = Summer 1974; dashed line = Spring 1976.

Moos (1974) studied the relationship between the "ward atmosphere," as rated by patients and staff, and the frequency of rehospitalizations. His data indicated that highly interactive wards encourage rapid discharge and discourage too much expression. His data, like Rapoport's, show that on more interactive wards patients whose perceptions of the ward are deviant, or who would prefer the ward to be different than it is, tend to do worse after discharge. On less interactive wards, although overall results are not as good, there is less difference between the outcomes of patients who agree with ward norms and those who do not. Similarly, Almond (1974) has shown that patients on a therapeutic community ward tended to adopt the community ideology while undergoing treatment but returned to their old values after discharge. He was unable to relate adoption of ward ideology to positive outcome.

The implication of these studies is that highly interactive programs effectively exclude certain patients from treatment while providing a setting in which many others can benefit. These studies did not address the processes of oscillatory cycles—their contribution to treatment or whether more effective management of these cycles and of other large group processes have a measurable effect on outcome. We believe that they do and anticipate that future studies will confirm this impression.

As we review our experiences with this approach, we discover a variety of leadership implications which have proven useful to us. As we became aware of recurrent cycles of tension we were able to pinpoint more exactly what modes of leadership various staff members had contributed during the different phases of each cycle.

During phase A we tend to rely primarily on leaders who are comfortable with contact and closeness, and who can help legitimize the articulation of important areas of concern in a public setting, in order to help establish a mood of seriousness and work. These leaders are particularly helpful in being able to speak reflectively about highly charged or previously avoided problems. Some discussions assume a spontaneous emotional intensity, and there are staff members who are effective and comfortable with these dramatic moments. Patient leaders also are an indispensable part of phase A. The patients who came through the previous cycle and learned from it became positive leaders. In addition new patients, who are fresh to the areas of potential community conflict, often take over and allow the positive aspects of the phase to be asserted.

There is a complication during phase A which requires a somewhat different shading of leadership. At times during this phase there is a certain amount of ritualized attendance to platitudes about openness, harmony, and love. In the midst of all of this, there must be staff who are able to find the authentic moments, who are able to form genuinely deep relationships with patients and to follow through on them. This can be difficult, because along with the great potential of this phase there is a sense of fatigue from the previous cycle. There is a reluctance on the part of some to confront and involve themselves deeply in the sickness of new patients. These features contribute to the sense of staff withdrawal, which generally accompanies the rise of new tensions toward phase B.

The rising tension of phase B often involves a number of new patients whom no one knows very well; one of our best leaders is a psychiatric technician who is particularly good at confronting and exercising authority over them. The best phase B leaders can express genuine anger rather than the impotent rage which gradually increases and comes to dominate the staff during this time. Another leadership task during this phase is to be able to confront the general cynicism which arises along with the community tensions and continue to articulate the community's ideals in the face of it. This often means presenting those ideals at moments when they are doomed to fall flat and appear meaningless. However, it is essential that even though no one seems to believe in those ideals it is made clear that the leaders really still do. There is still a clear commitment to the building of personal relationships with patients. This is a link from the relative successes of the earlier, more harmonious phase to the time of trouble which lies ahead. A particularly important area which must be dealt with at this time is staff conflict and withdrawal. This can be very difficult to accomplish in the frustration and potentially cynical atmosphere of this phase. We believe that we will be able to prevent some of the more destructive forms of collective disturbance to the extent that we are able to be more effective at working within the staff itself in these areas.

During phase C there is a sharp constriction as leadership and power become concentrated in the top leadership of the community. The community leadership has three central tasks. First, it must take the administrative actions necessary to restore order if disruption is severe. We have relied on a system of rules and privileges which, while carrying a clear threat of exclusion, offers an opportunity to negotiate on each patient's behalf. The leaders must be able to exercise authority firmly and in cooperation with others and to express genuine anger with those patients who can tolerate it.

The second task is to continue to uphold the community ideals in the face of massive assault. If tension is high, almost no one believes that action can still be based on ideal rather than on mere survival. Core leaders again continue to express ideals in the face of apparently being ignored. In phase C, the very strongest leader will feel as though he or she is just barely maintaining a self-esteem through these attempts, and the less powerful leader will feel complete helplessness. Here the effective leader must draw upon his most personal qualities, expose them to public view, and emerge still respected. For example, the director's style under pressure tends toward the dramatic solo performance. During phase C he is perceived by some as being a prima donna; but at the same time the entire community relies upon his leadership when others are reluctant to assume the burden of leading community meetings. The evening supervisor, who is exceptional at setting limits and controlling very disruptive patients, comes to be seen by some as an ogre, but he, too, during this phase is seen as indispensable. It is still important, despite the law-and-order mood, that staff seek opportunities for genuine emotional encounters which are often most dramatic and unique during these personal and community crises.

The third and most sophisticated leadership task is the diagnosis and management of the fragmentation of staff relationships. This fragmentation generally begins in the relations within the core leadership group itself and is mirrored downward through other staff to impinge upon patients. For example, the nurse coordinator may feel as though she has been abandoned by the salaried psychiatrists. This will be reflected in difficulties in taking care of conflicts among the nursing-staff members, some of whom then take out their frustrations on misbehaving patients, thus contributing to further staff-patient split. Looking at it from another point of view, a core leader's perception of a colleague's poor performance may lead to withdrawal from interaction with that colleague, contributing again to a sense of abandonment and ultimately to staff-patient split. One test of our effectiveness as a therapeutic community is whether we are able to perceive, and actively confront, some of the organizational and staff problems which have complicated periods of community tension. This is one key to remaining a vigorous, growing community rather than a stagnant, routinized one. A therapeutic corollary to coping with staff fragmentation is the need to protect the patients who are vulnerable (commonly psychotic patients) to the destructive effects of this kind of social chaos. We have found no simple system for doing this. Individual staff members and patients have taken responsibility for particular patients, one of whom often does become upset and is a focus of attention during the next phase.

Phase D is a time of coming together. One of our most effective leaders, the nurse coordinator, is able to make contact with a variety of patients who have been outside the community (especially the recent troublemakers) and help them find ways of coming inside. Other staff may help patients follow through on contractual agreements, either by enforcing rules or by providing inspiration. An especially important reconnection often occurs between the top staff leadership and the reformed outlaws. The leaders must seek and remain open to this connection. The hallmark of effective work in this phase is a paradigm for much of therapy: engage the most problematic side of patients (primarily the character-disordered patient in this context), confront them with authentic feelings and authority, and then allow the relationship to be transformed to an alliance toward constructive outcome. The time is then ripe for an infusion of trust (even unearned trust) and a softer closeness. The best leaders take unusual risks and reap at least some small success. We have spent less time and energy explicitly resolving conflicts among staff members, perhaps less than we should. The feeling of renewed vitality often emerges nevertheless.

From this perspective, it has become clear that a variety of leadership skills and styles is essential to the management and shaping of these recurrent cycles in the community life. These skills must be selected, taught, cultivated, and nurtured in individuals, in many instances independent of the official leadership hierarchy. One problem of the past, which this conceptualization has helped to resolve, is that individuals with the natural skills needed and useful during the different cycles tend to be disrespectful, at times rejecting, of one another. For example, a natural straightforward phase B person will tend to find the activity and experiences of a competent phase A person distasteful or false, whereas a natural loving stage A person will tend to experience an effective stage B leader or stage C experience as inhuman or sadistic. Teaching this schema for the cycles has been invaluable in helping staff appreciate these necessary differences in leadership contribution, leading to greater overall respect and diminished competition and unwarranted criticism.

Conclusions

We have presented two conceptualizations which have emerged from our therapeutic community work with hospitalized adolescents. The first, stages of organizational development, addresses the inevitable struggle of the therapeutic community to integrate the need for spontaneity and creativity with the need for structure, order, and routine. The second, cycles of tension, addresses the inevitable waxing and waning of interpersonal tensions and ward disruptions present on an interactive unit for hospitalized adolescents. These two conceptualizations have proven useful to us in predicting and anticipating a variety of large and small group phenomena, and we are, therefore, better prepared to plan and manage our community and a variety of its recurrent needs. Being able to do this has led to improved overall staff-patient morale and sense of mastery and has decreased the likelihood of participants to personalize or scapegoat themselves or others for these inevitable, recurrent phenomena.

REFERENCES

Almond, R. 1974. *The Healing Community*. New York: Aronson.

Boyd, R. W.; Kageles, S. S.; and Greenblatt, M. 1954. Outbreak of gang destructive behavior on a psychiatric ward. *Journal of Nervous and Mental Disease* 120:338–342.

Caudill, W. 1958. *The Psychiatric Hospital as a Small Society*. Cambridge, Mass.: Harvard University Press.

Crabtree, L. H., Jr., and Cox, J. L. D. 1972. The overthrow of a therapeutic community. *International Journal of Group Psychotherapy* 22(1): 31–41.

Crabtree, L. H., Jr., and Grossman, W. K. 1974. Administrative clarity and redefinition for an open adolescent unit. *Psychiatry* 37:350–359.

Henry, J. 1957. Types of institutional structure. In M. Greenblatt, D. J.

Levinson, and R. H. Williams, eds. *The Patient and the Mental Hospital.* Glencoe, Ill.: Free Press.

Jones, M. 1953. *The Therapeutic Community.* New York: Basic.

Miller, D. 1957. The etiology of an outbreak of delinquence in a group of hospitalized adolescents. In M. Greenblatt, D. J. Levinson, and R. H. Williams, eds. *The Patient and the Mental Hospital.* Glencoe, Ill.: Free Press.

Moos, R. H. 1974. Role, theory and the treatment of antisocial acting out disorders. *British Journal of Delinquency* 7:285–300.

Rapoport, R. 1960. *Community as Doctor.* London: Tavistock.

Stanton, A., and Schwartz, M. 1954. *The Mental Hospital.* New York: Basic.

40   ADOLESCENT PSYCHODYNAMICS AND THE THERAPY GROUP

REED BROCKBANK

The crucial stage of adolescence is of such importance in every individual's development that it is necessary to be clear about the major tasks which confront both males and females during this period between childhood and adulthood. Boys and girls do not reach puberty with the same psychological and developmental accomplishments, and the tasks for girls are, therefore, not exactly the same as those for boys.

Puberty for girls represents special problems which begin with the adaptation to secondary sex characteristics followed by anticipation and management of the menarche with all of its complex psychological implications. Menarche brings an intensification of attention on both external and internal genitalia. Vaginal sensations are intensified and are the forerunners of orgastic experience as described by Kestenberg (1975). Boys masturbate, explore, and experiment with genitals much more frequently than do girls. Girls rely more on and have more confidence in their intuition than do boys. As adolescence progresses, both sexes try out in thought, fantasy, and action their increasing sense of themselves as sexual provokers while closely observing the reactions in peers and adults of their self-conscious powers.

The achievement of orgastic potency is more than the simple discharge of sexual products in the male and more than a peak of sexual excitement and its physiological correlates. It consists of a full ripening of sexual intimacy and mutuality as described by Erikson (1968)—the essence of what psychoanalysts call genitality. This accomplishment brings with it the possibility for a more accurate and integrated sense of one's self (Erikson refers to it as an "inner continuity and sameness") modified from old and conflictive attachments to one's parents. The center of these attachments is, of course, the oedipal conflict. The degree to which these tasks are achieved makes it possible for eventual termination of the adolescent phase. In Western culture this may occur anywhere from the end of the teens up to the mid-twenties. In the course of this development, the conflicts between reality and fantasy and between object relationships and narcissism are paramount. Narcissism is a particular issue which is evident and observable in group behavior, and we will focus on this in detail in our look at adolescent therapy groups.

Group Formation in Adolescents

The importance of the group to the adolescent has been known by those who have observed and worked with children and youth for many years. However, it was not until Erikson's (1968) studies of individual and group identity in adolescence that theoreticians could conceptualize the factors that have made adolescent group formation such an essential aspect of adolescent developmental psychology. We now recognize that group formation makes it possible for the adolescent to do a number of important things which are necessary for the resolution of certain conflicts which must be accomplished during this period of life. The adolescent achieves this conflict resolution in the group first by displacement of much unresolved childhood dependency on parents onto the peer group. This displacement makes possible the beginning of decathexis of parents as the exclusive focus upon which infantile and latency conflicts are acted out. This, of course, makes the adolescent peer group crucial for adolescent development. It also sets the stage for certain group dynamic phenomena to occur in the adolescent therapy group.

The second step necessary for conflict resolution during adolescence provided by the therapy group is the possibility for elaboration of both homosexual and heterosexual object ties which are now age congruent and yet contain leftover conflicts with parental objects of the past. The fact that now both libidinal and aggressive infantile drives are directed toward one's agemates makes possible further resolution of the oedipal conflicts of childhood.

The third significant factor in adolescent group formation is the use of the peer group for reworking and full flowering of both group and individual identity. As Erikson (1968) has shown, it is essential that one's individual identity have some reasonable congruence and synthesis with his group identity. The peer group offers multiple opportunities to validate consensually and repeatedly the values, judgments, and eccentricities consistent with each individual's unique past as well as with his ancestral origins and cultural linkages. The conflict which every adolescent struggles with between his

530

need for maintenance of his unique self-sameness, separate and distinct, and his need to be the same as others in thought, dress, values, and actions can be seen in clear perspective in any adolescent group. How this conflict is finally resolved determines whether identity diffusion is the result or whether the adolescent can pass on to commitment and intimacy with a greater satisfaction about his sense of himself as a unified, autonomous adult.

Adolescent Group-Therapy Behavior

When observing an adolescent therapy group which has developed a degree of cohesiveness and object ties to one another, the observer is struck by the amount of action taking place in rapid-fire order, all of highly symbolic character and all seeming to be pleasurable and compelling. Any attempt to frustrate and slow down the action is met with resistance and defiance. It is as though each patient in the group is more interested in acting than in thinking, and more concerned with interactions for their own sake than for meaning or self-reflection, at least on a conscious level. Yet each such action exchange or piece of verbal interaction appears to have the same communicative value as children's play. Zeligs's (1957) use of the term "acting in" appears to be typical of adolescent behavior in such a therapy group. He describes postural attitudes and other nonverbal behavior of patients in analysis as a type of action which lies midway between acting out at one extreme and verbalizing and remembering at the other. The group therapist who attempts to understand these action communications for purposes of clarification and interpretation usually finds himself unable to keep pace with the action and quickly falls behind what is happening. The complaint that one often hears about adult group therapy—namely, that it is difficult enough to know what is going on with one patient at a time, let alone with a group of patients all interacting with each other with multiple transference reactions— is even more the case with adolescents or children in group therapy. The propensity for action and for acting out as part of adolescent psychodynamics can be seen most clearly in adolescent groups. The question is whether this symbolic action or these so-called symptomatic acts can be utilized for therapeutic benefit or whether they will get out of control in a group setting so that through contagion (always present in all group behavior, but more so in adolescents) acting out overwhelms the effort to achieve insight and therapeutic effect.

It may be possible to expand our understanding so that it may be utilized for therapeutic effect by asking, What is the nature and purpose of this propensity for action and acting out? Several psychoanalysts (Shafer 1976; Valenstein 1962; and Wheelis 1950) have expressed their views that insight is therapeutic only when it is "worked through toward the action system" (Wallerstein 1965).

Ekstein is quoted as saying, "It is possible to overemphasize the resistance aspects of action such as acting out and to minimize the communicative value in the analytic situation" (Atkins 1970). This is certainly an accurate statement of the situation in group psychotherapy. Nonetheless, deterioration of the analytic group into repetitive action in the service of resistance must always be kept in mind.

Group Dynamics

As Erikson (1968) has further shown, the problem of the sense of one's identity is a central issue throughout all stages of development. Yet at no time is its importance more evident than during adolescence. Also, as I have indicated, the adolescent group provides the most clear opportunity to observe the various aspects of individual and group identity. We have learned from clinical experience that during a crisis or when the individual is under stress one can see most clearly those issues which are of particular significance to normal psychology as well as to pathology.

The developmental crisis of adolescence, therefore, provides us with some of the best occasions to understand both individual conflict and group dynamics. The motivation and need for group belongingness, present in all of us, can be seen in clear perspective in the adolescent's excessive and slavish devotion to his group. Yet the conflict he experiences as he struggles both to free himself from his family group and, at the same time, to maintain a sense of belongingness is the essence of the adolescent's dilemma. In his peer group, this need to identify with every aspect of other adolescents' thinking and behavior is countered by a fear of losing a unique sense of himself by total immersion in the group culture. If we ask ourselves why humans develop this ever-present need to belong, we would have to relate it to the relatively prolonged dependency on parental objects, particularly the mother, during infancy and childhood. Therefore, the need to belong to the mother, even to be part of her in a symbiotic sense, is the fundamental source of this need for belongingness which is the major drive toward group formation and also toward group identity.

Balint (1959) pointed out that this regressive pull and the ego's defensive struggle against it form a central part of the patient's struggle on the couch in formal psychoanalysis. He coined two terms to describe this conflict situation, "philobatism" and "oconophilia." The oconophile adheres and clings to his object, where he feels safe and secure. The philobat reaches out (like the acrobat) into objectless space, which excites his pleasure, while objects are felt to be treacherous and hazardous. It is my contention that this same dynamic situation exists in all group-therapy situations where cohesiveness, group identity, and belongingness have developed. As regression occurs in such a group situation, the need to belong becomes the need to belong to the mother, to be part of her, to be one and the same. Therefore, the group as a whole becomes for the patient a substitute for the symbiotic mother. The fear that many incipient schizophrenic patients have of groups arises from their intense fear of loss of their sense of identity and of ego boundaries that might result from such a further disintegration of their already regressed and threatened egos. Their defenses against this regression tend to keep them from group formations. Therefore, the intense anxiety and panic which are aroused by the group must be defended against by distancing and isolation.

Freud (1921) stated that the major dynamic process occuring in the member of a group is the projection and giving up of the individual superego and ego ideal in favor of that of the group and/or the group leader. With patients who have weak ego structures, a tightly closed and intense group experience associated with the propensity toward ego regression makes the patient very vulnerable indeed. This does not mean that I believe group therapy to be contraindicated in patients with weak ego structures and ego-boundary problems. But group therapy with such patients needs to be carefully considered and monitored, so that it does not become more of a hindrance than a help. Also, observations of particularly narcissistic patients show that they become quite threatened and their narcissistic defenses become exaggerated in a group-therapy situation. Typically, such patients tend to withdraw their object interest in other members of the group and to retreat to a self-absorbed preoccupation, often leading to grandiose and even megalomanic defenses. They may become demanding and dominating of the group time, with little awareness that they are putting themselves in the center of the group and have become intolerant or disdainfully indifferent to other group members' problems.

To illustrate, I will report briefly on such a patient, who came for psychotherapy at a clinic setting. He was included in group psychotherapy with four other patients. John was in his twenties and was highly intelligent and perceptive, but had little or no empathy for other people. He was almost totally self-absorbed, was contemptuously disdainful of all of the other patients in the group, and—on the few occasions that he paid any attention to them at all—made fun of them. The other patients were about the same age and socioeconomic status, but he regarded them as intellectually and personally inferior to himself. He made it clear that he had very little use for their communications to him. He would alternate between sitting with his back to the others and sitting near the center of the group circle. He either dominated the discussion or would look out the window in boredom when others of the group spoke. As this continued, the other patients predictably became angry with him and began refusing to talk to him. Some fell silent and started missing group sessions. This clearly pleased John, who openly admitted that he preferred having the therapists to himself. At about the same time, however, John began showing what appeared to be even more severely regressive behavior and threatened suicide. His personal problems in living were more than he could handle, so an individual session was scheduled with him by the two male cotherapists. During that session he sucked his thumb, writhed on the floor, sobbed incoherently, and curled up in a fetal position.

Since he had no prior history of psychosis and had shown no evidence of psychotic thinking during the initial diagnostic interviews, it was clear that his severe borderline and narcissistic personality structure was too fragile to deal with the group's threat to his narcissistic defenses. He was referred for individual therapy and removed from the group.

The significance of these observations of a young adult patient in group psychotherapy can tell us something about what may also be happening in the adolescent in a therapy group. First, we know that an adolescent's ego identity is frequently in a state of lability or even confusion. Because of this lack of solidity, he seeks a group experience and group identification in order to bolster his uncertain sense of himself. For him, in contrast to the adult schizophrenic or schizoid personality, the group represents a haven, or refuge, or at least an opportunity for growth. Indeed, it generally does serve this purpose, provided that his ego development up to this point has not succumbed to inherent or acquired weaknesses which have forced pathological defensive structures to develop. Second, we know that adolescents have difficulty in resolving narcissistic conflicts and yet adolescence is a crucial period for such resolution; if it does not occur during this time of life, then future, more severe problems with narcissism will be in the offing. Hence, parents as well as therapists watch their older adolescents with anxious concern about their degree of resolution of self-centered and seemingly calloused indifference to the needs and feelings of others.

A third observation is that imitation and contagion of emotion are characteristic features of adolescents, of all groups, and of collective mental life at all ages. McDougall (1920) wrote of the positive and creative effect of imitation: "Imitation is the great agency through which the child is led on from the life of mere animal impulse to a life of self control, deliberation, and true volition; and it has played a similar part in the development of the human race and of human society. Imitation is the prime condition of all collective mental life."

The fact that adolescents imitate one another and that they seek out group relations in order to accomplish this gives us another hint of the importance of group experiences for them. Hence, such therapy groups are meaningful both to the adolescent and for our understanding of group psychology as well.

Therapeutic Implications

As indicated, adolescents tend to act out their struggles and conflicts in their peer groups and in therapy groups in such a way that a group experience offers a unique opportunity to study these conflicts and to intervene in their resolution. Another advantage of group therapy is that these young people tend to bring their action potential and symptomatic acts directly into the treatment situation, so that it is more in the nature of acting in rather than acting out. Relatively undisguised sexual approaches combined with highly symbolic sexual and aggressive discharges are common. The latter may include striking matches and throwing them at each other, having water fights with obvious sexual symbolism, riding piggyback, and playing peekaboo with doors and one-way mirrors—all used to decrease sexual and aggressive passions.

Within the transference, joking innuendos about others' secret fantasies, sexual behavior, or the therapist's private life are common. As regression deepens and cohesiveness increases, multiple sibling identifications occur as the patients recreate a family setting. Diminution of superego and ego controls over aggressive drives occurs because of the giving up and projection of superego and ego ideals onto the group leaders. This regular feature of group dynamics produces in older adolescents an intensification of narcissistic elements and narcissistic defenses. These defenses can be seen in withdrawal from group interaction in favor of self-preoccupation on the one hand or, on the other, insistence on being in the center of the action and refusal to relate to the problems and concerns of the other group participants. Adolescents will say frequently, "I won't talk to the group about my problems. I will discuss these things with my individual therapist and only then when he talks to me and not when he just sits and listens. I don't know what's going on in this group anyway. I don't think anything happens here."

At this point other patients in the group will often attack this narcissistic withdrawal by accusing such a fellow patient of being selfish and insensitive to the others' problems. Opportunities for therapeutic intervention and interpretation by the therapist of the patient's fears of anger and aggression or fear of losing one's sense of uniqueness by participation with others in the group process adds insight to the action and behavior of such adolescents, results in modification of such fears, and furthers the therapeutic potential of the group.

These interpretations will usually lead to group exploration of the conflicts between needs for belongingness versus fear of loss of uniqueness and autonomy. As a part of the working-through aspects of the group experience, consensual validation occurs and patients recognize the similarity of their conflicts with those of others. A consequent decrease in fears of isolation and aloneness occurs. In this way, the adolescent patient comes to recognize that he is not an island, even though at times he may behave as if he wished to be one.

One of the most significant effects on patients of all ages in a group is the reduction of narcissistic cathexis in favor of object cathexis. This arises from the multiple transferences that occur, especially in therapeutic groups. As mentioned, this may result in a complication for those patients with weak ego boundaries whose loss of narcissistic cathexis causes a diminution of cathexis of their ego boundaries. On the other hand, with less disturbed adolescents, the encouragement of object cathexis in a group represents an important therapeutic advantage insofar as it results in less narcissism and a consequent strengthening and broadening of the ego.

As has long been recognized, identification plays a prominent role in the therapeutic encounter with patients, whether in individual psychotherapy, psychoanalysis, or in group psychotherapy. The muliple identifications between the patients and with the therapist in a group begin with what Weiss (1960) called "resonance identification." These identifications occur in a group because of a transference-determined love or hate that group members secretly share for the group leader (Freud 1921). This results in the binding quality and cohesiveness among patients in a group therapeutic setting. It is also because of identification, as Sterba (1934) described, that a so-called therapeutic split occurs in the ego which allows patients to experience as well as to observe intrapsychic processes occurring in themselves. This therapeutic split in the ego can readily be observed in adolescents in group therapy. Empathic identifications also occur in the group therapist, and he utilizes this in his interpretations and his understanding of each patient in the group. It is essential for the curative process that the group therapist be able to lend himself as an object for both identification and projection. His relaxed, accepting, and participating neutrality are essential for these processes to occur in the patients and in himself.

Conclusions

Group and individual psychodynamics can be seen in clear perspective in adolescent therapy groups. This makes possible a further understanding of narcissistic development during adolescence. In addition, the group setting provides an opportunity to offer therapeutic assistance in the resolution of typical adolescent conflicts. However, not all adolescents are candidates for group psychotherapy. The danger of a loss of narcissistic cathexis in group therapy can, for some especially vulnerable patients (both adult and adolescent), cause regression to psychotic levels of functioning. Such a regression in an adult patient has been described to illustrate this same kind of threat to especially vulnerable adolescent patients. It is also possible to relate this group-provoked regression in a therapeutic setting with the psychodynamic situation in less disturbed and normal adolescents as they struggle with conflicts between reality and fantasy and between more mature object relations and narcissistic object ties.

REFERENCES

Atkins, N. B. 1970. Acting, acting out and the symptomatic act. *Journal of the American Psychoanalytic Association* 18:631–643.
Balint, M. 1959. *Thrills and Regressions*. New York: International Universities Press.
Erikson, E. H. 1968. *Identity, Youth and Crisis*. New York: Norton.

Freud, S. 1921. Group psychology and the analysis of the ego. *Standard Edition* 18:67–143. London: Hogarth, 1955.

Kestenberg, J. S. 1975. *Children and Parents: Psychoanalytic Studies in Development*. New York: Aronson.

McDougall, W. 1920. *The Group Mind*. Reprint. New York: Cambridge University Press, 1969.

Shafer, R. 1976. *A New Language for Psychoanalysis*. New Haven, Conn.: Yale University Press.

Sterba, R. 1934. The fate of the ego in analytic therapy. *International Journal of Psychoanalysis* 15:117–126.

Valenstein, A. 1962. Affects, emotional reliving and insight in the psychoanalytic process. *International Journal of Psychoanalysis* 43:315–324.

Wallerstein, R. 1965. The goals of psychoanalysis. *Journal of the American Psychoanalytic Association* 13:748–770.

Weiss, E. 1960. *The Structure and Dynamics of the Human Mind*. New York: Grune & Stratton.

Wheelis, A. 1950. The place of action in personality change. *Psychiatry* 13:135–148.

Zeligs, M. A. 1957. Acting in: a contribution to the meaning of some postural attitudes observed during analysis. *Journal of the American Psychoanalytic Association* 5:685–705.

THE AUTHORS

ROBERT L. ARNSTEIN is Clinical Professor of Psychiatry, Yale School of Medicine, and Chief Psychiatrist, Yale University Health Services.

JUDITH A. ASHWAY is a Staff Member of the Clinic for Children and Adolescents, Postgraduate Center for Mental Health, New York.

PETER BARGLOW is Associate Professor of Psychiatry, Northwestern University Medical School, and Clinical Director, Psychosomatic and Psychiatric Institute, Michael Reese Hospital and Medical Center.

RONALD M. BENSON is Clinical Associate Professor of Psychiatry, and Associate Director, Child Analytic Study Program, University of Michigan.

IRVING N. BERLIN is Professor of Psychiatry and Director, Division of Child and Adolescent Psychiatry and the Children's Psychiatric Center, University of New Mexico School of Medicine.

SIDNEY BERMAN is Clinical Professor of Psychiatry, George Washington University School of Medicine, and on the Senior Advisory Staff, Children's Hospital, National Medical Center, Washington, D.C.

PETER BLOS is Lecturer, New York Psychoanalytic Institute and Columbia Psychoanalytic Clinic for Training and Research. He received the 1969 William A. Schonfeld Distinguished Service Award of the American Society for Adolescent Psychiatry.

MARK J. BLOTCKY is Clinical Instructor of Psychiatry, University of Texas Health Science Center at Dallas, and Director, Children's Unit, Child and Adolescent Service, Timberlawn Psychiatric Center, Dallas.

539

REED BROCKBANK is Associate Clinical Professor of Psychiatry, University of California School of Medicine at San Francisco.

DOYLE I. CARSON is Clinical Assistant Professor of Psychiatry, University of Texas Health Science Center at Dallas, and Medical Director, Timberlawn Hospital.

JOHN CAWELTI is Professor of English, University of Chicago.

LOREN H. CRABTREE, JR., is Director, Young Adult Program, Horsham Clinic and Hospital, Ambler, Pennsylvania.

LEON EISENBERG is Maude and Lillian Presley Professor of Psychiatry, Harvard Medical School, and Senior Associate in Psychiatry, Children's Hospital Medical Center, Boston, Massachusetts.

MIRIAM ELSON is Social Work Consultant, Student Mental Health Clinic, University of Chicago, and Faculty Member, Teacher Education Program, Chicago Institute for Psychoanalysis.

AARON H. ESMAN is Professor of Clinical Psychiatry, Cornell University Medical College, and Faculty Member, New York Psychoanalytic Institute.

SHERMAN C. FEINSTEIN is Clinical Professor of Psychiatry, Pritzker School of Medicine, University of Chicago, and Director, Child Psychiatry Research, Michael Reese Hospital and Medical Center. He is the Coordinating Editor of this volume.

SUSAN M. FISHER is Professorial Lecturer, Pritzker School of Medicine, University of Chicago.

PETER L. GIOVACCHINI is Clinical Professor of Psychiatry, Abraham Lincoln School of Medicine, University of Illinois, and a Senior Editor of this volume.

JOHN T. GOSSETT is Associate Director, Timberlawn Psychiatric Research Foundation, and Director of Evaluation Services, Timberlawn Psychiatric Center, Dallas.

PHILIP M. HAUSER is Lucy Flower Professor Emeritus of Urban Sociology and Director Emeritus, Population Research Center, University of Chicago.

PHILIP S. HOLZMAN is Professor of Psychology, Harvard University, and Training and Supervising Analyst, Boston Psychoanalytic Society and Institute.

PHILIP KATZ is Associate Professor of Psychiatry, University of Manitoba Faculty of Medicine, and Past-President, Canadian Society for Youth Psychiatry.

540

CLARICE J. KESTENBAUM is Clinical Professor of Psychiatry, Columbia University, and Director, Division of Child and Adolescent Psychiatry, St. Luke's Hospital, New York.

GERALD L. KLERMAN is Administrator, Alcohol, Drug Abuse, and Mental Health Administration, Department of Health and Human Services, Washington, D.C.

HEINZ KOHUT is a Professorial Lecturer in Psychiatry at the University of Chicago, and Training Analyst, Chicago Institute for Psychoanalysis. A former President of the American Psychoanalytic Association, he is the 1979 recipient of the William A. Schonfeld Distinguished Service Award of the American Society for Adolescent Psychiatry.

JOHN F. KRAMER is Associate Professor of Psychiatry, Pritzker School of Medicine, and Director, Student Mental Health Clinic, University of Chicago.

MOSES LAUFER is Director, Centre for Research into Adolescent Breakdown, Brent Consultation Centre, and Training and Supervising Analyst, British Psycho-Analytical Society, London. He received the 1976 William A. Schonfeld Memorial Award of the American Society for Adolescent Psychiatry.

EDWARD M. LEVINE is Professor of Sociology, Loyola University of Chicago.

SAUL V. LEVINE is Professor of Psychiatry and Associate Director, Child in the City Program, University of Toronto, and Senior Psychiatrist, Hospital for Sick Children.

DOUGLAS F. LEVINSON is a Fellow in Child and Adolescent Psychiatry, Albert Einstein College of Medicine.

JOHN G. LOONEY is Clinical Assistant Professor, University of Texas Health Science Center at Dallas; Director, Child and Adolescent Service, Timberlawn Psychiatric Center, Dallas; Research Psychiatrist, Timberlawn Foundation; and a Senior Editor of this volume.

RICHARD C. MAROHN is Director, Adolescent and Forensic Services, Illinois State Psychiatric Institute, and Attending Psychiatrist, Michael Reese Hospital and Medical Center.

DEREK MILLER is Professor of Psychiatry and Director of Adolescent Psychiatry Services, Northwestern University School of Medicine, Chicago.

JEFFREY R. MITCHELL is a Fellow in Child Psychiatry, University of Washington School of Medicine.

SOL NICHTERN is Assistant Clinical Professor of Psychiatry, New York Medical College, and Director of Psychiatric Services, Jewish Child Care Association.

OTTO POLLAK is Professor of Sociology, University of Pennsylvania.

ELIZABETH PHILLIPS is Senior Psychiatric Social Worker, Hill Health Center, New Haven, Connecticut.

VIVIAN M. RAKOFF is Professor of Psychiatry, and Head, Department of Psychiatry, Sunnybrook Medical Centre, University of Toronto.

LILLIAN H. ROBINSON is Professor of Psychiatry and Pediatrics and faculty member, Psychoanalytic Medicine Program, Tulane University School of Medicine, New Orleans, Louisiana.

CARLOS SALGUERO is Assistant Professor of Pediatrics and Psychiatry, Yale Child Study Center, Yale University School of Medicine and Child Psychiatrist, Hill Health Center, New Haven, Connecticut.

KATHLEEN RUDD SCHARF is with the Department of Socio-Medical Sciences and Community Medicine, Boston University School of Medicine.

NANCY SCHLESINGER is Coordinator, Teenage Pregnancy and Parenting Program, Hill Health Center, New Haven, Connecticut.

ALLAN Z. SCHWARTZBERG is Associate Clinical Professor of Psychiatry, Georgetown University School of Medicine, and a Senior Editor of this volume.

ARTHUR D. SOROSKY is Associate Clinical Professor of Psychiatry, Division of Child Psychiatry, University of California at Los Angeles Center for the Health Sciences, and a Senior Editor of this volume.

MARLIS B. STICHER is a Fellow in Child Psychiatry, Division of Child Psychiatry, University of California at Los Angeles Center for the Health Sciences.

JOHN TOEWS is Associate Professor of Psychiatry, University of Manitoba, and Director of Adult Psychiatry Services, Health Sciences Centre, Winnipeg, Manitoba, Canada.

SIDNEY WEISSMAN is Director of Residency Training and Education, Psychosomatic and Psychiatric Institute, Michael Reese Hospital and Medical Center, and Assistant Professor of Psychiatry, Pritzker School of Medicine, University of Chicago.

ERNEST S. WOLF is Assistant Professor of Psychiatry, Northwestern University, and Training and Supervising Analyst, Chicago Institute for Psychoanalysis.

EDILMA YEARWOOD is Director, Parent-Infant Center, Hill Health Center, New Haven, Connecticut.

IRVING I. ZARETSKY is President, New York Anthropology Research Institute, New York.

CONTENTS OF VOLUMES I–VII

548

554

555

556

NAME INDEX

Abse, D. W., 439, 441
Adatto, C., 423
Adelson, J., 191, 193, 204, 208, 259
Aichhorn, A., 46, 149, 180, 471
Allsopp, M. 347
Almond, R., 523
Angst, J., 349
Annell, A., 347
Anthony, E. J., 203, 209, 333, 341, 345, 346, 379, 380, 389
Aries, P., 26
Arieti, S., 333
Arnstein, R. L., 157
Ashway, J. A., 458

Bach, J. R., 389
Baittle, B, 173, 174, 175
Baker, G., 333
Baker, M., 350
Bales, R., 502
Balint, M., 533
Barglow, P., 158
Baron, M., 349
Bartsch, E., 440, 441
Bateson, G., 401
Beavers, W. R., 502
Bemporard, B., 362
Benedek, T., 219, 227
Benson, R. M., 159
Berg, C., 437
Berg, I., 347
Berger, B., 139, 140
Berlin, I. N., 158
Berman, S., 318
Bertelson, A., 348
Bibring, G., 411
Bettleheim, B., 174
Bleuler, E., 345
Blos, P., 3, 164, 174, 180, 185, 189, 214, 215, 253, 258, 320, 322, 334, 382, 428, 449
Blotcky, M. J., 158, 458
Bowlby, J., 380
Boyd, R. W., 517
Brazelton, T. B., 412
Brockbank, R., 458
Bunney, W. E., 333, 350, 362
Burlingham, D., 389
Busch, F., 260
Buxbaum, E., 438, 441

Cadoret, R. J., 348, 350
Canino, I., 346
Carkhuff, R. R., 499
Carlson, G. E., 345, 362
Carson, D. I., 458
Castellano, M. B., 106
Caudill, W., 517
Cawelti, J., 268, 311
Chadwick, O., 194
Chafetz, M. E., 432
Chambers, J., 109
Church, J., 162
Clayton, P. J., 344
Coelho, G. V., 192
Cohen, M. D., 333
Cohen, R. A., 333
Coleman, J. S., 31, 35
Crabtree, L. H., 458
Cytryn, L., 344, 347, 350

Darrow, C. N., 163
Darwin, C., 302, 303
Davis, J. M., 333
Davis, R. E., 340, 347
DeFries, Z., 427, 428
Delgado, R. A., 439
DelGaudio, A., 194, 206
Despert, J. L., 381
Deutsch, A., 114, 117
Deutsch, H., 21, 380
Deutsch, J., 215
Dietz, S. G., 344
Dorzab, J., 350
Douvan, E., 191, 193, 204, 208, 259
Dunner, D., 350, 362
Durkheim, E., 92

Efron, A. M., 350
Einstein, A., 25
Eisenberg, L., 4, 25
Eissler, K. R., 329
Engel, G. L., 303, 305
Erikson, E. H., 37, 42, 48, 87, 93, 101, 109, 162, 163, 220, 245, 246, 301, 304, 310, 382, 427, 529, 530, 532
Escoll, P., 101
Esman, A. H., 317
Eysenck, H. J., 508

557

SUBJECT INDEX